CALCULATION OF DRUG DOSAGES

A Work Text

CALCULATION OF DRUG DOSAGES

A Work Text

TENTH EDITION

Sheila J. Ogden, MSN, RN
President and CEO
SJOgden Consulting, Inc.
Indianapolis, Indiana

Linda K. Fluharty, MSN, RN
Professor
School of Nursing
Ivy Tech Community College
Indianapolis, Indiana

ELSEVIER

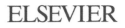

ELSEVIER

3251 Riverport Lane
St. Louis, Missouri 63043

CALCULATION OF DRUG DOSAGES: ISBN: 978-0-323-31069-7
A WORK TEXT, TENTH EDITION

International Standard Book Number: 978-0-323-31069-7

Senior Content Strategist: Yvonne Alexopoulos
Traditional Content Development Manager: Jean Sims Fornango
Senior Content Development Specialist: Danielle M. Frazier
Publishing Services Manager: Deborah L. Vogel
Senior Project Manager: Jodi M. Willard
Design Direction: Julia Dummitt

Printed in Canada

Last digit is the print number: 9   8   7   6   5   4

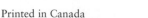

To David, my husband and best friend, for your patience, support, and love;
and to our wonderful family, John, Shannon, Kate, Claire,
Amy, Ryan, Connor, Justin, Maya, and Celeste.
Love, Sheila, Mom, and Nana.

S.J.O.

To my parents, Richard and Arlene Duke,
for their love and support when I said I wanted to be a nurse.
Love, Linda.

L.K.F.

Bret Alan Barker, MSN, RN, CCRN, PHN
Adjunct Faculty, Nursing Instructor
Gavilan College
Gilroy, California

Pricilla Clark, MSN, RN
Nursing Programs Coordinator/Professor
Central Texas College
Killeen, Texas

Janie Corbitt, RN, MLS
Former Instructor, Health Technology Core
Central Georgia Technical College
Milledgeville, Georgia

Marge Gingrich, RN, MSN, CRNP
Professor, Nursing
Harrisburg Area Community College
Harrisburg, Pennsylvania

Jessica Gonzales ARNP, MSN, RN
Nursing Instructor
Lake Washington Institute of Technology
Redmond, Washington

Bobbi Steelman, B.S. Ed, MA. Ed, CPhT
Adjunct Allied Health Instructor
Daymar Colleges Group
Bowling Green, Kentucky

Ann Thurman, BSN, RN
Coordinator, Allied Health/Practical Nursing
Tennessee Technology Center at Hartsville
Hartsville, Tennessee

Laura Warner, MSN, RN, CNE
Associate Professor of Nursing
Ivy Tech Community College
Indianapolis, Indiana

We are grateful to the students and instructors who have chosen to use this book; we continue to learn so much from each of you. You have helped us understand the problems that students have with basic mathematics and with the calculation of drug dosages. We appreciate the physicians, nurses, pharmacists, and representatives of various health care agencies who took the time to discuss topics with us. We hope this book will provide readers with a feeling of confidence when working with a variety of mathematical problems.

We want to give special thanks to the reviewers of this text. Your sincere evaluation and critique played an integral part in the revision of this edition, and your attention to detail was most helpful.

We would also like to acknowledge Danielle Frazier and Yvonne Alexopoulos for their help and support during the writing of this tenth edition. Danielle supplied answers to many questions, pushed to meet deadlines, and offered her services as needed. She also remained calm and offered guidance during the entire revision process. Yvonne has been diligent in providing clarity on the needs of students, faculty, and hospitals as the scope and use of the book continue to grow.

Thank you all so much!

Sheila J. Ogden

Linda K. Fluharty

This work text is designed for students in professional and vocational schools of nursing and for nurses returning to practice after being away from the clinical setting. It can be used in the classroom or for individual study. The work text contains an extensive review of basic mathematics to assist students who have not mastered the subject in previous educational experiences. It can also be used by those who have not attended school for a number of years and feel a lack of confidence in the area of mathematics computations.

ORGANIZATION OF MATERIAL

A pretest precedes each chapter in Parts One and Two and may be used for evaluating present skills. For those students who are comfortable with basic mathematics, a quick assessment of each area will confirm their competency in the subject matter.

Part Two begins with the use of the metric system, which is predominant in the medical field. The apothecary system continues to decline in use to the point of being almost extinct. However, in remembering that differences in practice exist throughout the United States and the world, it was felt that some of that content should remain in the book. Therefore it has been placed in the Appendix for reference. A new Chapter 7 has been added with the emphasis on calculations used in patient assessments.

Part Three helps students prepare for the actual calculation of drug dosages. The new Chapter 8 has combined material from all previous chapters and discusses various points concerning patient safety as it relates to medication administration. This chapter also includes safety issues for the nurse in the dispensing of medication. The case scenarios really emphasize the importance of delivering the correct medication to the patient as ordered. Chapter 9 provides an emphasis on the interpretation of the physician's orders, and Chapter 10 explains how to read medication labels.

Part Four has been renamed the Calculation of Drug Dosages. As students begin their clinical experiences, they start with basic medical surgical patients. Therefore the content moves from oral to parenteral, units, reconstitution and, finally, intravenous flow rates. Beginning in Part Four, we have added substantial content on dimensional analysis as a method for solving problems of drug calculations. This method has become the preferred method of use by numerous schools of nursing.

However, many schools are remaining with the ratio/proportion or formula methods. Examples of each type of calculation are now shown first with dimensional analysis followed by the proportion and formula methods. The division of the three methods will allow instructors to target the area of study they prefer for their students and/or schools.

The actual drug labels have been updated and increased in number in all chapters that discuss the calculation of drug dosages. Also in Part Four, we have separated and expanded the content for dosages measured in units (Chapter 13) and the reconstitution of medications (Chapter 14). These are two separate concepts and are sometimes difficult for students to understand. This separation allows for extended practice and attention to each chapter's content.

More medications are being delivered to patients via the intravenous route, not only in intensive care units, but in progressive care and medical surgical areas as well. Therefore, in addition to Chapter 15, Intravenous Flow Rates, a new Chapter 16, Intravenous Flow Rates for Dosages Measured in Units, has been added. Chapter 17 remains focused on Critical Care Intravenous Flow Rates. Chapter 18, Pediatric Dosages, continues to include oral, parenteral, and intravenous flow rate problems. Chapter 19, Obstetric Dosages, remains to address the calculation in regards to obstetric patients.

The majority of the calculation problems relating to drug dosages continue to represent actual physicians' orders in various health care settings.

FEATURES IN THE TENTH EDITION

- **Learning objectives** are listed at the beginning of each chapter so students will know the goals that must be achieved.
- Chapter **work sheets** provide the opportunity to practice solving realistic problems.
- Almost every chapter contains two **posttests** designed to evaluate the student's learning.
- A **comprehensive posttest** at the end of the book will help students assess their total understanding of the process of calculation of drug dosages.
- A **glossary** is included to define important terms.
- Numerous **full-color drug labels** continue to provide a more realistic representation of medication administration.
- **NEW! Chapter 13, Dosages Measured in Units, and Chapter 14, Reconstitution of Medications,** have been divided into two separate chapters.

ANCILLARIES

Evolve resources for instructors and students can be found online at http://evolve.elsevier.com/Ogden/calculation/

The instructor resources are designed to help instructors present the material in this text and include the following:

- Drug Label glossary
- TEACH Lesson Plan
- TEACH Lecture Outlines
- TEACH PowerPoint Slides
- Test Bank

*NEW VERSION! **Drug Calculations Comprehensive Test Bank, version 4.*** This generic test-bank contains over 700 questions on general mathematics, converting within the same system of measurements, converting between different systems of measurement, oral dosages, parenteral dosages, flow rates, pediatric dosages, IV calculations, and more.

Student Resources provide students with additional tools for learning and include the following:

- Student Practice Problems and Learning Activities
- Flash Cards

*NEW VERSION! **Drug Calculations Companion, version 5.*** This is a completely updated, interactive student tutorial that includes an extensive menu of various topic areas within drug calculations, such as oral, parenteral, pediatric, and intravenous calculations. it contains over 600 practice problems covering ratio and proportion, formula, and dimensional analysis methods.

DESCRIPTION AND FEATURES

Calculation of Drug Dosages is an innovative drug calculation work text designed to provide you with a systematic review of mathematics and a simplified method of calculating drug dosages. It affords you the opportunity to move at a comfortable pace to ensure success. It includes information on the dimensional analysis, ratio and proportion, and formula methods of drug calculation, as well as numerous practice problems. Take a look at the following features so that you may familiarize yourself with this text and maximize its value.

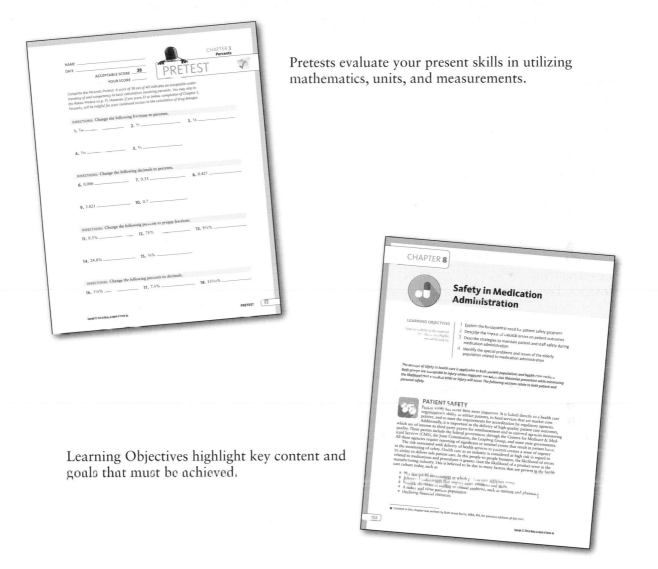

Pretests evaluate your present skills in utilizing mathematics, units, and measurements.

Learning Objectives highlight key content and goals that must be achieved.

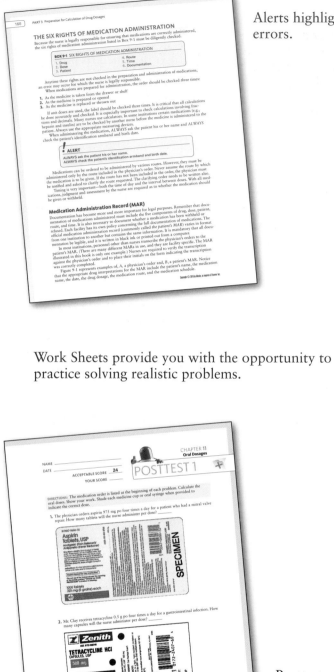

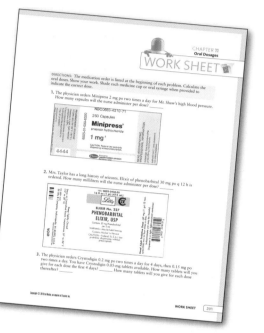

Alerts highlight potential and common drug calculation errors.

Work Sheets provide you with the opportunity to practice solving realistic problems.

Posttests are designed to assess your learning and identify your strengths and weaknesses.

NEW VERSION! **Drug Calculations Companion, version 5.** This is a completely updated, interactive student tutorial that includes an extensive menu of various topic areas within drug calculations, such as oral, parenteral, pediatric, and intravenous calculations. it contains over 600 practice problems covering ratio and proportion, formula, and dimensional analysis methods.

evolve   Look for this icon at the end of the chapters. It will refer to *Drug Calculations Companion, version 5* for additional practice problems and content information.

A pretest precedes each chapter in Parts One and Two to assess previous learning. If your grade on the pretest is acceptable (an acceptable score is noted at the top of the test), you may continue to the next pretest. If your score on the pretest indicates a need for further study, read the introduction to the chapter, study the method of solving the problems, and complete the work sheet. If you have difficulty with a problem, refer to the examples in the introduction.

On completion of the work sheet, refer to the answer key at the end of each chapter to verify that your answers are correct. Rework all the incorrect problems to find your errors. It may be necessary to refer again to the examples in each chapter. Then proceed to the first posttest and grade the test. if your grade is acceptable, as indicated at the top of the test, continue to the next chapter. If your grade is less than acceptable, rework all incorrect problems to find your errors. Review as necessary before completing the second posttest. Again, verify that your answers are correct. At this point, if you have followed the system of study, your grade on the second posttest should be more than acceptable. Follow the same system of study in each of the chapters.

When all the chapters in the work text are completed with acceptable scores (between 95% and 100%), you should be proficient in solving problems relating to drug dosages; more important, you will have completed the first step toward becoming a safe practitioner of medication administration.

On completion of the material provided in this work text, you will have mastered the following mathematical concepts for use in the accurate performance of computations:

1. Solving problems using fractions, decimals, percents, ratios, proportions, and dimensional analysis
2. Solving problems involving the apothecary, metric, and household systems of measurements
3. Solving problems measured in units and milliequivalents
4. Solving problems related to oral and parenteral dosages
5. Solving problems involving intravenous flow rates and critical care intravenous flow rates
6. Solving problems confirming the correct dosage of pediatric medications
7. Solving problems confirming the correct dosages of OB medications
8. Solving problems by using the or dimensional analysis, ratio and proportion, and formula methods.

You are now ready to begin Chapter 1!

CONTENTS

REVIEW of MATHEMATICS

A solid knowledge base of general mathematics is necessary before you will be able to use these concepts in the more complicated calculations of drug dosages. It is this knowledge that allows for the safe administration of medications to your patients and prevents medication errors.

For students who have been away from basic mathematics awhile, please take the time and effort to review the multiplication tables of one through twelve. These tables must be memorized to allow ease in the computation of all problems found in this textbook.

As you prepare to learn how to calculate drug dosages, an assessment of your current basic mathematics understanding and competency is essential. A general mathematics pretest is provided. Allow 1 to 2 hours in a quiet study area to complete the pretest without the use of a calculator. This is your opportunity to assess your true capability of performing basic math problems. Calculators are very useful tools. In most areas of health care, the use of a calculator is actually required to ensure accuracy in the delivery of medications. Follow the direction of your instructor as to the acceptable use of calculators while using this text on your path to safe administration of medications.

The pretest allows you to assess your need for a more extensive review. After completion of the test, check your answers with the key provided. A score of 95%, or 48 out of 50 problems correct, indicates a firm foundation in basic mathematics. You may then skip to Part II, Units and Measurements for the Calculation of Drug Dosages. However, a score of 47 or below indicates a need to review fraction, decimal, percent, ratio, and/or proportion calculations. Chapters 1 through 5 allow you to work on these basic mathematical skills at your leisure.

The pretest and review chapters are provided to ensure your success in the calculation and administration of your future patients' medications. Begin now, and good luck!

NAME _____

DATE _____

ACCEPTABLE SCORE ___**48**___

YOUR SCORE _____

PRETEST

DIRECTIONS: Perform the indicated computations. Reduce fractions to lowest terms.

1. $\frac{3}{8} + \frac{1}{3} = $ _____

2. $2\frac{3}{7} + 1\frac{2}{3} = $ _____

3. $1\frac{3}{5} + \frac{7}{8} / \frac{1}{3} = $ _____

4. $1.03 + 2.2 + 1.134 = $ _____

5. $1.479 + 28.68 + 4.5 = $ _____

6. $\frac{14}{15} - \frac{1}{6} = $ _____

7. $2\frac{1}{3} - \frac{1}{2} = $ _____

8. $2.04 - 0.987 = $ _____

9. $8.53 - 7.945 = $ _____

10. $3 \times \frac{4}{7} = $ _____

11. $2\frac{1}{2} \times 3\frac{3}{5} = $ _____

12. $0.315 \times 5.8 = $ _____

13. $4.884 \times 6.51 = $ _____

14. $\frac{3}{5} \div \frac{5}{6} = $ _____

15. $\frac{1}{150} \div \frac{1}{20} = $ _____

16. $2\frac{3}{4} \div 6\frac{2}{3} = $ _____

17. $241.73 \div 3.6 = $ _____

18. $22.68 \div 4.2 = $ _____

DIRECTIONS: Circle the decimal fraction that has the *least* value.

19. 0.3, 0.03, 0.003

20. 0.9, 0.45, 0.66

21. 0.72, 0.721, 0.0072

DIRECTIONS: Circle the decimal fraction that has the *greatest* value.

22. 0.1, 0.15, 0.155

23. 0.249, 0.1587, 0.00633

24. 2.913, 2.99, 2.9

DIRECTIONS: Change the following fractions to decimals.

25. $5/8 =$ _____ **26.** $17/25 =$ _____

DIRECTIONS: Change the following decimals to fractions reduced to lowest terms.

27. $0.375 =$ _____ **28.** $0.05 =$ _____

DIRECTIONS: Perform the indicated computations.

29. Express 0.432 as a percent. **30.** Express 65% as a proper fraction and reduce to the lowest terms.

31. Express 0.3% as a ratio. **32.** What percent of 2.5 is 0.5?

33. What is ¼% of 60? **34.** What is 65% of 450?

DIRECTIONS: Change the following fractions and decimals to ratios reduced to lowest terms.

35. $9/42 =$ _____ **36.** $1½/2⅔ =$ _____ **37.** $0.34 =$ _____

DIRECTIONS: Find the value of x.

38. $7 : 7/100 :: x : 4$ **39.** $x : 40 :: 7 : 56$ **40.** $2.5 : 6 :: 10 : x$

41. $x : ¼\% :: 9.6 : 1/300$ **42.** $1/150 : 1/100 :: x : 30$ **43.** $0.10 : 0.20 :: x : 200$

44. $\frac{1}{200} : \frac{1}{40} :: 100 : x$ **45.** $x : 85 :: 6 : 10$ **46.** $\frac{1}{20}/\frac{1}{5} : 5 :: x : 50$

47. $100 : 5 :: x : 3.4$ **48.** $75 : x :: 36 : 6$ **49.** $\frac{1}{3} : \frac{2}{5} :: x : 30$

50. $x : 9 :: 98 : 7$

ANSWERS ON P. 6.

ANSWERS

REVIEW OF MATHEMATICS PRETEST, pp. 3–5

1. $^{17}/_{24}$
2. $4^2/_{21}$
3. $4^9/_{40}$
4. 4.364
5. 34.659
6. $^{23}/_{30}$
7. $1^5/_6$
8. 1.053
9. 0.585
10. $1^5/_7$
11. 9
12. 1.827
13. 31.79484

14. $^{18}/_{25}$
15. $^2/_{15}$
16. $^{33}/_{80}$
17. 67.14722
18. 5.4
19. 0.003
20. 0.45
21. 0.0072
22. 0.155
23. 0.249
24. 2.99
25. 0.625
26. 0.68

27. $^3/_8$
28. $^1/_{20}$
29. 43.2%
30. $^{13}/_{20}$
31. 3:1000
32. 20%
33. 0.15
34. 292.5
35. 3:14
36. 9:16
37. 17:50
38. 400
39. 5

40. 24
41. $7^1/_5$ or 7.2
42. 20
43. 100
44. 500
45. 51
46. $2^1/_2$ or 2.5
47. 68
48. 12.5
49. 25
50. 126

NAME _____

DATE _____

ACCEPTABLE SCORE ___29___

YOUR SCORE _____

PRETEST

Complete the Fractions Pretest. A score of 29 out of 30 indicates an acceptable under-standing of and competency in basic calculations involving fractions. You may skip to the Decimals Pretest on p. 31. However, if you scored 28 or below, completion of Chapter 1, Fractions, will be helpful for your continued success in the calculation of drug dosages.

DIRECTIONS: Perform the indicated calculations and reduce fractions to lowest terms.

1. $5/7 + 4/9 =$ _____

2. $2\frac{1}{2} + 8\frac{1}{6} =$ _____

3. $3^{13}/_{20} + 1^{3}/_{10} + 4^{4}/_{5} =$ ___

4. $2^{5}/_{16} + 3\frac{1}{4} =$ _____

5. $5^{6}/_{11} + 3\frac{1}{2} =$ _____

6. $3^{2}/_{3} + 4^{2}/_{9} =$ _____

7. $1\frac{3}{4} + 2\frac{3}{8} + 1^{5}/_{6} =$ _____

8. $9/_{10} - 3/_{5} =$ _____

9. $2\frac{1}{4} - 1\frac{3}{8} =$ _____

10. $6\frac{1}{8} - 3\frac{1}{2} =$ _____

11. $4^{5}/_{6} - 2\frac{1}{8} =$ _____

12. $3\frac{3}{4} - 1^{11}/_{12} =$ _____

13. $7\frac{1}{2} - 5^{7}/_{10} =$ _____

14. $6\frac{1}{2} - 4^{2}/_{3} =$ _____

15. $4/_{5} \times 1/_{12} =$ _____

16. $1^{1}/_{3} \times 3\frac{3}{4} =$ _____

17. $3^{3}/_{7} \times 2^{2}/_{6} =$ _____

18. $5/_{8} \times 1^{5}/_{7} =$ _____

19. $1/_{1000} \times 1/_{10} =$ _____

20. $2^{4}/_{9} \times 1\frac{3}{4} =$ _____

21. $4\frac{1}{6} \times 2^{9}/_{10} =$ _____

22. $1\frac{1}{8} \times 2^{4}/_{7} =$ _____

23. $1/_{4} \div 4/_{5} =$ _____

24. $2\frac{1}{6} \div 1^{5}/_{8} =$ _____

25. $\frac{1}{3} \div \frac{1}{100} = $ _____   **26.** $1\frac{3}{4} \div 2 = $ _____   **27.** $\frac{4}{5}/\frac{3}{5} = $ _____

28. $\frac{1}{3}/\frac{3}{5} = $ _____   **29.** $2\frac{5}{6}/1\frac{2}{3} = $ _____   **30.** $4\frac{1}{2}/2\frac{1}{4} = $ _____

ANSWERS ON P. 29.

Fractions

LEARNING OBJECTIVES

Upon completion of the materials provided in this chapter, you will be able to perform computations accurately by mastering the following mathematical concepts:

1 Changing an improper fraction to a mixed number

2 Changing a mixed number to an improper fraction

3 Changing a fraction to an equivalent fraction with the lowest common denominator

4 Changing a mixed number to an equivalent fraction with the lowest common denominator

5 Adding fractions having the same denominator, having unlike denominators, or involving whole numbers and unlike denominators

6 Subtracting fractions having the same denominator, having unlike denominators, or involving whole numbers and unlike denominators

7 Multiplying fractions and mixed numbers

8 Dividing fractions and mixed numbers

9 Reducing a complex fraction

10 Reducing a complex fraction involving mixed numbers

Study the introductory material for fractions. The processes for the calculation of fraction problems are listed in steps. Memorize the steps for each type of calculation before beginning the work sheet. Complete the work sheet at the end of this chapter, which provides extensive practice in the manipulation of fractions. Check your answers. If you have difficulties, go back and review the steps for that type of calculation. When you feel ready to evaluate your learning, take the first posttest. Check your answers. An acceptable score (number of answers correct) as indicated on the posttest signifies that you are ready for the next chapter. An unacceptable score signifies a need for further study before you take the second posttest.

A **fraction** indicates the number of equal parts of a whole. For example, ¾ means three of four equal parts.

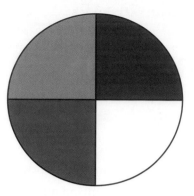

The **denominator** indicates the number of parts into which a whole has been divided. The denominator is the number *below* the fraction line. The **numerator** designates the number of parts that you have of a divided whole. It is the number *above* the fraction line. The line also indicates division to be performed and can be read as "divided by." The example ¾, or three fourths, can therefore be read as "three divided by four." In other words the numerator is "divided by" the denominator. The numerator is the **dividend,** and the denominator is the **divisor.** When numbers are multiplied, the answer is the **product.** When numbers are divided, the answer is the **quotient.**

A fraction can often be expressed in smaller numbers without any change in its real value. This is what is meant by the direction "Reduce to lowest terms." The reduction is accomplished by dividing both numerator and denominator by the same number.

EXAMPLE 1: ⁶⁄₈

a. $6 \div 2 = 3$

b. $8 \div 2 = 4$

c. $\dfrac{6}{8} = \dfrac{3}{4}$

EXAMPLE 2: ³⁄₉

a. $3 \div 3 = 1$

b. $9 \div 3 = 3$

c. $\dfrac{3}{9} = \dfrac{1}{3}$

EXAMPLE 3: ⁴⁄₁₀

a. $4 \div 2 = 2$

b. $10 \div 2 = 5$

c. $\dfrac{4}{10} = \dfrac{2}{5}$

There are several different types of fractions. A **proper fraction** is one in which the numerator is smaller than the denominator. A proper fraction is sometimes called a *common* or *simple fraction.*

EXAMPLES: ⅔, ⅛, ⁵⁄₁₂

An **improper fraction** is a fraction in which the numerator is larger than or equal to the denominator.

EXAMPLES: ⁸⁄₇, ⁶⁄₆, ⁴⁄₂

A **complex fraction** is one that contains a fraction in its numerator, its denominator, or both.

EXAMPLES: 2⅓/3, 2/1½, ¾/⅜

Sometimes a fraction is seen in conjunction with a whole number. This combination is called a **mixed number.**

EXAMPLES: 2⅜, 4⅓, 6½

IMPROPER FRACTIONS

Changing an Improper Fraction to a Mixed Number

1. Divide the numerator by the denominator.
2. Place any remainder over the denominator and write this proper fraction beside the whole number found in step 1.

EXAMPLE 1: $^5/_3$ **EXAMPLE 2:** $^7/_2$

$$3\overline{)5} \quad 1 \text{ remainder } 2 = 1\frac{2}{3}$$
$$\underline{3}$$
$$2$$

$$2\overline{)7} \quad 3 \text{ remainder } 1 = 3\frac{1}{2}$$
$$\underline{6}$$
$$1$$

When an improper fraction is reduced, it will *always* result in a mixed number or a whole number.

Changing a Mixed Number to an Improper Fraction

1. Multiply the denominator of the fraction by the whole number.
2. Add the product to the numerator of the fraction.
3. Place the sum over the denominator.

EXAMPLE 1: $3\frac{1}{4}$ **EXAMPLE 2:** $1\frac{3}{8}$ **EXAMPLE 3:** $2^7/_{10}$

a. $4 \times 3 = 12$ **a.** $8 \times 1 = 8$ **a.** $10 \times 2 = 20$

b. $12 + 1 = 13$ **b.** $8 + 3 = 11$ **b.** $20 + 7 = 27$

c. $3\frac{1}{4} = \frac{13}{4}$ **c.** $1\frac{3}{8} = \frac{11}{8}$ **c.** $2\frac{7}{10} = \frac{27}{10}$

! ALERT

If fractions are to be added or subtracted, it is necessary for their *denominators to be the same.*

LOWEST COMMON DENOMINATOR

Computations are facilitated when the lowest common denominator is used. The term **lowest common denominator** is defined as the smallest whole number that can be divided evenly by all denominators within the problem.

When trying to determine the lowest common denominator, first observe whether one of the denominators in the problem is evenly divisible by each of the other denominators. If so, this will be the lowest common denominator for the problem.

EXAMPLE 1: $^2/_3$ and $^5/_{12}$
You find that 12 is evenly divisible by 3; therefore 12 is the lowest common denominator.

EXAMPLE 2: $^1/_2$ and $^3/_8$
You find that 8 is evenly divisible by 2; therefore 8 is the lowest common denominator.

EXAMPLE 3: $^2/_7$ and $^5/_{14}$ and $^1/_{28}$
You find that 28 is evenly divisible by 7 and 14; therefore 28 is the lowest common denominator.

Changing a Fraction to an Equivalent Fraction with the Lowest Common Denominator

1. Divide the lowest common denominator by the denominator of the fraction to be changed.
2. Multiply the quotient by the numerator of the fraction to be changed.
3. Place the product over the lowest common denominator.

EXAMPLE 1: $\frac{2}{3} = \frac{?}{12}$

   a. $12 \div 3 = 4$

   b. $4 \times 2 = 8$

   c. $\dfrac{2}{3} = \dfrac{8}{12}$

EXAMPLE 2: $\frac{1}{2} = \frac{?}{8}$

   a. $8 \div 2 = 4$

   b. $4 \times 1 = 4$

   c. $\dfrac{1}{2} = \dfrac{4}{8}$

EXAMPLE 3: $\frac{2}{7} = \frac{?}{14}$

   a. $14 \div 7 = 2$

   b. $2 \times 2 = 4$

   c. $\dfrac{2}{7} = \dfrac{4}{14}$

Changing a Mixed Number to an Equivalent Fraction with the Lowest Common Denominator

1. Change the mixed number to an improper fraction.
2. Divide the lowest common denominator by the denominator of the fraction.
3. Multiply the quotient by the numerator of the improper fraction.
4. Place the product over the lowest common denominator.

EXAMPLE 1: $1\frac{3}{4}$ and $\frac{5}{12}$

   a. $1\dfrac{3}{4} = \dfrac{?}{12}$

       $4 \times 1 = 4$

       $4 + 3 = 7$

   b. $\dfrac{7}{4} = \dfrac{?}{12}$

       $12 \div 4 = 3$

   c. $3 \times 7 = 21$

   d. $1\dfrac{3}{4} = \dfrac{21}{12}$

EXAMPLE 2: $3\frac{2}{3}$ and $\frac{4}{9}$

   a. $3\dfrac{2}{3} = \dfrac{?}{9}$

       $3 \times 3 = 9$

       $9 + 2 = 11$

   b. $\dfrac{11}{3} = \dfrac{?}{9}$

       $9 \div 3 = 3$

   c. $3 \times 11 = 33$

   d. $3\dfrac{2}{3} = \dfrac{33}{9}$

If one of the denominators in the problem is not the lowest common denominator for all, you must look further. One suggestion is to multiply two of the denominators together and if possible use that number as the lowest common denominator.

EXAMPLE: $3\frac{1}{2}$ and $\frac{2}{3}$

   Multiply the two denominators: $2 \times 3 = 6$

   a. $3\dfrac{1}{2} = \dfrac{?}{6}$

       $2 \times 3 = 6$

       $6 + 1 = 7$

   b. $\dfrac{7}{2} = \dfrac{?}{6}$

   c. $6 \div 2 = 3$

   d. $3 \times 7 = 21$

   e. $3\dfrac{1}{2} = \dfrac{21}{6}$

   a. $\dfrac{2}{3} = \dfrac{?}{6}$

   b. $6 \div 3 = 2$

   c. $2 \times 2 = 4$

   d. $\dfrac{2}{3} = \dfrac{4}{6}$

Another method is to multiply one of the denominators by 2, 3, or 4. Determine whether the resulting number can be used as a common denominator.

EXAMPLE: ¾ and ⅛ and ⁵⁄₁₂

Multiply the denominator 8 by 3: $8 \times 3 = 24$

a. $\dfrac{3}{4} = \dfrac{?}{24}$

b. $24 \div 4 = 6$

c. $6 \times 3 = 18$

d. $\dfrac{3}{4} = \dfrac{18}{24}$

a. $\dfrac{1}{8} = \dfrac{?}{24}$

b. $24 \div 8 = 3$

c. $3 \times 1 = 3$

d. $\dfrac{1}{8} = \dfrac{3}{24}$

a. $\dfrac{5}{12} = \dfrac{?}{24}$

b. $24 \div 12 = 2$

c. $2 \times 5 = 10$

d. $\dfrac{5}{12} = \dfrac{10}{24}$

ADDITION OF FRACTIONS

Addition of Fractions with the Same Denominator

1. Add the numerators.
2. Place the sum over the common denominator.
3. Reduce to lowest terms.

EXAMPLE 1: ⅟₇ + ²⁄₇ = _____

a. $\dfrac{1}{7} + \dfrac{2}{7} =$

b. $\dfrac{1+2}{7} =$

c. $\dfrac{3}{7}$

EXAMPLE 2: ⅛ + ⅜ = _____

a. $\dfrac{1}{8} + \dfrac{3}{8} =$

b. $\dfrac{1+3}{8} =$

c. $\dfrac{4}{8} = \dfrac{1}{2}$

Addition of Fractions with Unlike Denominators

1. Change the fractions to equivalent fractions with the lowest common denominator.
2. Add the numerators.
3. Place the sum over the lowest common denominator.
4. Reduce to lowest terms.

EXAMPLE 1: ⅔ + ⅕ = _____

To find the lowest common denominator, multiply the two denominators together.

$3 \times 5 = 15$

Change each fraction to an equivalent fraction with 15 as the denominator.

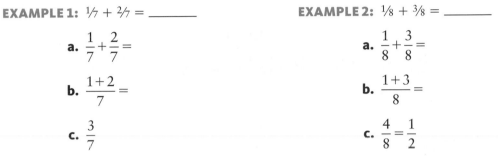

a. $\dfrac{2}{3} = \dfrac{?}{15}$

$15 \div 3 = 5$

$5 \times 2 = 10$

$\dfrac{2}{3} = \dfrac{10}{15}$

a. $\dfrac{1}{5} = \dfrac{?}{15}$

$15 \div 5 = 3$

$3 \times 1 = 3$

$\dfrac{1}{5} = \dfrac{3}{15}$

b. $\dfrac{10}{15} + \dfrac{3}{15} =$

c. $\dfrac{10+3}{15} = \dfrac{13}{15}$

EXAMPLE 2: $\frac{1}{6} + \frac{1}{4} + \frac{1}{3} =$ _____

To find a common denominator, try multiplying two of the denominators together and check to see whether that number is divisible by the other denominator.

$$4 \times 3 = 12$$

Is 12 divisible by the other denominator, 6? The answer is YES.

a. $\frac{1}{6} = \frac{?}{12}$

$12 \div 6 = 2$

$2 \times 1 = 2$

$\frac{1}{6} = \frac{2}{12}$

a. $\frac{1}{4} = \frac{?}{12}$

$12 \div 4 = 3$

$3 \times 1 = 3$

$\frac{1}{4} = \frac{3}{12}$

a. $\frac{1}{3} = \frac{?}{12}$

$12 \div 3 = 4$

$4 \times 1 = 4$

$\frac{1}{3} = \frac{4}{12}$

b. $\frac{2}{12} + \frac{3}{12} + \frac{4}{12} =$

c. $\frac{2+3+4}{12} = \frac{9}{12}$

d. $\frac{9}{12} = \frac{3}{4}$ (reduced to lowest terms)

Addition of Fractions Involving Whole Numbers and Unlike Denominators

1. Change the fractions to equivalent fractions with the lowest common denominator.
2. Add the numerators.
3. Place the sum over the lowest common denominator.
4. Reduce to lowest terms.
5. Write the reduced fraction next to the sum of the whole numbers.

EXAMPLE 1: $1\frac{1}{3} + 2\frac{3}{8} =$ _____

To find the lowest common denominator, multiply the two denominators together.

$$3 \times 8 = 24$$

Change the fractions $\frac{1}{3}$ and $\frac{3}{8}$ to equivalent fractions with 24 as their denominators.

a. $\frac{1}{3} = \frac{?}{24}$

$24 \div 3 = 8$

$8 \times 1 = 8$

$\frac{1}{3} = \frac{8}{24}$

a. $\frac{3}{8} = \frac{?}{24}$

$24 \div 8 = 3$

$3 \times 3 = 9$

$\frac{3}{8} = \frac{9}{24}$

b. $1\frac{8}{24} + 2\frac{9}{24} =$

c. $1\frac{8}{24}$

$+2\frac{9}{24}$

d. $3\frac{17}{24}$

EXAMPLE 2: $5\frac{1}{2} + 3\frac{3}{10} = $ _____

Because 10 is evenly divisible by 2, 10 is the lowest common denominator. Therefore ½ needs to be changed to an equivalent fraction with 10 as the denominator.

a. $\dfrac{1}{2} = \dfrac{?}{10}$

$10 \div 2 = 5$

$5 \times 1 = 5$

$\dfrac{1}{2} = \dfrac{5}{10}$

b. $5\dfrac{5}{10} + 3\dfrac{3}{10} =$

c.
$$5\dfrac{5}{10}$$
$$+3\dfrac{3}{10}$$
_____
$$8\dfrac{8}{10} = 8\dfrac{4}{5} \text{ (reduced to lowest terms)}$$

SUBTRACTION OF FRACTIONS

Subtraction of Fractions with the Same Denominator

1. Subtract the numerator of the **subtrahend** (the number being subtracted) from the numerator of the **minuend** (the number from which another number is subtracted).
2. Place the difference over the common denominator.
3. Reduce to lowest terms.

EXAMPLE 1: $\frac{6}{8} - \frac{4}{8} = $ _____

a. $\dfrac{6}{8} - \dfrac{4}{8} =$

b. $\dfrac{6-4}{8} =$

c. $\dfrac{2}{8} = \dfrac{1}{4}$ (reduced to lowest terms)

EXAMPLE 2: $\frac{7}{12} - \frac{1}{12} = $ _____

a. $\dfrac{7}{12} - \dfrac{1}{12} =$

b. $\dfrac{7-1}{12} =$

c. $\dfrac{6}{12} = \dfrac{1}{2}$ (reduced to lowest terms)

Subtraction of Fractions with Unlike Denominators

1. Change the fractions to equivalent fractions with the lowest common denominator.
2. Subtract the numerator of the subtrahend from that of the minuend.
3. Place the difference over the lowest common denominator.
4. Reduce to lowest terms.

EXAMPLE 1: $\frac{2}{3} - \frac{1}{6} = $ _____

The lowest common denominator is 6, because 6 is evenly divisible by 3. Therefore the fraction ⅔ needs to be changed to an equivalent fraction with 6 as the denominator.

a. $\dfrac{2}{3} = \dfrac{?}{6}$

$6 \div 3 = 2$

$2 \times 2 = 4$

$\dfrac{2}{3} = \dfrac{4}{6}$

b. $\dfrac{4}{6} - \dfrac{1}{6} =$

c. $\dfrac{4-1}{6} =$

d. $\dfrac{3}{6} = \dfrac{1}{2}$ (reduced to lowest terms)

EXAMPLE 2: $\frac{7}{10} - \frac{3}{5} = $ _____

The lowest common denominator is 10, because 10 is evenly divisible by 5. Therefore the fraction $\frac{3}{5}$ needs to be changed to an equivalent fraction with 10 as the denominator.

a. $\frac{3}{5} = \frac{?}{10}$

$10 \div 5 = 2$

$2 \times 3 = 6$

$\frac{3}{5} = \frac{6}{10}$

b. $\frac{7}{10} - \frac{6}{10} =$

c. $\frac{7-6}{10} = \frac{1}{10}$

Subtraction of Fractions Involving Whole Numbers and Unlike Denominators

1. Change the fractions to equivalent fractions with the lowest common denominator.
2. Subtract the numerator of the subtrahend from that of the minuend, borrowing 1 from the whole number if necessary.
3. Place the difference over the lowest common denominator.
4. Reduce to lowest terms.
5. Write the reduced fraction next to the difference of the whole numbers.

EXAMPLE 1: $3\frac{2}{3} - 1\frac{1}{4} = $ _____

The lowest common denominator is 12 (determined by multiplying 3×4). Each fraction needs to be changed to an equivalent fraction with 12 as the common denominator.

a. $\frac{2}{3} = \frac{?}{12}$

$12 \div 3 = 4$

$4 \times 2 = 8$

$\frac{2}{3} = \frac{8}{12}$

a. $\frac{1}{4} = \frac{?}{12}$

$12 \div 4 = 3$

$3 \times 1 = 3$

$\frac{1}{4} = \frac{3}{12}$

b. $3\frac{8}{12} - 1\frac{3}{12} =$

c. $\quad 3\frac{8}{12}$

$\quad -1\frac{3}{12}$

$\quad\quad 2\frac{5}{12}$

EXAMPLE 2: $8\frac{1}{2} - 3\frac{4}{7} =$ _____

The lowest common denominator is 14 (determined by multiplying 2×7). Each fraction needs to be changed to an equivalent fraction with 14 as the common denominator.

a. $\dfrac{1}{2} = \dfrac{?}{14}$

$14 \div 2 = 7$

$7 \times 1 = 7$

$\dfrac{1}{2} = \dfrac{7}{14}$

a. $\dfrac{4}{7} = \dfrac{?}{14}$

$14 \div 7 = 2$

$2 \times 4 = 8$

$\dfrac{4}{7} = \dfrac{8}{14}$

b. $8\dfrac{7}{14} - 3\dfrac{8}{14} =$

To perform the subtraction, it is necessary to borrow 1 from the whole number. "One" for this problem can be expressed as $\frac{14}{14}$. Therefore $8\frac{7}{14} = 7\frac{21}{14}$. Now the mathematics may be completed.

c. $8\dfrac{7}{14}$

$-3\dfrac{8}{14}$

=

d. $7\dfrac{21}{14}$

$-3\dfrac{8}{14}$

$4\dfrac{13}{14}$

MULTIPLICATION OF FRACTIONS

1. Multiply the numerators.
2. Multiply the denominators.
3. Place the product of the numerators over the product of the denominators.
4. Reduce to lowest terms.

EXAMPLE 1: $\frac{2}{3} \times \frac{3}{5} =$ _____

$\dfrac{2}{3} \times \dfrac{3}{5} =$

a. $\dfrac{2 \times 3}{3 \times 5} = \dfrac{6}{15}$

b. $\dfrac{6}{15} = \dfrac{2}{5}$ (reduced to lowest terms)

EXAMPLE 2: $\frac{4}{9} \times \frac{4}{5} =$ _____

$\dfrac{4}{9} \times \dfrac{4}{5} =$

a. $\dfrac{4 \times 4}{9 \times 5} = \dfrac{16}{45}$ (reduced to lowest terms)
b.

The process of multiplying fractions may be shortened by **canceling.** In other words, numbers common to the numerators and denominators may be divided or canceled out.

EXAMPLE 1: $\frac{2}{3} \times \frac{3}{5} =$ _____

$\dfrac{2}{\cancel{3}_1} \times \dfrac{\cancel{3}^1}{5} = \dfrac{2 \times 1}{1 \times 5} = \dfrac{2}{5}$

EXAMPLE 2: $\frac{7}{20} \times \frac{2}{5} \times \frac{3}{14} =$ _____

$\dfrac{\cancel{7}^1}{\cancel{20}_{10}} \times \dfrac{\cancel{2}^1}{5} \times \dfrac{3}{\cancel{14}_2} =$

$\dfrac{1 \times 1 \times 3}{10 \times 5 \times 2} = \dfrac{3}{100}$

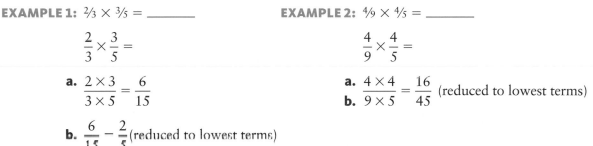

EXAMPLE 3: $\frac{2}{6} \times \frac{3}{4} =$ _____

$$\frac{\overset{1}{\cancel{2}}}{\underset{2}{\cancel{6}}} \times \frac{\overset{1}{\cancel{3}}}{\underset{2}{\cancel{4}}} = \frac{1 \times 1}{2 \times 2} = \frac{1}{4}$$

Multiplication of Mixed Numbers

1. Change each mixed number to an improper fraction.
2. Multiply the numerators.
3. Multiply the denominators.
4. Place the product of the numerators over the product of the denominators.
5. Reduce to lowest terms.

> **! ALERT**
>
> *Remember the denominator of a whole number is *always* 1.

$$6 = \frac{6}{1}$$

$$12 = \frac{12}{1}$$

EXAMPLE 1: $1\frac{1}{2} \times 2\frac{1}{4} =$ _____

a. $\dfrac{3}{2} \times \dfrac{9}{4} =$

b. $\dfrac{3 \times 9}{2 \times 4} = \dfrac{27}{8} = 3\dfrac{3}{8}$ (reduced to lowest terms)

EXAMPLE 2: $2 \times 3\frac{5}{6} =$ _____

a. $\dfrac{2}{1} \times \dfrac{23}{6} =$

b. $\dfrac{\overset{1}{\cancel{2}}}{1} \times \dfrac{23}{\underset{3}{\cancel{6}}} =$

c. $\dfrac{1 \times 23}{1 \times 3} = \dfrac{23}{3} = 7\dfrac{2}{3}$ (reduced to lowest terms)

DIVISION OF FRACTIONS

1. Invert (or turn upside down) the divisor.
2. Multiply the two fractions.
3. Reduce to lowest terms.

EXAMPLE 1: $\frac{2}{3} \div \frac{6}{8} =$ _____

$$\frac{2}{3} \div \frac{6}{8} =$$

a. $\dfrac{2}{3} \times \dfrac{8}{6} =$

b. c. $\dfrac{\overset{1}{\cancel{2}}}{3} \times \dfrac{8}{\underset{3}{\cancel{6}}} = \dfrac{1 \times 8}{3 \times 3} = \dfrac{8}{9}$

EXAMPLE 2: $\frac{3}{4} \div \frac{8}{9} =$ _____

$$\frac{3}{4} \div \frac{8}{9} =$$

a. $\dfrac{3}{4} \times \dfrac{9}{8} =$

b. c. $\dfrac{3 \times 9}{4 \times 8} = \dfrac{27}{32}$

Division of Mixed Numbers

1. Change each mixed number to an improper fraction.
2. Invert (or turn upside down) the divisor.
3. Multiply the two fractions.
4. Reduce to lowest terms.

EXAMPLE 1: $1\frac{3}{4} \div 2\frac{1}{8} =$ _____   **EXAMPLE 2:** $\frac{1}{7} \div 7 =$ _____

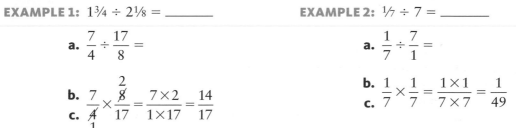

a. $\dfrac{7}{4} \div \dfrac{17}{8} =$ **a.** $\dfrac{1}{7} \div \dfrac{7}{1} =$

b.
c. $\dfrac{7}{\cancel{4}_{1}} \times \dfrac{\cancel{8}^{2}}{17} = \dfrac{7 \times 2}{1 \times 17} = \dfrac{14}{17}$ **b.**
c. $\dfrac{1}{7} \times \dfrac{1}{7} = \dfrac{1 \times 1}{7 \times 7} = \dfrac{1}{49}$

REDUCTION OF A COMPLEX FRACTION

1. Rewrite the complex fraction as a division problem.
2. Invert (or turn upside down) the divisor.
3. Multiply the two fractions.
4. Reduce to lowest terms.

EXAMPLE 1: $\frac{3}{8} / \frac{1}{4} =$ _____   **EXAMPLE 2:** $\frac{1}{2} / \frac{2}{7} =$ _____

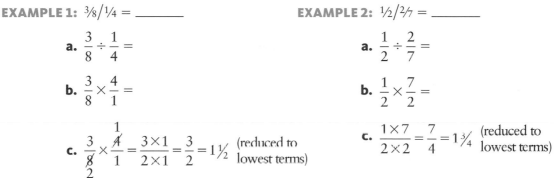

a. $\dfrac{3}{8} \div \dfrac{1}{4} =$ **a.** $\dfrac{1}{2} \div \dfrac{2}{7} =$

b. $\dfrac{3}{8} \times \dfrac{4}{1} =$ **b.** $\dfrac{1}{2} \times \dfrac{7}{2} =$

c. $\dfrac{3}{\cancel{8}_{2}} \times \dfrac{\cancel{4}^{1}}{1} = \dfrac{3 \times 1}{2 \times 1} = \dfrac{3}{2} = 1\frac{1}{2}$ (reduced to lowest terms)

c. $\dfrac{1 \times 7}{2 \times 2} = \dfrac{7}{4} = 1\frac{3}{4}$ (reduced to lowest terms)

Reduction of a Complex Fraction with Mixed Numbers

1. Rewrite the complex fraction as a division problem.
2. Change the mixed numbers to improper fractions.
3. Invert (or turn upside down) the divisor.
4. Multiply the two fractions.
5. Reduce to lowest terms.

EXAMPLE 1: $2\frac{1}{2} / 1\frac{1}{3} =$ _____   **EXAMPLE 2:** $3\frac{3}{4} / 2\frac{1}{6} =$ _____

a. $2\dfrac{1}{2} \div 1\dfrac{1}{3} =$ **a.** $3\dfrac{3}{4} \div 2\dfrac{1}{6} =$

b. $\dfrac{5}{2} \div \dfrac{4}{3} =$ **b.** $\dfrac{15}{4} \div \dfrac{13}{6} =$

c. $\dfrac{5}{2} \times \dfrac{3}{4} =$ **c.** $\dfrac{15}{4} \times \dfrac{6}{13} =$

d. $\dfrac{5 \times 3}{2 \times 4} = \dfrac{15}{8} = 1\dfrac{7}{8}$ (reduced to lowest terms)

d. $\dfrac{15 \times \cancel{6}^{3}}{\cancel{4}_{2} \times 13} = \dfrac{45}{26} = 1\dfrac{19}{26}$ (reduced to lowest terms)

WORK SHEET

DIRECTIONS: Change the following improper fractions to mixed numbers.

1. $4/3 =$ _____   **2.** $6/2 =$ _____   **3.** $16/5 =$ _____   **4.** $13/4 =$ _____

5. $15/10 =$ _____   **6.** $9/8 =$ _____   **7.** $10/6 =$ _____   **8.** $26/12 =$ _____

9. $21/6 =$ _____   **10.** $11/8 =$ _____   **11.** $7/2 =$ _____   **12.** $112/100 =$ _____

DIRECTIONS: Change the following mixed numbers to improper fractions.

1. $1\frac{1}{2} =$ _____   **2.** $3\frac{3}{4} =$ _____   **3.** $2\frac{2}{3} =$ _____   **4.** $2\frac{5}{6} =$ _____

5. $1\frac{3}{5} =$ _____   **6.** $3\frac{4}{7} =$ _____   **7.** $4\frac{7}{8} =$ _____   **8.** $3\frac{7}{100} =$ _____

9. $2\frac{7}{10} =$ _____   **10.** $6\frac{5}{8} =$ _____   **11.** $1\frac{3}{25} =$ _____   **12.** $4\frac{1}{4} =$ _____

DIRECTIONS: Add and reduce fractions to lowest terms.

1. $2/3 + 5/6 =$ _____   **2.** $2/5 + 3/7 =$ _____   **3.** $3\frac{1}{8} + 2/3 =$ _____

4. $2\frac{1}{2} + 3/4 =$ _____   **5.** $2\frac{1}{4} + 3\frac{2}{5} =$ _____   **6.** $1\frac{6}{13} + 1\frac{2}{3} =$ _____

7. $1\frac{1}{2} + 3\frac{3}{4} + 2\frac{3}{8} =$ _____ **8.** $4\frac{3}{11} + 2\frac{1}{2} =$ _____ **9.** $2\frac{2}{3} + 3\frac{7}{9} =$ _____

10. $1\frac{3}{10} + 4\frac{2}{5} + \frac{2}{3} =$ _____ **11.** $3\frac{1}{2} + 2\frac{5}{6} + 2\frac{2}{3} =$ _____ **12.** $5\frac{5}{6} + 2\frac{2}{5} =$ _____

DIRECTIONS: Subtract and reduce fractions to lowest terms.

1. $\frac{2}{3} - \frac{3}{7} =$ _____ **2.** $\frac{7}{8} - \frac{5}{16} =$ _____ **3.** $\frac{9}{16} - \frac{5}{12} =$ _____

4. $1\frac{1}{3} - \frac{5}{6} =$ _____ **5.** $2\frac{17}{20} - 1\frac{3}{4} =$ _____ **6.** $5\frac{1}{4} - 3\frac{5}{16} =$ _____

7. $5\frac{3}{8} - 4\frac{3}{4} =$ _____ **8.** $3\frac{1}{4} - 1\frac{11}{12} =$ _____ **9.** $6\frac{1}{2} - 3\frac{7}{8} =$ _____

10. $4\frac{1}{6} - 2\frac{3}{4} =$ _____ **11.** $5\frac{2}{3} - 3\frac{7}{8} =$ _____ **12.** $2\frac{5}{16} - 1\frac{3}{8} =$ _____

DIRECTIONS: Multiply and reduce fractions to lowest terms.

1. $\frac{1}{3} \times \frac{4}{5} =$ _____ **2.** $\frac{7}{8} \times \frac{2}{3} =$ _____ **3.** $6 \times \frac{2}{3} =$ _____

4. $\frac{3}{8} \times 4 =$ _____ **5.** $2\frac{1}{3} \times 3\frac{3}{4} =$ _____ **6.** $4\frac{3}{8} \times 2\frac{5}{7} =$ _____

7. $2\frac{5}{12} \times 5\frac{1}{4} =$ _____ **8.** $\frac{3}{4} \times 2\frac{3}{8} =$ _____ **9.** $\frac{3}{8} \times \frac{4}{5} \times \frac{2}{3} =$ _____

10. $\frac{1}{10} \times \frac{3}{100} =$ _____ **11.** $3\frac{1}{2} \times 1\frac{5}{6} =$ _____ **12.** $2\frac{4}{9} \times 1\frac{3}{11} =$ _____

DIRECTIONS: Divide and reduce fractions to lowest terms.

1. $1\frac{2}{3} \div 3\frac{1}{2} = $ _____

2. $5\frac{1}{2} \div 2\frac{1}{2} = $ _____

3. $3\frac{1}{2} \div 2\frac{1}{4} = $ _____

4. $4\frac{3}{8} \div 1\frac{3}{4} = $ _____

5. $3\frac{1}{2} \div 1\frac{6}{7} = $ _____

6. $\frac{9}{10} \div \frac{2}{3} = $ _____

7. $3 \div 1\frac{5}{6} = $ _____

8. $6\frac{2}{3} \div 1\frac{7}{10} = $ _____

9. $\frac{7}{8} / \frac{1}{4} = $ _____

10. $6\frac{1}{2} / 2\frac{5}{6} = $ _____

11. $5\frac{1}{2} / 2\frac{2}{3} = $ _____

12. $2\frac{2}{3} / 1\frac{7}{9} = $ _____

ANSWERS ON P. 29.

NAME _____

DATE _____

ACCEPTABLE SCORE __**29**__

YOUR SCORE _____

DIRECTIONS: Perform the indicated calculations and reduce fractions to lowest terms.

1. $^2\!/_3 + {}^4\!/_9 =$ _____

2. $^3\!/_8 + {}^1\!/_3 =$ _____

3. $2^3\!/_4 + 2^1\!/_3 =$ _____

4. $2^2\!/_3 + {}^3\!/_7 =$ _____

5. $^3\!/_4 + {}^3\!/_{100} =$ _____

6. $4^2\!/_5 + 3^3\!/_4 =$ _____

7. $4^1\!/_6 + {}^2\!/_3 + 2^3\!/_4 =$ _____

8. $1^3\!/_{10} - {}^2\!/_5 =$ _____

9. $2^1\!/_2 - 1^2\!/_3 =$ _____

10. $^5\!/_7 - {}^1\!/_2 =$ _____

11. $3^1\!/_2 - 1^9\!/_{16} =$ _____

12. $2^5\!/_7 - 1^2\!/_9 =$ _____

13. $9^1\!/_5 - 3^1\!/_2 =$ _____

14. $2^1\!/_4 - {}^7\!/_9 / {}^2\!/_3 =$ _____

15. $^3\!/_4 \times {}^6\!/_7 =$ _____

16. $3 \times {}^4\!/_5 =$ _____

17. $^2\!/_9 \times 9 =$ _____

18. $2^3\!/_4 \times 1^1\!/_6 =$ _____

19. $1^1\!/_4 \times 2^2\!/_3 =$ _____

20. $10^1\!/_2 \times 1^2\!/_3 =$ _____

21. $5^6\!/_7 \times {}^3\!/_5 =$ _____

22. $^1\!/_4 \times 3^1\!/_2 =$ _____

23. $^2\!/_3 \div {}^5\!/_8 =$ _____

24. $^1\!/_5 \div {}^1\!/_{50} =$ _____

25. $\frac{1}{3} \div \frac{1}{2} =$ _____

26. $\frac{5}{6} \div \frac{2}{3} =$ _____

27. $\frac{1}{5} / \frac{1}{3} =$ _____

28. $1\frac{1}{5} / \frac{8}{9} =$ _____

29. $\frac{3}{4} / \frac{1}{6} =$ _____

30. $3\frac{1}{8} / 2\frac{3}{4} =$ _____

ANSWERS ON P. 29.

NAME _____

DATE _____

ACCEPTABLE SCORE **29**

YOUR SCORE _____

POSTTEST 2

DIRECTIONS: Perform the indicated calculations and reduce fractions to lowest terms.

1. $\frac{1}{4} + \frac{5}{6} =$ _____

2. $2\frac{3}{5} + 1\frac{1}{2} =$ _____

3. $\frac{2}{3} + 2\frac{3}{7} =$ _____

4. $1\frac{7}{8} + 3\frac{2}{5} =$ _____

5. $1\frac{3}{4} + \frac{5}{8} + 2\frac{5}{12} =$ _____

6. $10\frac{1}{2} + 1\frac{3}{10} =$ _____

7. $1\frac{5}{14} + 2\frac{3}{21} =$ _____

8. $\frac{4}{9} - \frac{1}{3} =$ _____

9. $2\frac{3}{4} - \frac{7}{8} =$ _____

10. $3\frac{1}{2} - 1\frac{2}{3} =$ _____

11. $3\frac{5}{8} - 1\frac{5}{16} =$ _____

12. $7\frac{1}{3} - 5\frac{5}{6} =$ _____

13. $7\frac{7}{10} - 3\frac{4}{5} =$ _____

14. $3\frac{4}{15} - 2\frac{2}{3} =$ _____

15. $\frac{2}{7} \times \frac{2}{3} =$ _____

16. $3\frac{4}{9} \times 1\frac{4}{5} =$ _____

17. $2 \times \frac{2}{3} =$ _____

18. $\frac{5}{6} \times 2\frac{1}{3} =$ _____

19. $\frac{1}{100} \times \frac{1}{10} -$ _____

20. $6\frac{3}{4} \times 5\frac{1}{3} =$

21. $2\frac{5}{8} \times 1\frac{1}{3} -$ _____

22. $3\frac{1}{2} \times 3\frac{3}{14} =$ _____

23. $\frac{3}{4} \div \frac{8}{9} =$ _____

24. $1\frac{1}{2} \div 1\frac{6}{7} =$ _____

25. $2\frac{1}{3} \div \frac{3}{8} =$ _____

26. $\frac{1}{7} \div 7 =$ _____

27. $\frac{5}{6} / 1\frac{1}{3} =$ _____

28. $1\frac{1}{2}/2\frac{2}{7} =$ _____

29. $2\frac{1}{4}/1\frac{1}{3} =$ _____

30. $\frac{3}{8}/\frac{3}{9} =$ _____

ANSWERS ON P. 29.

evolve   For additional practice problems, refer to the Mathematics Review
section of *Drug Calculations Companion,* Version 5, on Evolve.

ANSWERS

CHAPTER 1 Fractions—Pretest, pp. 7–8

1. $1\frac{10}{63}$	7. $5\frac{23}{24}$	12. $1\frac{5}{6}$	17. $7\frac{19}{63}$	21. $12\frac{1}{12}$	26. $\frac{7}{8}$
2. $10\frac{2}{3}$	8. $\frac{3}{10}$	13. $1\frac{4}{5}$	18. $1\frac{1}{14}$ or $\frac{15}{14}$	22. $2\frac{25}{28}$	27. $1\frac{1}{3}$
3. $9\frac{3}{4}$	9. $\frac{1}{8}$	14. $1\frac{5}{6}$		23. $\frac{5}{16}$	28. $\frac{5}{9}$
4. $5\frac{9}{16}$	10. $2\frac{5}{8}$	15. $\frac{1}{15}$	19. $\frac{1}{10,000}$, 0.0001	24. $1\frac{1}{3}$	29. $1\frac{7}{10}$
5. $9\frac{1}{22}$	11. $2\frac{17}{24}$	16. 5	20. $4\frac{5}{18}$	25. $33\frac{1}{3}$	30. 2
6. $7\frac{8}{9}$					

CHAPTER 1 Fractions—Work Sheet, pp. 21–23

Improper Fractions to Mixed Numbers, *p. 21*

1. $1\frac{1}{3}$	3. $3\frac{1}{5}$	5. $1\frac{1}{2}$	7. $1\frac{2}{3}$	9. $3\frac{1}{2}$	11. $3\frac{1}{2}$
2. 3	4. $3\frac{1}{4}$	6. $1\frac{1}{8}$	8. $2\frac{1}{6}$	10. $1\frac{3}{8}$	12. $1\frac{3}{25}$

Mixed Numbers to Improper Fractions, *p. 21*

1. $\frac{3}{2}$	3. $\frac{8}{3}$	5. $\frac{8}{5}$	7. $\frac{39}{8}$	9. $\frac{27}{10}$	11. $\frac{28}{25}$
2. $\frac{15}{4}$	4. $\frac{17}{6}$	6. $\frac{25}{7}$	8. $\frac{307}{100}$	10. $\frac{53}{8}$	12. $\frac{17}{4}$

Addition, *pp. 21–22*

1. $1\frac{1}{2}$	3. $3\frac{19}{24}$	5. $5\frac{13}{20}$	7. $7\frac{5}{8}$	9. $6\frac{4}{9}$	11. 9
2. $\frac{29}{35}$	4. $3\frac{1}{4}$	6. $3\frac{5}{39}$	8. $6\frac{17}{22}$	10. $6\frac{11}{30}$	12. $8\frac{7}{30}$

Subtraction, *p. 22*

1. $\frac{5}{21}$	3. $\frac{7}{48}$	5. $1\frac{1}{10}$	7. $\frac{5}{8}$	9. $2\frac{5}{8}$	11. $1\frac{19}{24}$
2. $\frac{9}{16}$	4. $\frac{1}{2}$	6. $1\frac{15}{16}$	8. $1\frac{1}{3}$	10. $1\frac{5}{12}$	12. $\frac{15}{16}$

Multiplication, *p. 22*

1. $\frac{4}{15}$	3. 4	5. $8\frac{3}{4}$	7. $12\frac{11}{16}$	9. $\frac{1}{5}$	11. $6\frac{5}{12}$
2. $\frac{7}{12}$	4. $1\frac{1}{2}$	6. $11\frac{7}{8}$	8. $1\frac{25}{32}$	10. $\frac{3}{1000}$	12. $3\frac{1}{9}$

Division, *p. 23*

1. $\frac{10}{21}$	3. $1\frac{5}{9}$	5. $1\frac{23}{26}$	7. $1\frac{7}{11}$	9. $3\frac{1}{2}$	11. $2\frac{1}{16}$
2. $2\frac{1}{5}$	4. $2\frac{1}{2}$	6. $1\frac{7}{20}$	8. $3\frac{47}{51}$	10. $2\frac{5}{17}$	12. $1\frac{1}{2}$

CHAPTER 1 Fractions—Posttest 1, pp. 25–26

1. $1\frac{1}{9}$	6. $8\frac{3}{20}$	11. $1\frac{15}{16}$	16. $2\frac{2}{5}$	21. $3\frac{18}{35}$	26. $1\frac{1}{4}$
2. $\frac{17}{24}$	7. $7\frac{7}{12}$	12. $1\frac{31}{63}$	17. 2	22. $\frac{7}{8}$	27. $\frac{3}{5}$
3. $5\frac{1}{12}$	8. $\frac{9}{10}$	13. $5\frac{7}{10}$	18. $3\frac{5}{24}$	23. $1\frac{1}{15}$	28. $1\frac{7}{20}$
4. $3\frac{2}{21}$	9. $\frac{5}{6}$	14. $1\frac{1}{12}$	19. $3\frac{1}{3}$	24. 10	29. $4\frac{1}{2}$
5. $\frac{39}{50}$	10. $\frac{3}{14}$	15. $\frac{9}{14}$	20. $14\frac{7}{10}$	25. $\frac{2}{3}$	30. $1\frac{3}{22}$

CHAPTER 1 Fractions—Posttest 2, pp. 27–28

1. $1\frac{1}{12}$	6. $11\frac{4}{5}$	11. $2\frac{5}{16}$	16. $6\frac{1}{5}$	21. $3\frac{1}{2}$	26. $\frac{1}{49}$
2. $4\frac{1}{10}$	7. $3\frac{1}{2}$	12. $1\frac{1}{2}$	17. $1\frac{1}{3}$	22. $11\frac{1}{4}$	27. $\frac{5}{8}$
3. $3\frac{2}{21}$	8. $\frac{1}{9}$	13. $3\frac{9}{10}$	18. $1\frac{17}{18}$	23. $\frac{27}{32}$	28. $\frac{21}{32}$
4. $5\frac{11}{40}$	9. $1\frac{7}{8}$	14. $\frac{3}{5}$	19. $\frac{1}{1000}$	24. $\frac{21}{26}$	29. $1\frac{11}{16}$
5. $4\frac{19}{24}$	10. $1\frac{5}{6}$	15. $\frac{4}{21}$	20. 36	25. $6\frac{2}{9}$	30. $1\frac{1}{8}$

ACCEPTABLE SCORE ___**36**___

YOUR SCORE _____

PRETEST

Complete the Decimals Pretest. A score of 36 out of 38 indicates an acceptable understanding of and competency in basic calculations involving decimals. You may skip to the Percents Pretest on p. 53. However, if you score 35 or below, completion of Chapter 2, Decimals, will be helpful for your continued success in the calculation of drug dosages.

DIRECTIONS: Write the following numbers in words.

1. 0.04 _____

2. 1.6 _____

3. 16.06734 _____

_____

4. 1.015 _____

5. 0.009 _____

DIRECTIONS: Circle the decimal with the *least value.*

6. 0.2, 0.25, 0.025, 0.02   **7.** 0.4, 0.48, 0.04, 0.004

8. 1.6, 1.64, 1.682, 1.69   **9.** 2.8, 2.82, 2.082, 2.822

10. 0.3, 0.33, 0.003, 0.033

DIRECTIONS: Perform the indicated calculations.

11. 6.8 + 2.986 +
14.7 + 0.89 = _____

12. 141.71 + 84.98 +
9.98 + 87.63 = _____

13. 1006.48 + 0.008 +
6.2 + 0.179 = _____

14. 47.21 + 48.496 +
0.2976 + 54.67 = _____

15. 5.971 + 63.1 +
8.264 + 7.23 = _____

16. 2.176 − 1.098 = _____

17. 2.006 − 0.998 = _____

18. 836.2 − 76.8 = _____

19. 100.3 − 98.6 = _____

20. 12.6 − 1.654 = _____   **21.** 0.63 × 0.09 = _____   **22.** 41.545 × 0.16 = _____

23. 5.25 × 0.37 = _____   **24.** 44.08 × 0.67 = _____   **25.** 56.7 × 3.29 = _____

26. 0.89 ÷ 4.32 = _____   **27.** 1.436 ÷ 0.08 = _____   **28.** 0.689 ÷ 62.8 = _____

29. 12.54 ÷ 0.02 = _____   **30.** 23 ÷ 1236 = _____

DIRECTIONS: Change the following decimal fractions to proper fractions.

31. 0.008 = _____   **32.** 0.25 = _____   **33.** 0.322 = _____ **34.** 0.004 = _____

DIRECTIONS: Change the following proper fractions to decimal fractions.

35. 3/5 = _____   **36.** 2/3 = _____   **37.** 3/500 = _____ **38.** 7/20 = _____

ANSWERS ON P. 49.

CHAPTER 2

Decimals

LEARNING OBJECTIVES

Upon completion of the materials provided in this chapter, you will be able to perform computations accurately by mastering the following mathematical concepts:

1 Reading and writing decimal numbers
2 Determining the value of decimal fractions
3 Adding, subtracting, multiplying, and dividing decimals
4 Rounding decimal fractions to an indicated place value
5 Multiplying and dividing decimals by 10 or a power of 10
6 Multiplying and dividing decimals by 0.1 or a multiple of 0.1
7 Converting a decimal fraction to a proper fraction
8 Converting a proper fraction to a decimal fraction

Study the introductory material for decimals. The processes for the calculation of decimal problems are listed in steps. Memorize the steps for each calculation before beginning the work sheet. Complete the work sheet at the end of this chapter, which provides for extensive practice in the manipulation of decimals. Check your answers. If you have difficulties, go back and review the steps for that type of calculation. When you feel ready to evaluate your learning, take the first posttest. Check your answers. An acceptable score as indicated on the posttest signifies that you are ready for the next chapter. An unacceptable score signifies a need for further study before you take the second posttest.

Decimals are used in the metric system of measurement. **Nurses use the metric system in the calculation of drug dosages. Therefore it is essential for nurses to be able to manipulate decimals easily and accurately.**

Each **decimal fraction** consists of a numerator that is expressed in numerals; a decimal point placed to designate the value of the denominator; and the denominator, which is understood to be 10 or some power of 10. **In writing a decimal fraction, always place a zero to the left of the decimal point so that the decimal point can readily be seen. The omission of the zero may result in a critical medication error.** Some examples are as follows:

Fraction	Decimal fraction
$\frac{7}{10}$	0.7
$\frac{13}{100}$	0.13
$\frac{227}{1000}$	0.227

Decimal numbers include an integer (or whole number), a decimal point, and a decimal fraction. The value of the combined integer and decimal fraction is determined by the placement of the decimal point. Whole numbers are written to the *left* of the decimal point, and decimal fractions to the *right*. Figure 2-1 illustrates the place occupied by the numeral that has the value indicated.

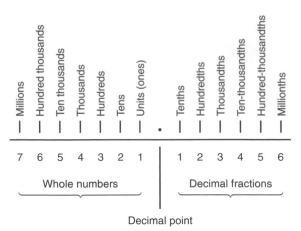

FIGURE 2-1   Decimal place values.

READING DECIMAL NUMBERS

The reading of a decimal number is determined by the place value of the integers and decimal fractions.

1. Read the whole number.
2. Read the decimal point as "and" or "point."
3. Read the decimal fraction.

EXAMPLES:		
	0.4	four tenths
	0.86	eighty-six hundredths
	3.659	three and six hundred fifty-nine thousandths
	182.0012	one hundred eighty-two and twelve ten-thousandths
	9.47735	nine and forty-seven thousand seven hundred thirty-five hundred-thousandths

DETERMINING THE VALUES OF DECIMAL FRACTIONS

1. Place the numbers in a vertical column with the decimal points in a vertical line.
2. Add zeros on the right in the decimal fractions to make columns even.
3. The largest number in the first column to the right of the decimal point has the *greatest* value.
4. If two numbers in a column are of equal value, examine the next column to the right, and so on.
5. The smallest number in the first column to the right of the decimal point has the *least* value. If two numbers in the first column are of equal value, examine the second column to the right, and so on.

> **EXAMPLE 1:**   Of the following fractions (0.623, 0.841, 0.0096, 0.432), which has the greatest value? the least value?
>
> 0.6320
> 0.8410
> 0.0096
> 0.4320
>
> 0.841 has the greatest value; 0.0096 has the least value.
>
> NOTE: In mixed numbers the values of both the integer and the fraction are considered.

EXAMPLE 2: Which decimal number (0.4, 0.25, 1.2, 1.002) has the greatest value? the least value?

> 0.400
> 0.250
> 1.200
> 1.002

1.2 has the greatest value; 0.25 has the least value.

ADDITION AND SUBTRACTION OF DECIMALS

1. Write the numerals in a vertical column with the decimal points in a straight line.
2. Add zeros as needed to complete the columns.
3. Add or subtract each column as indicated by the symbol.
4. Place the decimal point in the sum or difference directly below the decimal points in the column.
5. Place a zero to the left of the decimal point in a decimal fraction.

EXAMPLE 1: Add: $14.8 + 6.29 + 3.028$

```
   14.800
    6.290
 +  3.028
   ──────
   24.118
```

EXAMPLE 2: Subtract: $5.163 - 4.98$

```
   5.163
 - 4.980
 ───────
   0.183
```

MULTIPLICATION OF DECIMALS

1. Place the shorter group of numbers under the longer group of numbers.
2. Multiply.
3. Add the number of places to the right of the decimal point in the **multiplicand** and the **multiplier** (i.e., the numbers being multiplied). The sum determines the placement of the decimal point within the product.
4. Count from right to left of the value of the sum and place the decimal point.

EXAMPLE 1: 0.19×0.2

```
    0.19   two place values
 ×  0.2    one place value
 ──────
    038
    000
 ──────
  0.038   three place values
```

EXAMPLE 2: 0.459×0.52

```
    0.459   three place values
 ×   0.52   two place values
 ────────
    0918
    2295
    0000
 ─────────
  0.23868   five place values
```

EXAMPLE 3: 8.265×4.36

```
    8.265   three place values
 ×   4.36   two place values
 ────────
   49590
   24795
   33060
 ─────────
  36.03540   five place values
```

EXAMPLE 4: 160.41×3.527

```
   160.41   two place values
 ×   3.527   three place values
 ─────────
   112287
    32082
    80205
    48123
 ──────────
  565.76607   five place values
```

Multiplying a Decimal by 10 or a Power of 10 (100, 1000, 10,000, 100,000)

1. Move the decimal point to the right the *same number of places as there are zeros in the multiplier.*
2. Zeros may be added as indicated.

    EXAMPLE 1: $0.132 \times 10 = 1.32$ **EXAMPLE 2:** $0.053 \times 100 = 5.3$

    EXAMPLE 3: $2.64 \times 1000 = 2640$ **EXAMPLE 4:** $49.6 \times 10{,}000 = 496{,}000$

Multiplying a Whole Number or Decimal by 0.1 or a Multiple of 0.1 (0.01, 0.001, 0.0001, 0.00001)

1. Move the decimal point to the left the *same number of spaces as there are numbers to the right of the decimal point in the multiplier.*
2. Zeros may be added as indicated.

    EXAMPLE 1: $354.86 \times 0.0001 = 0.035486$ **EXAMPLE 2:** $0.729 \times 0.1 = 0.0729$

    EXAMPLE 3: $12.73 \times 0.01 = 0.1273$ **EXAMPLE 4:** $5.752 \times 0.001 = 0.005752$

ROUNDING A DECIMAL FRACTION

1. Find the number to the right of the place value desired.
2. If the number is 5, 6, 7, 8, or 9, add 1 to the number in the place value desired and drop the rest of the numbers.
3. If the number is 0, 1, 2, 3, or 4, remove all numbers to the right of the desired place value.

    EXAMPLE 1: Round the following decimal fractions to the nearest tenth.

        a. 0.268

           0.2)68   6 is the number to the right of the tenths place. Therefore 1 should be added to the number 2 and the 68 dropped.

           0.3   correct answer

        b. 4.374

           4.3)74   7 is the number to the right of the tenths place. Therefore 1 should be added to the number 3 and the 74 dropped.

           4.4   correct answer

        c. 5.723

           5.7)23   2 is the number to the right of the tenths place. Therefore all numbers to the right of the tenths place should be removed.

           5.7   correct answer

    EXAMPLE 2: Round the following decimal fractions to the nearest hundredth.

        a. 0.876

           0.87)6   6 is the number to the right of the hundredths place. Therefore 1 should be added to the number 7 and the 6 dropped.

           0.88   correct answer

        b. 2.3249

           2.32)49   4 is the number to the right of the hundredths place. Therefore all numbers to the right of the hundredths place should be removed.

           2.32   correct answer

EXAMPLE 3: Round the following decimal fractions to the nearest thousandth.

    a. 3.1325

      3.132)5   5 is the number to the right of the thousandths place. Therefore 1 should be added to the number 2 and the 5 dropped.

      3.133   correct answer

    b. 0.4674

      0.467)4   4 is the number to the right of the thousandths place. Therefore all numbers to the right of the thousandths place should be removed.

      0.467   correct answer

Rounding numbers helps to estimate values, compare values, have more realistic and workable numbers, and spot errors. Decimal fractions may be rounded to any designated place value.

DIVISION OF DECIMALS

1. Place a caret ($\wedge$) to the right of the last number in the divisor, signifying the movement of the decimal point that will make the divisor a whole number.
2. Count the number of spaces that the decimal point is moved in the divisor.
3. Count to the right an equal number of spaces in the dividend and place a caret to signify the movement of the decimal.
4. Place a decimal point on the quotient line directly above the caret.
5. Divide, extending the decimal fraction three places to the right of the decimal point.
6. Zeros may be added as indicated to extend the decimal fraction dividend.
7. Round the quotient to the nearest hundredth.

EXAMPLE 1: 8.326 ÷ 1.062

```
                  7 . 839  or 7.84
     1.062 ∧)8.326 ∧ 000
            7 434
            ‾‾‾‾‾
              892 0
              849 6
              ‾‾‾‾‾
               42 40
               31 86
               ‾‾‾‾‾
               10 540
                9 558
```

EXAMPLE 2: 386 ÷ 719

```
              0.536  or 0.54
      719)386.000
          359 5
          ‾‾‾‾‾
           26 50
           21 57
           ‾‾‾‾‾
            4 930
            4 314
```

NOTE: The decimal fraction is emphasized by the placement of a zero to the left of the decimal point.

Dividing a Decimal by 10 or a Multiple of 10 (100, 1000, 10,000, 100,000)

1. Move the decimal point to the left the same number of places as there are zeros in the divisor.
2. Zeros may be added as indicated.

EXAMPLE 1: 6.41 ÷ 10 = 0.641

EXAMPLE 2: 358.0 ÷ 100 = 3.58

Dividing a Whole Number or a Decimal Fraction by 0.1 or a Multiple of 0.1 (0.01, 0.001, 0.0001, 0.00001)

1. Move the decimal point to the right as many places as there are numbers in the divisor.
2. Zeros may be added as indicated.

EXAMPLE 1: $5.897 \div 0.01 = 589.7$ **EXAMPLE 2:** $46.31 \div 0.001 = 46{,}310$

CONVERSION

Converting a Decimal Fraction to a Proper Fraction

1. Remove the decimal point and the zero preceding it.
2. The numerals are the numerator.
3. The placement of the decimal point indicates what the denominator will be.
4. Reduce to lowest terms.

EXAMPLE 1: 0.3   **EXAMPLE 2:** 0.86   **EXAMPLE 3:** 0.375

$$\frac{3}{10}$$ $$\frac{86}{100} = \frac{43}{50}$$ $$\frac{375}{1000} = \frac{3}{8}$$

Converting a Proper Fraction to a Decimal Fraction

1. Divide the numerator by the denominator.
2. Extend the decimal the desired number of places (often three).
3. Place a zero to the left of the decimal point in a decimal fraction.

EXAMPLE 1: $\frac{4}{5}$ **EXAMPLE 2:** $\frac{7}{8}$

$$
\begin{array}{r}
0.8 \\
5\overline{)4.0} \\
4\,0 \\
\hline
\end{array}
$$

$\frac{4}{5} = 0.8$

$$
\begin{array}{r}
0.875 \\
8\overline{)7.000} \\
6\,4 \\
\hline
60 \\
56 \\
\hline
40 \\
40 \\
\hline
\end{array}
$$

$\frac{7}{8} = 0.875$

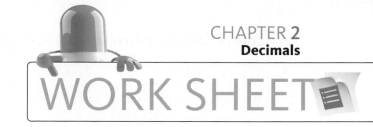

WORK SHEET

DIRECTIONS: Write the following numbers in words.

1. 0.2 _____

2. 9.68 _____

3. 0.0003 _____

4. 1,968.342 _____

_____

5. 0.02 _____

DIRECTIONS: Circle the decimal numbers with the *greatest value*.

1. 0.2, 0.15, 0.1, 0.25   **2.** 0.4, 0.45, 0.04, 0.042   **3.** 0.9, 0.09, 0.95, 0.98

4. 0.5, 0.065, 0.58, 0.68   **5.** 1.8, 1.08, 1.18, 1.468   **6.** 7.4, 7.42, 7.423, 7.44

DIRECTIONS: Circle the decimal numbers with the *least value*.

1. 0.6, 0.66, 0.666, 0.6666   **2.** 0.3, 0.03, 0.003, 0.0003   **3.** 1.2, 1.22, 1.022, 1.0022

4. 0.8, 0.08, 0.868, 0.859   **5.** 0.75, 0.07, 0.007, 0.0075   **6.** 3.015, 3.1, 3.006, 3.02

DIRECTIONS: Add the following decimal problems.

1. 1.080 + 31.2 +
0.065 + 9.41 = _____

2. 2.2 + 355.6 +
8.125 + 6.75 = _____

3. 24.684 + 5.3697 +
8.025 + 2.9 = _____

4. 18.95 + 1.903 +
8.82 + 9.4 = _____

5. 56.93 + 765.7 +
64.882 + 7.33 = _____

6. 0.3 + 0.874 +
2.763 + 63.2 = _____

7. 13.5 + 1.023 +
8.83 + 3.267 = _____

8. 3.6 + 8.25 +
2.05 + 24 = _____

9. 0.6 + 0.985 +
1.432 + 52.1 = _____

DIRECTIONS: Subtract the following decimal problems.

1. 1321.52 − 63.65 = _____   **2.** 4.745 − 2.896 = _____   **3.** 1.8 − 1.09 = _____

4. 250.7 − 75.896 = _____   **5.** 24.186 − 16.768 = _____   **6.** 6.33 − 2.186 = _____

7. 0.486 − 0.025 = _____   **8.** 1 − 0.012 = _____   **9.** 63 − 0.978 = _____

DIRECTIONS: Multiply the following decimal problems.

1. $1.3 \times 12.5 =$ _____   **2.** $127 \times 4.8 =$ _____   **3.** $1.69 \times 30.8 =$ _____

4. $9.08 \times 6.18 =$ _____   **5.** $52.4 \times 0.8 =$ _____   **6.** $420 \times 0.08 =$ _____

7. $2.3 \times 45.21 =$ _____   **8.** $7.46 \times 54.83 =$ _____   **9.** $1.19 \times 0.127 =$ _____

DIRECTIONS: Multiply the following numbers by 10 by moving the decimal point.

1. 0.09 _____   **2.** 0.2 _____   **3.** 0.18 _____

4. 0.3 _____   **5.** 0.625 _____   **6.** 2.33 _____

DIRECTIONS: Multiply the following numbers by 100 by moving the decimal point.

1. 0.023 _____
2. 1.5 _____
3. 0.004 _____
4. 0.125 _____
5. 8.65 _____
6. 76.4 _____

DIRECTIONS: Multiply the following numbers by 1000 by moving the decimal point.

1. 0.2 _____
2. 0.005 _____
3. 0.187 _____
4. 9.65 _____
5. 0.46 _____
6. 0.489 _____

DIRECTIONS: Multiply the following numbers by 0.1 by moving the decimal point.

1. 30.0 _____
2. 0.69 _____
3. 1.7 _____
4. 0.95 _____
5. 0.138 _____
6. 5.67 _____

DIRECTIONS: Multiply the following numbers by 0.01 by moving the decimal point.

1. 0.26 _____
2. 90.8 _____
3. 5.5 _____
4. 11.2 _____
5. 0.875 _____
6. 63.3 _____

DIRECTIONS: Multiply the following numbers by 0.001 by moving the decimal point.

1. 56.0 _____
2. 12.55 _____
3. 126.5 _____
4. 33.3 _____
5. 9.684 _____
6. 241 _____

DIRECTIONS: Round the following decimal fractions to the nearest tenth.

1. 0.33 _____
2. 0.913 _____
3. 2.359 _____
4. 0.66 _____
5. 58.36 _____
6. 8.092 _____

DIRECTIONS: Round the following decimal fractions to the nearest hundredth.

1. 2.555 _____
2. 4.275 _____
3. 0.284 _____
4. 3.923 _____
5. 6.534 _____
6. 2.988 _____

DIRECTIONS: Round the following decimal fractions to the nearest thousandth.

1. 27.86314 _____
2. 5.9246 _____
3. 2.1574 _____
4. 0.8493 _____
5. 321.0869 _____
6. 455.7682 _____

DIRECTIONS: Divide. Round the quotient to the nearest hundredth.

1. $7.02 \div 6 =$ _____

2. $124.2 \div 0.03 =$ _____

3. $5.46 \div 0.7 =$ _____

4. $24 \div 0.06 =$ _____

5. $24 \div 1500 =$ _____

6. $4.6 \div 35.362 =$ _____

7. $4.13 \div 0.05 =$ _____

8. $9.08 \div 2.006 =$ _____

9. $63 \div 132.3 =$ _____

DIRECTIONS: Divide the following numbers by 10 by moving the decimal point.

1. 6.0 _____

2. 0.2 _____

3. 9.8 _____

4. 0.05 _____

5. 0.375 _____

6. 0.99 _____

DIRECTIONS: Divide the following numbers by 100 by moving the decimal point.

1. 0.7 _____

2. 8.11 _____

3. 700.0 _____

4. 0.19 _____

5. 12.0 _____

6. 30.2 _____

DIRECTIONS: Divide the following numbers by 1000 by moving the decimal point.

1. 1.8 _____

2. 360.0 _____

3. 0.25 _____

4. 54.6 _____

5. 7.5 _____

6. 7140 _____

DIRECTIONS: Divide the following numbers by 0.1 by moving the decimal point.

1. 2.8 _____

2. 0.1 _____

3. 0.65 _____

4. 0.987 _____

5. 15.0 _____

6. 8.25 _____

DIRECTIONS: Divide the following numbers by 0.01 by moving the decimal point.

1. 36.0 _____

2. 0.16 _____

3. 0.48 _____

4. 9.59 _____

5. 0.8 _____

6. 0.097 _____

DIRECTIONS: Divide the following numbers by 0.001 by moving the decimal point.

1. 6.2 _____

2. 839.0 _____

3. 5.0 _____

4. 0.86 _____

5. 13.8 _____

6. 0.0156 _____

DIRECTIONS: Change the following decimal fractions to proper fractions.

1. 0.06 _____   **2.** 0.8 _____   **3.** 0.68 _____   **4.** 0.0025 _____

5. 0.625 _____   **6.** 0.25 _____   **7.** 0.64 _____   **8.** 0.005 _____

DIRECTIONS: Change the following proper fractions to decimal fractions.

1. $\frac{1}{8}$ _____   **2.** $\frac{2}{3}$ _____   **3.** $\frac{16}{25}$ _____   **4.** $\frac{3}{5}$ _____

5. $\frac{8}{200}$ _____   **6.** $\frac{1}{3}$ _____   **7.** $\frac{4}{5}$ _____   **8.** $\frac{7}{8}$ _____

ANSWERS ON PP. 49–51.

NAME _____

DATE _____

ACCEPTABLE SCORE __31__

YOUR SCORE _____

POSTTEST 1

DIRECTIONS: Write the following numbers in words.

1. 634.18 _____

_____

2. 0.9 _____

3. 64.231 _____

_____

DIRECTIONS: Circle the decimal fractions with the *greatest value*.

4. 0.1, 0.01, 0.15, 0.015   **5.** 0.666, 0.068, 0.006, 0.66

DIRECTIONS: Perform the indicated calculations.

6. 1.342 + 0.987 +
8.062 + 44.269 = _____

7. 0.6 + 0.45 +
2.9 + 4.94 = _____

8. 3.004 + 0.848 +
0.9 + 1.6 = _____

9. 2.875 + 0.75 +
0.094 + 2.385 = _____

10. 1981.62 + 4.876 +
146.35 + 19.78 = _____

11. 1 − 0.661 = _____

12. 2.46 − 1.0068 = _____

13. 844.6 − 521.52 = _____

14. 43.69 − 0.0823 = _____

15. 0.9 − 0.689 = _____

16. 72.8 × 9.649 = _____

17. 1.58 × 0.088 = _____

18. $360 \times 0.45 =$ _____   **19.** $26.2 \times 1.69 =$ _____   **20.** $1.5 \times 0.39 =$ _____

21. $268.8 \div 16 =$ _____   **22.** $8.89 \div 0.006 =$ _____   **23.** $12.54 \div 0.02 =$ _____

24. $56.4 \div 40 =$ _____   **25.** $165.9 \div 3.006 =$ _____

DIRECTIONS: Change the following decimal fractions to proper fractions.

26. 0.09 _____   **27.** 0.0025 _____   **28.** 0.375 _____   **29.** 0.4 _____

DIRECTIONS: Change the following proper fractions to decimal fractions.

30. $5/7$ _____   **31.** $1/100$ _____   **32.** $1/250$ _____   **33.** $1/8$ _____

ANSWERS ON P. 51.

NAME _____

DATE _____

ACCEPTABLE SCORE __**31**__

YOUR SCORE _____

POSTTEST 2

DIRECTIONS: Write the following numbers in words.

1. 0.516 _____

_____

2. 4.0002 _____

3. 123.69 _____

_____

DIRECTIONS: Circle the decimal with the *greatest value*.

4. 0.04, 0.45, 0.8, 0.86   **5.** 1.202, 1.22, 1.2, 1.222

DIRECTIONS: Perform the indicated calculations.

6. $1.2791 + 327.8 + 123.07 + 4.67 =$ _____

7. $6.95 + 0.8 + 0.625 + 7.68 =$ _____

8. $19.29 + 3.5 + 5.869 + 4.55 =$ _____

9. $1.5 + 6.3 + 10.46 + 29.465 =$ _____

10. $322 + 0.95 + 6.45 + 9.6 =$ _____

11. $632.838 - 19.869 =$ _____

12. $1.572 - 0.985 =$ _____

13. $6.4 - 3.634 =$ _____

14. $2.6 - 0.087 =$ _____

15. $4.819 - 3.734 =$ _____

16. $57.6 \times 2.9 =$ _____

17. $149.36 \times 700 =$ _____

18. $56.43 \times 0.018 =$ _____

19. $12.8 \times 6.5 =$ _____

20. $27.5 \times 5.89 =$ _____

21. $5.9 \div 5.3 =$ _____   **22.** $0.295 \div 0.059 =$ _____   **23.** $124 \div 0.008 =$ _____

24. $0.7 \div 2.3 =$ _____   **25.** $5.928 \div 2.4 =$ _____

DIRECTIONS: Change the following decimal fractions to proper fractions.

26. 0.005 _____   **27.** 0.35 _____   **28.** 0.125 _____   **29.** 0.85 _____

DIRECTIONS: Change the following proper fractions to decimal fractions.

30. $\frac{1}{6}$ _____   **31.** $\frac{1}{400}$ _____   **32.** $\frac{7}{8}$ _____   **33.** $\frac{1}{150}$ _____

ANSWERS ON P. 52.

evolve   For additional practice problems, refer to the Mathematics Review
section of *Drug Calculations Companion,* Version 5, on Evolve.

ANSWERS

CHAPTER 2 Decimals—Pretest, pp. 31–32

1. Four hundredths
2. One and six tenths
3. Sixteen and six thousand seven hundred thirty-four hundred thousandths
4. One and fifteen thousandths
5. Nine thousandths

6. 0.02	15. 84.565	24. 29.5336	33. $161/500$
7. 0.004	16. 1.078	25. 186.543	34. $1/250$
8. 1.6	17. 1.008	26. 0.206	35. 0.6
9. 2.082	18. 759.4	27. 17.95	36. 0.67
10. 0.003	19. 1.7	28. 0.01097	37. 0.006
11. 25.376	20. 10.946	29. 627	38. 0.35
12. 324.3	21. 0.0567	30. 0.0186	
13. 1012.867	22. 6.6472	31. $1/125$	
14. 150.6736	23. 1.9425	32. $1/4$	

CHAPTER 2 Decimals—Work Sheet, pp. 39–43

Writing Numbers in Words, *p. 39*

1. Two tenths
2. Nine and sixty-eight hundredths
3. Three ten thousandths
4. One thousand nine hundred sixty-eight and three hundred forty-two thousandths
5. Two hundredths

Decimal Numbers with the Greatest Value, *p. 39*

1. 0.25	3. 0.98	5. 1.8
2. 0.45	4. 0.68	6. 7.44

Decimal Numbers with the Least Value, *p. 39*

1. 0.6	3. 1.0022	5. 0.007
2. 0.0003	4. 0.08	6. 3.006

Addition, *p. 39*

1. 41.755	4. 39.073	7. 26.62
2. 372.675	5. 894.842	8. 37.9
3. 40.9787	6. 67.137	9. 55.117

Subtraction, *p. 40*

1. 1257.87	4. 174.804	7. 0.461
2. 1.849	5. 7.418	8. 0.988
3. 0.71	6. 4.144	9. 62.022

Multiplication, *p. 40*

1. 16.25	4. 56.1144	7. 103.983
2. 609.6	5. 41.92	8. 409.0318
3. 52.052	6. 33.6	9. 0.15113

Multiply by 10, *p. 40*

1. 0.9	3. 1.8	5. 6.25
2. 2	4. 3	6. 23.3

Multiply by 100, *p. 41*

1. 2.3	3. 0.4	5. 865
2. 150	4. 12.5	6. 7640

Multiply by 1000, *p. 41*

1. 200	3. 187	5. 460
2. 5	4. 9650	6. 489

Multiply by 0.1, *p. 41*

1. 3	3. 0.17	5. 0.0138
2. 0.069	4. 0.095	6. 0.567

Multiply by 0.01, *p. 41*

1. 0.0026	3. 0.055	5. 0.00875
2. 0.908	4. 0.112	6. 0.633

Multiply by 0.001, *p. 41*

1. 0.056	3. 0.1265	5. 0.009684
2. 0.01255	4. 0.0333	6. 0.241

Round to the Nearest Tenth, *p. 41*

1. 0.3	3. 2.4	5. 58.4
2. 0.9	4. 0.7	6. 8.1

Round to the Nearest Hundredth, *p. 41*

1. 2.56	3. 0.28	5. 6.53
2. 4.28	4. 3.92	6. 2.99

Round to the Nearest Thousandth, *p. 41*

1. 27.863	3. 2.157	5. 321.087
2. 5.925	4. 0.849	6. 455.768

Division, *p. 42*

1. 1.17	4. 400	7. 82.6
2. 4140	5. 0.02	8. 4.53
3. 7.8	6. 0.13	9. 0.48

Divide by 10, *p. 42*

1. 0.6	3. 0.98	5. 0.0375
2. 0.02	4. 0.005	6. 0.099

ANSWERS

Divide by 100, *p. 42*

1. 0.007	3. 7	5. 0.12
2. 0.0811	4. 0.0019	6. 0.302

Divide by 1000, *p. 42*

1. 0.0018	3. 0.00025	5. 0.0075
2. 0.36	4. 0.0546	6. 7.14

Divide by 0.1, *p. 42*

1. 28	3. 6.5	5. 150
2. 1	4. 9.87	6. 82.5

Divide by 0.01, *p. 42*

1. 3600	3. 48	5. 80
2. 16	4. 959	6. 9.7

Divide by 0.001, *p. 42*

1. 6200	3. 5000	5. 13,800
2. 839,000	4. 860	6. 15.6

Decimal Fractions to Proper Fractions, *p. 43*

1. 3/50	4. 1/400	7. 16/25
2. 4/5	5. 5/8	8. 1/200
3. 17/25	6. 1/4	

Proper Fractions to Decimal Fractions, *p. 43*

1. 0.125	4. 0.6	7. 0.8
2. 0.67	5. 0.04	8. 0.875
3. 0.64	6. 0.33	

CHAPTER 2 Decimals—Posttest 1, pp. 45–46

1. Six hundred thirty-four and eighteen hundredths
2. Nine tenths
3. Sixty-four and two hundred thirty-one thousandths

4. 0.15	14. 43.6077	24. 1.41
5. 0.666	15. 0.211	25. 55.19
6. 54.66	16. 702.4472	26. 9/100
7. 8.89	17. 0.13904	27. 1/400
8. 6.352	18. 162	28. 3/8
9. 6.104	19. 44.278	29. 2/5
10. 2152.626	20. 0.585	30. 0.71
11. 0.339	21. 16.8	31. 0.01
12. 1.4532	22. 1481.67	32. 0.004
13. 323.08	23. 627	33. 0.125

CHAPTER 2 Decimals—Posttest 2, pp. 47–48

1. Five hundred sixteen thousandths
2. Four and two ten thousandths
3. One hundred twenty-three and sixty-nine hundredths

4.	0.86	14.	2.513	24.	0.30
5.	1.222	15.	1.085	25.	2.47
6.	456.8191	16.	167.04	26.	$\frac{1}{200}$
7.	16.055	17.	104,552	27.	$\frac{7}{20}$
8.	33.209	18.	1.01574	28.	$\frac{1}{8}$
9.	47.725	19.	83.2	29.	$\frac{17}{20}$
10.	339	20.	161.975	30.	0.17
11.	612.969	21.	1.11	31.	0.003
12.	0.587	22.	5	32.	0.875
13.	2.766	23.	15,500	33.	0.007

NAME _____

DATE _____

ACCEPTABLE SCORE ___38___

YOUR SCORE _____

PRETEST

Complete the Percents Pretest. A score of 38 out of 40 indicates an acceptable under-standing of and competency in basic calculations involving percents. You may skip to the Ratios Pretest on p. 71. However, if you score 37 or below, completion of Chapter 3, Percents, will be helpful for your continued success in the calculation of drug dosages.

DIRECTIONS: Change the following fractions to percents.

1. $\frac{1}{60}$ _____

2. $\frac{5}{7}$ _____

3. $\frac{1}{8}$ _____

4. $\frac{3}{10}$ _____

5. $\frac{4}{3}$ _____

DIRECTIONS: Change the following decimals to percents.

6. 0.006 _____

7. 0.35 _____

8. 0.427 _____

9. 3.821 _____

10. 0.7 _____

DIRECTIONS: Change the following percents to proper fractions.

11. 0.5% _____

12. 75% _____

13. $9\frac{1}{2}$% _____

14. 24.8% _____

15. $\frac{3}{8}$% _____

DIRECTIONS: Change the following percents to decimals.

16. $1\frac{1}{6}$% _____

17. 7.5% _____

18. $13\frac{3}{10}$% _____

19. $\frac{8}{9}$% _____   **20.** 63% _____

DIRECTIONS: What percent of

21. 1.60 is 6 _____   **22.** ¾ is ⅛ _____   **23.** 100 is 65 _____

24. 500 is 1 _____   **25.** 4.5 is 1.5 _____   **26.** 37.8 is 4.6 _____

27. 1$\frac{4}{9}$ is ⅝ _____   **28.** 1000 is 100 _____   **29.** 3½ is ¼ _____

30. 9.7 is ⅙ _____

DIRECTIONS: What is

31. 3% of 60 _____   **32.** ¼% of 60 _____   **33.** 4.5% of 57 _____

34. 2⅛% of 32 _____   **35.** 4% of 77 _____   **36.** 9.3% of 46 _____

37. $\frac{3}{7}$% of 14 _____   **38.** 22% of 88 _____   **39.** 7.6% of 156 _____

40. 5% of 300 _____

ANSWERS ON P. 67.

CHAPTER 3

Percents

LEARNING OBJECTIVES

Upon completion of the materials provided in this chapter, you will be able to perform computations accurately by mastering the following mathematical concepts:

1 Changing a fraction or decimal to a percent
2 Changing a percent to a fraction or decimal
3 Changing a percent containing a fraction to a decimal
4 Finding what percent one number is of another
5 Finding the given percent of a number

Study the introductory material on percents. The processes for the calculation of percent problems are listed in steps. Memorize the steps for each calculation before beginning the work sheet. Complete the work sheet at the end of this chapter, which provides for extensive practice in the manipulation of percents. Check your answers. If you have any difficulty, go back and review the steps for that type of calculation. When you feel ready to evaluate your learning, take the first posttest. Check your answers. An acceptable score as indicated on the posttest signifies that you are ready for the next chapter. An unacceptable score signifies a need for further study before taking the second posttest.

A **percent** is a third way of showing a fractional relationship. Fractions, decimals, and percents can all be converted from one form to the others. Conversions of fractions and decimals are discussed in Chapter 2. A percent indicates a value equal to the number of hundredths. Therefore when a percent is written as a fraction, the denominator is *always* 100. The number beside the percent sign (%) becomes the numerator.

> **! ALERT**
>
> - When a percent is written as a fraction, the denominator is ALWAYS 100.
> - The number beside the percent sign (%) is the numerator.
>
> $$\text{Example: } 59\% = \frac{59}{100}$$

CHANGING A FRACTION TO A PERCENT

1. Multiply by 100.
2. Add the percent sign (%).

EXAMPLE 1: $^2\!/_5$

a. $\dfrac{2}{\cancel{5}} \times \dfrac{\overset{20}{\cancel{100}}}{1} =$
$\quad\; 1$

b. $\dfrac{2 \times 20}{1 \times 1} = 40$

c. 40%

EXAMPLE 2: $^3\!/_{10}$

a. $\dfrac{3}{\cancel{10}} \times \dfrac{\overset{10}{\cancel{100}}}{1} =$
$\quad\; 1$

b. $\dfrac{3 \times 10}{1 \times 1} = 30$

c. 30%

EXAMPLE 3: $1\frac{1}{4}$

a. $\dfrac{5}{\cancel{4}} \times \dfrac{\overset{25}{\cancel{100}}}{1} =$
$\quad\; 1$

b. $\dfrac{5 \times 25}{1 \times 1} = 125$

c. 125%

EXAMPLE 4: $^1\!/_3$

a. $\dfrac{1}{3} \times \dfrac{100}{1} =$

b. $\dfrac{1 \times 100}{3 \times 1} = \dfrac{100}{3} = 33\dfrac{1}{3}$

c. $33\frac{1}{3}\%$

CHANGING A DECIMAL TO A PERCENT

1. Multiply by 100 (by moving the decimal point two places to the right).
2. Add the percent sign (%).

EXAMPLE 1: 0.421

a. $0.421 \times 100 = 42.1$

b. 42.1%

EXAMPLE 2: 0.98

a. $0.98 \times 100 = 98$

b. 98%

EXAMPLE 3: 0.2

a. $0.2 \times 100 = 20$

b. 20%

EXAMPLE 4: 1.1212

a. $1.1212 \times 100 = 112.12$

b. 112.12%

CHANGING A PERCENT TO A FRACTION

1. Drop the % sign.
2. Write the remaining number as the fraction's numerator.
3. Write 100 as the denominator. (The denominator will *always* be 100.)
4. Reduce to lowest terms.

EXAMPLE 1: 45%

a. $\dfrac{45}{100} = \dfrac{9}{20}$ (reduced to lowest terms)

EXAMPLE 2: 0.3%

a. $\dfrac{0.3}{100} =$

b. $\dfrac{\frac{3}{10}}{100}$

c. $\dfrac{3}{10} \div \dfrac{100}{1} =$

d. $\dfrac{3}{10} \times \dfrac{1}{100} = \dfrac{3}{1000}$

EXAMPLE 3: $3\frac{1}{2}\%$

a. $\dfrac{3\frac{1}{2}}{100} = \dfrac{7/2}{100}$

b. $\dfrac{7}{2} \div \dfrac{100}{1} =$

c. $\dfrac{7}{2} \times \dfrac{1}{100} = \dfrac{7}{200}$

CHANGING A PERCENT TO A DECIMAL

1. Drop the % sign.
2. Divide the remaining number by 100 (by moving the decimal point two places to the left).
3. Express the quotient as a decimal. Place a zero before the decimal if there are no whole numbers.

> **EXAMPLE 1:** 32%
>
> 0.32

> **EXAMPLE 2:** 125%
>
> 1.25

CHANGING A PERCENT CONTAINING A FRACTION TO A DECIMAL

1. Drop the % sign.
2. Change the mixed number to an improper fraction.
3. Divide by 100. Remember, the denominator of all whole numbers is 1.
4. Reduce to lowest terms.
5. Divide the numerator by the denominator, expressing the quotient as a decimal.

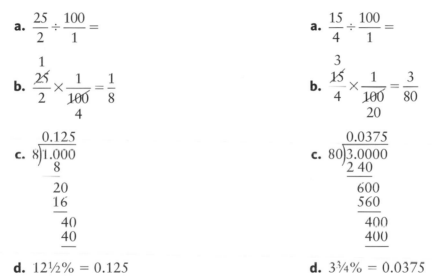

> **EXAMPLE 1:** 12½%
>
> a. $\dfrac{25}{2} \div \dfrac{100}{1} =$
>
> b. $\dfrac{\overset{1}{\cancel{25}}}{2} \times \dfrac{1}{\underset{4}{\cancel{100}}} = \dfrac{1}{8}$
>
> c. $\begin{array}{r} 0.125 \\ 8\overline{)1.000} \\ \underline{8} \\ 20 \\ \underline{16} \\ 40 \\ \underline{40} \end{array}$
>
> d. 12½% = 0.125

> **EXAMPLE 2:** 3¾%
>
> a. $\dfrac{15}{4} \div \dfrac{100}{1} =$
>
> b. $\dfrac{\overset{3}{\cancel{15}}}{4} \times \dfrac{1}{\underset{20}{\cancel{100}}} = \dfrac{3}{80}$
>
> c. $\begin{array}{r} 0.0375 \\ 80\overline{)3.0000} \\ \underline{2\,40} \\ 600 \\ \underline{560} \\ 400 \\ \underline{400} \end{array}$
>
> d. 3¾% = 0.0375

FINDING WHAT PERCENT ONE NUMBER IS OF ANOTHER

1. Write the number following the word *of* as the denominator of a fraction.
2. Write the other number as the numerator of the fraction.
3. Divide the numerator by the denominator, extending the decimal fraction four places to the right of the decimal point.
4. Multiply by 100.
5. Add the % sign.

EXAMPLE 1: What percent of 24 is 9?

a. $\dfrac{9}{24} = \dfrac{3}{8}$

b. $8\overline{)3.000}$ with quotient 0.375
$$\underline{2\,4}$$
$$60$$
$$\underline{56}$$
$$40$$
$$\underline{40}$$

c. $0.375 \times 100 = 37.5$

d. 37.5%

EXAMPLE 2: What percent of 5.4 is 1.2?

a. $\dfrac{1.2}{5.4} = 5.4\overline{)1.2\,0000}$ with quotient 0.2222
$$\underline{1\,0\,8}$$
$$1\,20$$
$$\underline{1\,08}$$
$$120$$
$$\underline{108}$$
$$120$$
$$\underline{108}$$

b. $0.2222 \times 100 = 22.22$

c. 22.22%

EXAMPLE 3: What percent of 2 is ¼?

a. $\tfrac{1}{4}/2$

b. $\dfrac{1}{4} \div 2 =$

c. $\dfrac{1}{4} \div \dfrac{2}{1} =$

d. $\dfrac{1}{4} \times \dfrac{1}{2} = \dfrac{1}{8}$

e. $\dfrac{1}{\underset{2}{\cancel{8}}} \times \dfrac{\overset{25}{\cancel{100}}}{1} = \dfrac{25}{2} = 12.5$

f. 12.5%

EXAMPLE 4: What percent of 8.7 is 3½?

a. $\dfrac{3\frac{1}{2}}{8.7} = \dfrac{3.5}{8.7}$

b. $8.7\overline{)3.5\,000}$ with quotient 0.402
$$\underline{3\,4\,8}$$
$$20$$
$$\underline{00}$$
$$200$$
$$\underline{174}$$

c. $0.402 \times 100 = 40.2$

d. 40.2%

FINDING THE GIVEN PERCENT OF A NUMBER

1. Write the percent as a decimal number.
2. Multiply by the other number.

EXAMPLE 1: What is 40% of 180?

a. $\dfrac{40}{100} = 100\overline{)40.0}$ with quotient 0.4
$$\underline{40\,0}$$

b. $\begin{array}{r} 180 \\ \times\,0.4 \\ \hline 72.0 \end{array}$

c. 40% of $180 = 72$

EXAMPLE 2: What is ³⁄₁₀% of 52?

a. $\dfrac{\frac{3}{10}}{100} = \dfrac{3}{10} \div \dfrac{100}{1} =$

b. $\dfrac{3}{10} \times \dfrac{1}{100} = \dfrac{3}{1000}$

c. $\dfrac{3}{1000} = 0.003$

d. $\begin{array}{r} 0.003 \\ \times\quad 52 \\ \hline 0\,006 \\ 00\,15 \\ \hline 00.156 \end{array}$

e. ³⁄₁₀% of $52 = 0.156$

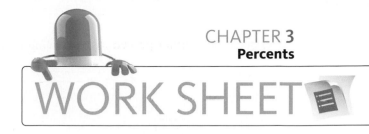

WORK SHEET

DIRECTIONS: Change each of the following proper fractions to a percent.

1. $3/4$ _____

2. $3/8$ _____

3. $4/5$ _____

4. $8/25$ _____

5. $3/1000$ _____

6. $7/200$ _____

7. $9/400$ _____

8. $3/20$ _____

9. $9/150$ _____

10. $11/16$ _____

11. $5/6$ _____

12. $75/10,000$ _____

DIRECTIONS: Change each of the following decimals to a percent.

1. 0.402 _____

2. 0.0367 _____

3. 0.163 _____

4. 0.98 _____

5. 0.3 _____

6. 0.145 _____

7. 0.7 _____

8. 0.42 _____

9. 0.159 _____

10. 0.673 _____

11. 0.3712 _____

12. 2.2 _____

DIRECTIONS: Change each of the following percents to a mixed number or a proper fraction.

1. 3.5% _____   **2.** ¾% _____   **3.** 0.125% _____   **4.** 10% _____

5. ⅔% _____   **6.** 20.2% _____   **7.** 12% _____   **8.** 0.25% _____

9. 2⅜% _____   **10.** 6¼% _____   **11.** 2.1% _____   **12.** 66⅔% _____

DIRECTIONS: Change each of the following percents to a decimal.

1. 37.5% _____   **2.** 3% _____   **3.** 6¾% _____   **4.** 0.42% _____

5. ¼% _____   **6.** 2½% _____   **7.** 0.23% _____   **8.** 72.6% _____

9. 16% _____   **10.** 5/16% _____   **11.** ½% _____   **12.** 7/12% _____

DIRECTIONS: What percent of

1. 40 is 22 _____   **2.** 80 is 6.3 _____   **3.** 200 is 4 _____   **4.** 500 is 60 _____

5. 20 is 1 _____   **6.** 24 is 3.6 _____   **7.** 275 is 55 _____   **8.** 1000 is 100 _____

9. 800 is 360 _____   **10.** 25 is ¼ _____   **11.** 250 is 5.2 _____   **12.** 35 is 7 _____

DIRECTIONS: What is

1. 25% of 478 _____

2. 10% of 34 _____

3. 2.8% of 510 _____

4. ½% of 28 _____

5. 33⅓% of 3000 _____

6. ⅕% of 65 _____

7. 2¼% of 26 _____

8. ⅜% of 32 _____

9. 62% of 871 _____

10. ¼% of 68 _____

11. 41% of 27 _____

12. 8.4% of 128 _____

ANSWERS ON PP. 67–68.

NAME _____

DATE _____

ACCEPTABLE SCORE ___**29**___

YOUR SCORE _____

POSTTEST 1

DIRECTIONS: Change the following fractions to percents.

1. $^{7}/_{8}$ _____

2. $^{11}/_{20}$ _____

3. $^{3}/_{1000}$ _____

DIRECTIONS: Change the following decimals to percents.

4. 0.256 _____

5. 0.004 _____

6. 0.9 _____

DIRECTIONS: Change the following percents to proper fractions.

7. 85% _____

8. 0.3% _____

9. $3^{1}/_{2}$% _____

DIRECTIONS: Change the following percents to decimals.

10. 86.3% _____

11. $4^{5}/_{8}$% _____

12. 0.36% _____

DIRECTIONS: What percent of

13. 70 is 7 _____

14. 24 is 1.2 _____

15. 300 is 1 _____

16. $66^{2}/_{3}$ is 8 _____

17. 3.5 is 1.5 _____

18. 2.5 is 0.5 _____

19. $^{3}/_{4}$ is $^{3}/_{8}$ _____

20. 160 is 12 _____

21. 250 is 20 _____

DIRECTIONS: What is

22. 65% of 800 _____

23. 90% of 40 _____

24. ⅛% of 72 _____

25. 8.5% of 2000 _____

26. 4½% of 940 _____

27. 65% of 450 _____

28. ¼% of 60 _____

29. 4.3% of 56 _____

30. 0.52% of 88 _____

ANSWERS ON P. 68.

NAME _____

DATE _____

ACCEPTABLE SCORE __**29**__

YOUR SCORE _____

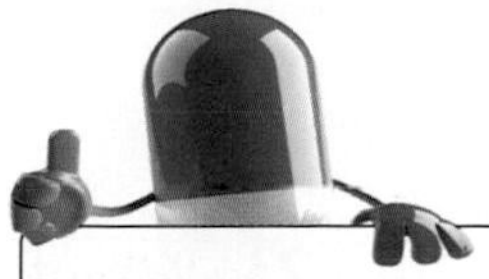

POSTTEST 2

DIRECTIONS: Change the following fractions to percents.

1. ⅛ _____   **2.** ⅖ _____   **3.** ⅙ _____

DIRECTIONS: Change the following decimals to percents.

4. 0.065 _____   **5.** 0.005 _____   **6.** 0.2 _____

DIRECTIONS: Change the following percents to proper fractions.

7. 0.3% _____   **8.** 16½% _____   **9.** 0.25% _____

DIRECTIONS: Change the following percents to decimals.

10. 3¾% _____   **11.** 7% _____   **12.** 5.55% _____

DIRECTIONS: What percent of

13. 5.4 is 1.2 _____   **14.** ¼ is ⅛ _____   **15.** 250 is 6 _____

16. 40 is 32 _____   **17.** 160 is 12 _____   **18.** 500 is 50 _____

19. 5¾ is 2⅜ _____   **20.** 120 is 15 _____   **21.** ⁹⁄₁₆ is ⁵⁄₇ _____

DIRECTIONS: What is

22. 35% of 650 _____

23. ¼% of 116 _____

24. 4½% of 940 _____

25. 11% of 88 _____

26. 16% of 90 _____

27. 7.5% of 261 _____

28. 45% of 24.27 _____

29. ⅞% of 64 _____

30. 82.4% of 118 _____

ANSWERS ON P. 69.

 For additional practice problems, refer to the Mathematics Review
section of *Drug Calculations Companion,* Version 5, on Evolve.

ANSWERS

CHAPTER 3 Percents—Pretest, pp. 53–54

Fractions to Percents, p. 53

1. 1⅔%, 1.6666%
2. 71³/₇%, 71.4285%
3. 12½%, 12.5%
4. 30%
5. 133⅓%, 133.3333%

Decimals to Percents, p. 53

6. 0.6%
7. 35%
8. 42.7%
9. 382.1%
10. 70%

Percents to Proper Fractions, p. 53

11. ¹/₂₀₀
12. ¾
13. ¹⁹/₂₀₀
14. ³¹/₁₂₅
15. ³/₈₀₀

Percents to Decimals, pp. 53–54

16. 0.0117
17. 0.075
18. 0.133
19. 0.0088
20. 0.63

What Percent of, p. 54

21. 375%
22. 16⅔%, 16.6666%
23. 65%
24. ⅕%, 0.2%
25. 33⅓%, 33.333%
26. 12³²/₁₈₉%, 12.1693%
27. 43⁷/₂₆%, 43.2692%
28. 10%
29. 7¹/₇%, 7.1428%
30. 1²⁰⁹/₂₉₁%, 1.7182%

What Is, p. 54

31. 1.8
32. 0.15
33. 2.565
34. 0.68
35. 3.08
36. 4.278
37. 0.06
38. 19.36
39. 11.856
40. 15

CHAPTER 3 Percents—Work Sheet, pp. 59–61

Fractions to Percents, p. 59

1. 75%
2. 37½%
3. 80%
4. 32%
5. ³/₁₀% or 0.3%
6. 3½%
7. 2¼% or 2.25%
8. 15%
9. 6%
10. 68¾% or 68.75%
11. 83⅓% or 83.3%
12. ¾% or 0.75%

Decimals to Percents, p. 59

1. 40.2%
2. 3.67%
3. 16.3%
4. 98%
5. 30%
6. 14.5%
7. 70%
8. 42%
9. 15.9%
10. 67.3%
11. 37.12%
12. 220%

Percents to Mixed Numbers or Proper Fractions, *p. 60*

1. $7/200$	5. $1/150$	9. $19/800$
2. $3/400$	6. $101/500$	10. $1/16$
3. $1/800$	7. $3/25$	11. $21/1000$
4. $1/10$	8. $1/400$	12. $2/3$

Percents to Decimals, *p. 60*

1. 0.375	5. 0.0025	9. 0.16
2. 0.03	6. 0.025	10. 0.003125
3. 0.0675	7. 0.0023	11. 0.005
4. 0.0042	8. 0.726	12. 0.0058

What Percent of, *p. 60*

1. 55%	5. 5%	9. 45%
2. $7\frac{7}{8}$%, 7.875%	6. 15%	10. 1%
3. 2%	7. 20%	11. $2\frac{2}{25}$%, 2.08%
4. 12%	8. 10%	12. 20%

What Is, *p. 61*

1. 119.5	5. 999.9 or 1000	9. 540.02
2. 3.4	6. 0.13	10. 0.17
3. 14.28	7. 0.585	11. 11.07
4. 0.14	8. 0.12	12. 10.752

CHAPTER 3 Percents—Posttest 1, pp. 63–64

Fractions to Percents, *p. 63*

1. $87\frac{1}{2}$%, 87.5%	2. 55%	3. $3/10$%, 0.3%

Decimals to Percents, *p. 63*

4. 25.6%	5. 0.4%	6. 90%

Percents to Proper Fractions, *p. 63*

7. $17/20$	8. $3/1000$	9. $7/200$

Percents to Decimals, *p. 63*

10. 0.863	11. 0.04625	12. 0.0036

What Percent of, *p. 63*

13. 10%	16. 12%	19. 50%
14. 5%	17. $42\frac{6}{7}$%, 42.8571%	20. $7\frac{1}{2}$%, 7.5%
15. $1/3$%, 0.33%	18. 20%	21. 8%

What Is, *p. 64*

22. 520	25. 170	28. 0.15
23. 36	26. 42.3	29. 2.408
24. 0.09	27. 292.5	30. 0.4576

ANSWERS

CHAPTER 3 Percents—Posttest 2, pp. 65–66

Fractions to Percents, *p. 65*

1. 12½%, 12.5%	2. 40%	3. 16⅔%, 16.6666%

Decimals to Percents, *p. 65*

4. 6.5%	5. 0.5%	6. 20%

Percents to Proper Fractions, *p. 65*

7. ³⁄₁₀₀₀	8. ³³⁄₂₀₀	9. ¹⁄₄₀₀

Percents to Decimals, *p. 65*

10. 0.0375	11. 0.07	12. 0.0555

What Percent of, *p. 65*

13. 22²⁄₉%, 22.2222%	16. 80%	19. 41⁷⁄₂₃%, 41.3043%
14. 50%	17. 7½%, 7.5%	20. 12½%, 12.5%
15. 2²⁄₅%, 2.4%	18. 10%	21. 126⁶²⁄₆₃%, 126.9841%

What Is, *p. 66*

22. 227.5	25. 9.68	28. 10.9215
23. 0.29	26. 14.4	29. 0.56
24. 42.3	27. 19.575	30. 97.232

NAME _____

DATE _____

ACCEPTABLE SCORE ___**29**___

YOUR SCORE _____

PRETEST

Complete the Ratios Pretest. A score of 29 out of 30 indicates an acceptable understanding of and competency in basic calculations involving ratios. You may skip to the Proportions Pretest on p. 87. However, if you score 28 or below, completion of Chapter 4, Ratios, will be helpful for your continued success in the calculation of drug dosages.

DIRECTIONS: Convert to equivalents.

	Ratio	Fraction	Decimal	Percent
1.	17 : 51			
2.			0.715	
3.		$8/20$		
4.				$12\frac{1}{2}\%$
5.	21 : 420			
6.		$5/32$		
7.			0.286	
8.				$71\frac{3}{7}\%$
9.				$16\frac{1}{4}\%$
10.			0.462	

ANSWERS ON P. 84.

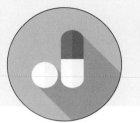

Ratios

LEARNING OBJECTIVES

Upon completion of the materials provided in this chapter, you will be able to perform computations accurately by mastering the following mathematical concepts:

1 Changing a proper fraction, decimal fraction, and percent to a ratio reduced to lowest terms
2 Changing a ratio to a proper fraction, a decimal fraction, and a percent

Study the introductory material on ratios. The processes for the calculation of ratio problems are listed in steps. Memorize the steps for each calculation before beginning the work sheet. Review previous chapters on fractions, decimals, and percents as necessary. Complete the work sheet at the end of this chapter, which provides for extensive practice in the manipulation of ratios. Check your answers. If you have difficulties, go back and review the steps for that type of calculation. When you feel ready to evaluate your learning, take the first posttest. Check your answers. An acceptable score as indicated on the posttest signifies that you are ready for the next chapter. An unacceptable score signifies a need for further study before taking the second posttest.

A **ratio** is another way of indicating a relationship between two numbers. In other words, it is another way to express a fraction. A ratio indicates *division*. The numerator is the first number listed.

> **! ALERT**
> - A ratio is another way to represent a fraction.
> - A ratio indicates DIVISION.
> - The numerator is the first number listed.

EXAMPLE 1: ¾ written as a ratio is 3 : 4
In reading a ratio, one reads the colon as "is to." The example would then be read as "three is to four."

EXAMPLE 2: 7 written as a ratio is 7 : 1
To express any whole number as a ratio, the number following the colon is *always* 1. The example would be read as "seven is to one."

CHANGING A PROPER FRACTION TO A RATIO REDUCED TO LOWEST TERMS

1. Reduce the fraction to lowest terms.
2. Write the numerator of the fraction as the first number of the ratio.

3. Place a colon after the first number.
4. Write the denominator of the fraction as the second number of the ratio.

EXAMPLE 1: $^4/_{12}$

    a. $^4/_{12}$ reduced to lowest terms equals $^1/_3$

    b. $^1/_3$ written as a ratio is 1 : 3

EXAMPLE 2: $^1/_{1000}/^1/_{10}$

    a. $\dfrac{1}{1000} \div \dfrac{1}{10} =$

    b. $\dfrac{1}{\underset{100}{\cancel{1000}}} \times \dfrac{\overset{1}{\cancel{10}}}{1} = \dfrac{1}{100}$

    c. $^1/_{1000}/^1/_{10}$ reduced to lowest terms equals $^1/_{100}$

    d. $^1/_{100}$ written as a ratio is 1 : 100

CHANGING A DECIMAL FRACTION TO A RATIO REDUCED TO LOWEST TERMS

1. Express the decimal fraction as a proper fraction reduced to lowest terms.
2. Write the numerator of the fraction as the first number of the ratio.
3. Place a colon after the first number.
4. Write the denominator of the fraction as the second number of the ratio.

EXAMPLE 1: 0.85

    a. $\dfrac{85}{100} = \dfrac{17}{20}$ (reduced to lowest terms)

    b. $\dfrac{17}{20}$ written as a ratio is 17 : 20

EXAMPLE 2: 0.125

    a. $\dfrac{125}{1000} = \dfrac{1}{8}$ (reduced to lowest terms)

    b. $\dfrac{1}{8}$ written as a ratio is 1 : 8

CHANGING A PERCENT TO A RATIO REDUCED TO LOWEST TERMS

1. Express the percent as a proper fraction reduced to lowest terms.
2. Write the numerator of the fraction as the first number of the ratio.
3. Place a colon after the first number.
4. Write the denominator of the fraction as the second number of the ratio.

EXAMPLE 1: 30%

    a. $\dfrac{30}{100} = \dfrac{3}{10}$ (reduced to lowest terms)

    b. $\dfrac{3}{10}$ written as a ratio is 3 : 10

EXAMPLE 2: ½%   **EXAMPLE 3:** 3⁹⁄₁₀%

a. $\dfrac{\frac{1}{2}}{100} =$ **a.** $\dfrac{3\frac{9}{10}}{100} =$

b. $\dfrac{1}{2} \div \dfrac{100}{1} =$ **b.** $\dfrac{39}{10} \div \dfrac{100}{1} =$

c. $\dfrac{1}{2} \times \dfrac{1}{100} = \dfrac{1}{200}$ **c.** $\dfrac{39}{10} \times \dfrac{1}{100} = \dfrac{39}{1000}$

d. $\dfrac{1}{200}$ written as a ratio is 1 : 200   **d.** $\dfrac{39}{1000}$ written as a ratio is 39 : 1000

CHANGING A RATIO TO A PROPER FRACTION REDUCED TO LOWEST TERMS

1. Write the first number of the ratio as the numerator.
2. Write the second number of the ratio as the denominator.
3. Reduce to lowest terms.

EXAMPLE 1: 9 : 15   **EXAMPLE 2:** 11 : 22

$\dfrac{9}{15} = \dfrac{3}{5}$ (reduced to lowest terms) $\dfrac{11}{22} = \dfrac{1}{2}$ (reduced to lowest terms)

CHANGING A RATIO TO A DECIMAL FRACTION

Divide the first number of the ratio by the second number of the ratio, using long division.

EXAMPLE 1: 4 : 5

a.
```
    0.8
 5)4.0
   4 0
```

b. 4 : 5 written as a decimal is 0.8

EXAMPLE 2: 3½ : 2¼

a. 3.5 : 2.25

b.
```
           1 . 555
 2.25 ʌ)3.50 ʌ000
        2 25
        1 25  0
        1 12  5
          12  50
          11  25
           1  250
           1  125
```

c. 3½ : 2¼ written as a decimal is 1.555

CHANGING A RATIO TO A PERCENT

1. Express the ratio as a proper fraction or a decimal fraction, whichever you prefer to work with.
2. Multiply by 100.
3. Add the percent sign (%).

EXAMPLE 1: 3 : 5

Changing to a proper fraction:

a. $\dfrac{3}{\cancel{5}} \times \dfrac{\overset{20}{\cancel{100}}}{1} = \dfrac{60}{1}$

b. 60%

Changing to a decimal fraction:

a. $5\overline{)3.0}$ → 0.6
$\quad\ \underline{3\,0}$

b. $0.6 \times 100 = 60$

c. 60%

EXAMPLE 2: 60 : 180

Changing to a proper fraction:

a. $\dfrac{60}{180} = \dfrac{1}{3}$

b. $\dfrac{1}{3} \times \dfrac{100}{1} = \dfrac{100}{3} = 33\tfrac{1}{3}$

c. 33⅓%

Changing to a decimal fraction:

a. $180\overline{)60.000}$ → 0.333
$\quad\ \ \underline{54\,0}$
$\quad\quad\ 6\,00$
$\quad\quad\ \underline{5\,40}$
$\quad\quad\ \ 600$
$\quad\quad\ \ \underline{540}$
$\quad\quad\ \ \ 600$
$\quad\quad\ \ \ \underline{540}$
$\quad\quad\ \ \ \ 60$

b. $0.333 \times 100 = 33.3$

c. 33.3%

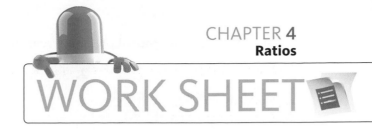

CHAPTER 4
Ratios

WORK SHEET

DIRECTIONS: Change the following fractions to ratios reduced to lowest terms.

1. ⁹⁄₁₂ _____   **2.** ⁴⁄₆ _____   **3.** ¹¹⁄₂₂ _____

4. ⁵⁶⁄₁₀₀ _____   **5.** ²⁰⁄₅₀ _____   **6.** ³¹⁰⁄₁₀₀₀ _____

7. ¹⁰⁄₁₆ _____   **8.** ⁵⁄₆/3⅓ _____   **9.** 1³⁄₅/2⁷⁄₁₀ _____

10. ¹⁄₁₀/¹⁄₁₀₀ _____   **11.** ¹⁴⁄₃₀/2 _____   **12.** 3⅓/3⅓ _____

DIRECTIONS: Change the following decimal fractions to ratios reduced to lowest terms.

1. 0.896 _____   **2.** 0.96 _____   **3.** 0.06 _____

4. 0.6 _____   **5.** 0.4032 _____   **6.** 0.74 _____

7. 0.166 _____   **8.** 0.26 _____   **9.** 0.492 _____

10. 0.95 _____   **11.** 0.235 _____   **12.** 0.172 _____

Copyright © 2016 by Mosby, an imprint of Elsevier Inc.

WORK SHEET 77

DIRECTIONS: Change the following percents to ratios reduced to lowest terms.

1. 10% _____

2. 33⅓% _____

3. ⅜% _____

4. 2⁷⁄₁₀% _____

5. 44% _____

6. 15.7% _____

7. 7¾% _____

8. 0.44% _____

9. 7.8% _____

10. 1% _____

11. ⅗% _____

12. 3³⁄₇% _____

DIRECTIONS: Change the following ratios to fractions reduced to lowest terms.

1. 4 : 64 _____

2. 4 : 800 _____

3. 3 : 150 _____

4. ⅜ : ¼ _____

5. ⁸⁄₁₂ : ⅔ _____

6. 2½ : 7½ _____

7. ⅘ : ¼ _____

8. ¹⁄₁₀ : ⁴⁄₂₀ _____

9. ⁴⁄₇₅ : ³⁄₁₀ _____

10. 0.68 : 0.44 _____

11. 1.85 : 3.35 _____

12. 1.64 : 2.54 _____

DIRECTIONS: Change the following ratios to decimal numbers.

1. 7 : 14 _____ **2.** 5 : 20 _____ **3.** 3 : 8 _____

4. 11 : 33 _____ **5.** $^5/_8$: $^1/_{10}$ _____ **6.** $^1/_{1000}$: $^1/_{500}$ _____

7. $^3/_4$: $^1/_2$ _____ **8.** $^3/_{1000}$: $^3/_{100}$ _____ **9.** 2 : 5 _____

10. $^1/_2$: $^5/_9$ _____ **11.** 7 : 259 _____ **12.** $1^2/_5$: $^{12}/_{30}$ _____

DIRECTIONS: Change the following ratios to percents.

1. 2 : 4 _____ **2.** 7 : 231 _____ **3.** 25 : 250 _____

4. 30 : 150 _____ **5.** $1^1/_4$: $3^3/_8$ _____ **6.** 1 . 1000 _____

7. 0.15 : 0.6 _____ **8.** $^5/_{16}$: $^3/_5$ _____ **9.** 1 : 500 _____

10. $1^8/_{12}$: $2^3/_6$ _____ **11.** 2.5 : 4.5 _____ **12.** 4 : $^3/_{16}$ _____

ANSWERS ON P. 84.

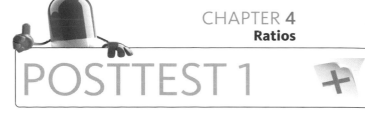

CHAPTER 4
Ratios

ACCEPTABLE SCORE **29**

YOUR SCORE _____

POSTTEST 1

DIRECTIONS: Convert to equivalents.

	Ratio	Fraction	Decimal	Percent
1.	42 : 48			
2.			0.004	
3.		13/20		
4.				2¼%
5.			0.35	
6.		6/25		
7.	⅜ : 5/9			
8.				0.3%
9.			0.205	
10.		4/11		

ANSWERS ON P. 84.

NAME _____

DATE _____

ACCEPTABLE SCORE ___29___

YOUR SCORE _____

PRETEST

DIRECTIONS: Change to equivalent metric or household measurements. Solve each problem and show your work.

1. 800,000 mcg = _____ g   **2.** 3 mg = _____ mcg   **3.** 255 mg = _____ g

4. 46 mg = _____ mcg   **5.** 3000 mcg = _____ mg   **6.** 0.68 g = _____ mg

7. 326 mL = _____ L   **8.** 33 kg = _____ lb   **9.** 2.1 g = _____ mg

10. 3000 g = _____ kg   **11.** 0.1 L = _____ mL   **12.** 53 kg = _____ lb

13. 0.005 mg = _____ mcg   **14.** 0.8 kg = _____ g   **15.** 250 mcg = _____ mg

16. 1¼ cups = _____ mL   **17.** 22 lb = _____ g   **18.** 0.63 L = _____ mL

19. 733 g = _____ kg   **20.** 1.25 g = _____ mcg   **21.** 60 mg = _____ g

22. 0.25 mg = _____ mcg   **23.** 0.25 L = _____ mL   **24.** 45 lb = _____ kg

25. 10,000 mcg = _____ g   **26.** 1.2 kg = _____ g   **27.** 1⅔ Tbsp = _____ mL

28. 0.71 g = _____ mg   **29.** 480 mL = _____ L   **30.** 650 g = _____ lb

ANSWERS ON P. 127.

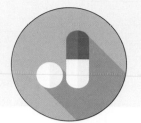

Metric and Household Measurements

LEARNING OBJECTIVES

Upon completion of the materials provided in this chapter, you will be able to perform computations accurately by mastering the following mathematical concepts:

1 Recalling the metric measures of weight, volume, and length

2 Computing equivalents within the metric system by using dimensional analysis or a proportion

3 Recalling approximate equivalents between metric and household measures

4 Computing equivalents between the metric and household systems of measure by using dimensional analysis or a proportion

METRIC MEASUREMENTS

The metric system has become the system of choice for dealing with the weights and measures involved in the calculation of drug dosages. This is a result of its accuracy and simplicity because it is based on the decimal system. The use of decimals tends to eliminate errors made when working with fractions. Therefore all answers within the metric system need to be expressed as decimals, not as fractions.

EXAMPLES: 0.5, not ½
0.75, not ¾
0.007, not ⁷⁄₁₀₀₀

Certain prefixes identify the multiples of 10 that are being used. The four most commonly used prefixes of the metric system involved with the calculation of drug dosages are the following:

micro = 0.000001 or one millionth

milli = 0.001 or one thousandth

centi = 0.01 or one hundredth

kilo = 1000 or one thousand

These prefixes may be used with any of the base units of weight (gram), volume (liter), or length (meter). The nurse most often uses the following list of metric measures (Box 6-1). Memorize all the entries in the list.

> **BOX 6-1** COMMON METRIC MEASURES
>
> **Metric Measure of Weight**
> 1,000,000 micrograms (mcg) = 1 gram (g)
> 1000 micrograms (mcg) = 1 milligram (mg)
> 1000 milligrams (mg) = 1 gram (g)
> 1000 grams (g) = 1 kilogram (kg)
>
> **Metric Measure of Volume**
> 1000 milliliters (mL) = 1 liter (L)
> 1 cubic centimeter (cc) = 1 milliliter (mL)
>
> **Metric Measure of Length**
> 1 meter (m) = 1000 mm or 100 cm
> 1 centimeter (cm) = 10 mm or 0.01 m
> 1 millimeter (mm) = 0.1 cm or 0.001 m

Sometimes, to compute drug dosages, the nurse must convert a metric measure to an equivalent measure within the system. This may be done easily by using dimensional analysis or a proportion.

DIMENSIONAL ANALYSIS

Dimensional analysis is one format for setting up problems to calculate equivalents or drug dosages. Dimensional analysis has been around for many years. It was first used in the sciences, such as advanced algebra, chemistry, and physics, to name a few. Recently dimensional analysis has become popular for the calculation of drug dosage problems.

The advantage of dimensional analysis is that only one equation is needed. This format allows a single equation to replace multiple calculations to find the answer.

Three items are required to set up the single equation. These are the desired answer, which goes on the left side of the equation; the equivalent between the two units in the problem; and the given quantity and the unit in which it is supplied.

Let's take a look at some examples that illustrate the dimensional analysis method.

Metric Conversions: Dimensional Analysis Method

EXAMPLE 1: 300 mg equals how many grams?

a. On the left side of the equation, place the name or abbreviation of the drug form of x, or what you are solving for.

$$x \text{ g} =$$

b. On the right side of the equation, place the available information related to the measurement or abbreviation that was placed on the left side. In this example that is g. This information is placed in the equation as a common fraction; match the appropriate abbreviation or measurement. Thus the abbreviation that matches the x quantity must be placed in the numerator. We also know there are 1000 mg in 1 g. This information is the denominator of our fraction.

$$x \text{ g} = \frac{1 \text{ g}}{1000 \text{ mg}}$$

c. Next, find the information that matches the measurement or abbreviation used in the denominator of the fraction you created. In this example mg is in the denominator and we have 300 mg. Therefore the full equation is

$$x \text{ g} = \frac{1 \text{ g}}{1000 \text{ mg}} \times \frac{300 \text{ mg}}{1}$$

d. Now cancel out the like abbreviations on the right side of the equation. If you have set up the problem correctly, the remaining measurement or abbreviation should match that used on the left side of the equation. You are now ready to solve for x.

$$x \text{ g} = \frac{1 \text{ g}}{\underset{10}{\cancel{1000} \text{ }\cancel{mg}}} \times \frac{\overset{3}{\cancel{300} \text{ }\cancel{mg}}}{1}$$

$$x = \frac{1 \times 3}{10 \times 1} = \frac{3}{10}$$

$$x = 0.3 \text{ g}$$

The answer to the problem is 0.3 g.

EXAMPLE 2: 2.5 L equals how many milliliters?

a. On the left side of the equation, place the name or abbreviation of the drug form of x, or what you are solving for.

$$x \text{ mL} =$$

b. On the right side of the equation, place the available information related to the measurement or abbreviation that was placed on the left side. In this example that is *mL*. This information is placed in the equation as a common fraction; match the appropriate abbreviation or measurement. Thus the abbreviation that matches the x quantity must be placed in the numerator. We also know there are 1000 mL in 1 L. This information is the denominator of our fraction.

$$x \text{ mL} = \frac{1000 \text{ mL}}{1 \text{ L}}$$

c. Next, find the information that matches the measurement or abbreviation used in the denominator of the fraction you created. In this example L is in the denominator and we have 2.5 L. Therefore the full equation is

$$x \text{ mL} = \frac{1000 \text{ mL}}{1 \text{ L}} \times \frac{2.5 \text{ L}}{1}$$

d. Now cancel out the like abbreviations on the right side of the equation. If you have set up the problem correctly, the remaining measurement or abbreviation should match that used on the left side of the equation. You are now ready to solve for x.

$$x \text{ mL} = \frac{1000 \text{ mL}}{1 \text{ }\cancel{L}} \times \frac{2.5 \text{ }\cancel{L}}{1}$$

$$x = \frac{1000 \times 2.5}{1 \times 1} = \frac{2500}{1}$$

$$x = 2500 \text{ mL}$$

The answer to the problem is 2500 mL.

EXAMPLE 3: 180 mcg equals how many grams?

a. On the left side of the equation, place the name or abbreviation of the drug form of x, or what you are solving for.

$$x \text{ g} =$$

b. On the right side of the equation, place the available information related to the measurement or abbreviation that was placed on the left side. In this example that is *g*. This information is placed in the equation as a common fraction; match the appropriate abbreviation or measurement. Thus the abbreviation that matches the *x* quantity must be placed in the numerator. We also know there are 1,000,000 mcg in 1 g. This information is the denominator of our fraction.

$$x \, g = \frac{1 \, g}{1{,}000{,}000 \, mcg}$$

c. Next, find the information that matches the measurement or abbreviation used in the denominator of the fraction you created. In this example *mcg* is in the denominator and we have 180 mcg. Therefore the full equation is

$$x \, g = \frac{1 \, g}{1{,}000{,}000 \, mcg} \times \frac{180 \, mcg}{1}$$

d. Now cancel out the like abbreviations on the right side of the equation. If you have set up the problem correctly, the remaining measurement or abbreviation should match that used on the left side of the equation. You are now ready to solve for *x*.

$$x \, g = \frac{1 \, g}{\underset{50{,}000}{1{,}000{,}000 \, \cancel{mcg}}} \times \frac{\overset{9}{\cancel{180} \, \cancel{mcg}}}{1}$$

$$x = \frac{1 \times 9}{50{,}000} = \frac{9}{50{,}000}$$

$$x = 0.00018 \, g$$

The answer to the problem is 0.00018 g.

EXAMPLE 4: 15 mm equals how many centimeters?

a. On the left side of the equation, place the name or abbreviation of the drug form of *x*, or what you are solving for.

$$x \, cm =$$

b. On the right side of the equation, place the available information related to the measurement or abbreviation that was placed on the left side. In this example that is *cm*. This information is placed in the equation as a common fraction; match the appropriate abbreviation or measurement. Thus the abbreviation that matches the *x* quantity must be placed in the numerator. We also know there is 1 cm in 10 mm. This information is the denominator of our fraction.

$$x \, cm = \frac{1 \, cm}{10 \, mm}$$

c. Next, find the information that matches the measurement or abbreviation used in the denominator of the fraction you created. In this example *mm* is in the denominator and the length we are given is 15 mm. Therefore the full equation is

$$x \, cm = \frac{1 \, cm}{10 \, mm} \times \frac{15 \, mm}{1}$$

d. Now cancel out the like abbreviations on the right side of the equation. If you have set up the problem correctly, the remaining measurement or abbreviation should match that used on the left side of the equation. You are now ready to solve for x.

$$x \text{ cm} = \frac{1 \text{ cm}}{\overset{}{\underset{2}{10 \text{ mm}}}} \times \frac{\overset{3}{15 \text{ mm}}}{1}$$

$$x = \frac{1 \times 3}{2 \times 1} = \frac{3}{2}$$

$$x = 1.5 \text{ cm}$$

The answer to the problem is 1.5 cm.

PROPORTION

Historically, the proportion method was taught as a means of calculating equivalents and also drug dosages. If this is the method you are comfortable with, we have continued to include many examples using this method. If you need a review of the steps in solving proportion problems, see Chapter 5, Proportions, on page 89.

Metric Conversions: Proportion Method

EXAMPLE 1: 300 mg equals how many grams?

a. On the left side of the proportion, place what you know to be an equivalent between milligrams and grams. From Box-1 we know that there are 1000 mg in 1 g. Therefore the left side of the proportion would be

$$1000 \text{ mg} : 1 \text{ g} ::$$

b. The right side of the proportion is determined by the problem and by the abbreviations used on the left side of the proportion. Only *two* different abbreviations may be used in a single proportion. The abbreviations must also be in the same position on the right as they are on the left.

$$1000 \text{ mg} : 1 \text{ g} :: \underline{\quad} \text{ mg} : \underline{\quad} \text{ g}$$

From the problem we know we have 300 mg.

$$1000 \text{ mg} : 1 \text{ g} :: 300 \text{ mg} : \underline{\quad} \text{ g}$$

We need to find the number of grams 300 mg equals, so we use the symbol x to represent the unknown. Therefore the full proportion would be

$$1000 \text{ mg} : 1 \text{ g} :: 300 \text{ mg} : x \text{ g}$$

c. Rewrite the proportion without using the abbreviations.

$$1000 : 1 :: 300 : x$$

d. Solve for x by multiplying the means and extremes. Write the answer as a decimal, because the metric system is based on decimals.

$$1000 : 1 :: 300 : x$$

$$1000x = 300$$

$$x = \frac{300}{1000}$$

$$x = 0.3$$

e. Label your answer, as determined by the abbreviation placed next to x in the original proportion.

$$300 \text{ mg} = 0.3 \text{ g}$$

EXAMPLE 2: 2.5 L equals how many milliliters?

  a. 1000 mL : 1 L ::

  b. 1000 mL : 1 L ::

      _____ mL : _____ L

    1000 mL : 1 L :: x mL : 2.5 L

  c. 1000 : 1 :: x : 2.5

  d. 1x = 2500

     x = 2500

  e. 2.5 L = 2500 mL

EXAMPLE 3: 180 mcg equals how many grams?

  a. 1,000,000 mcg : 1 g ::

  b. 1,000,000 mcg : 1 g ::

      _____ mcg : _____ g

    1,000,000 mcg : 1 g :: 180 mcg : x g

  c. 1,000,000 : 1 :: 180 : x

  d. 1,000,000x = 180

$$x = \frac{180}{1,000,000}$$

     x = 0.00018

  e. 180 mcg = 0.00018 g

EXAMPLE 4: 15 mm equals how many centimeters?

  a. 1 cm : 10 mm

  b. 1 cm : 10 mm :: _____ cm : _____ mm

    1 cm : 10 mm :: x cm : 15 mm

  c. 1 : 10 :: x : 15

  d. 10x = 1 × 15

    10x = 15

$$x = \frac{15}{10}$$

    x = 1.5

  e. 15 mm = 1.5 cm

HOUSEHOLD MEASUREMENTS

Household measures are not accurate enough for the nurse to use in the calculation of drug dosages in the hospital. However, their metric equivalents are used in keeping a written record of a patient's "I" and "O," or intake and output. Always use your institution's conversions when documenting intake.

Memorize the following list of approximate equivalents between metric and household measurements (Box 6-2).

BOX 6-2 METRIC HOUSEHOLD EQUIVALENTS

Metric Measure = Household Measure
5 milliliters (mL) = 1 teaspoon (tsp)
15 milliliters (mL) = 1 tablespoon (Tbsp)
30 milliliters (mL) = 1 ounce (oz)
240 milliliters (mL) = 1 standard measuring cup
1 kilogram (kg) or 1000 grams (g) = 2.2 pounds (lb)
2.5 cm = 1 inch
1 foot = 12 inches

Metric   Household

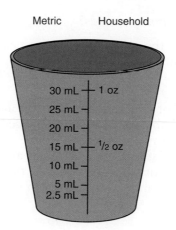

30 mL ─┼─ 1 oz
25 mL ─┤
20 mL ─┤
15 mL ─┼─ ½ oz
10 mL ─┤
 5 mL ─┤
2.5 mL ─┤

Conversion of measures between the metric and household systems of measure may also be done by using dimensional analysis or a proportion, as has been illustrated.

Household Conversions: Dimensional Analysis Method

EXAMPLE 1: 1½ cups equals how many milliliters?

a. On the left side of the equation, place the name or abbreviation of the drug form of x, or what you are solving for.

$$x \text{ mL} =$$

b. On the right side of the equation, place the available information related to the measurement or abbreviation that was placed on the left side. In this example that is mL. This information is placed in the equation as a common fraction; match the appropriate abbreviation or measurement. Thus the abbreviation that matches the x quantity must be placed in the numerator. We also know there are 240 mL in 1 cup. This information is the denominator of our fraction.

$$x \text{ mL} = \frac{240 \text{ mL}}{1 \text{ cup}}$$

c. Next, find the information that matches the measurement or abbreviation used in the denominator of the fraction you created. In this example *cup* is in the denominator and we have 1½ cups. Therefore the full equation is

$$x \text{ mL} = \frac{240 \text{ mL}}{1 \text{ cup}} \times \frac{1.5 \text{ cups}}{1}$$

d. Now cancel out the like abbreviations on the right side of the equation. If you have set up the problem correctly, the remaining measurement or abbreviation should match that used on the left side of the equation. You are now ready to solve for x.

$$x \text{ mL} = \frac{240 \text{ mL}}{1 \text{ cup}} \times \frac{1.5 \text{ cups}}{1}$$

$$x = \frac{240 \times 1.5}{1 \times 1} = \frac{360}{1}$$

$$x = 360 \text{ mL}$$

The answer to the problem is 360 mL.

EXAMPLE 2: 35 kg equals how many pounds?

    a. On the left side of the equation, place the name or abbreviation of the drug form of x, or what you are solving for.

$$x \text{ lb} =$$

    b. On the right side of the equation, place the available information related to the measurement or abbreviation that was placed on the left side. In this example that is *lb*. This information is placed in the equation as a common fraction; match the appropriate abbreviation or measurement. Thus the abbreviation that matches the x quantity must be placed in the numerator. We also know there are 2.2 lb in each kilogram. This information is the denominator of our fraction.

$$x \text{ lb} = \frac{2.2 \text{ lb}}{1 \text{ kg}}$$

    c. Next, find the information that matches the measurement or abbreviation used in the denominator of the fraction you created. In this example *kg* is in the denominator and the weight we are given is 35 kg. Therefore the full equation is

$$x \text{ lb} = \frac{2.2 \text{ lb}}{1 \text{ kg}} \times \frac{35 \text{ kg}}{1}$$

    d. Now cancel out the like abbreviations on the right side of the equation. If you have set up the problem correctly, the remaining measurement or abbreviation should match that used on the left side of the equation. You are now ready to solve for x.

$$x \text{ lb} = \frac{2.2 \text{ lb}}{1 \ \cancel{\text{kg}}} \times \frac{35 \ \cancel{\text{kg}}}{1}$$

$$x = \frac{2.2 \times 35}{1 \times 1} = \frac{77}{1}$$

$$x = 77 \text{ lb}$$

    The answer to the problem is 77 lb.

EXAMPLE 3: 18 inches equals how many centimeters?

    a. On the left side of the equation, place the name or abbreviation of the drug form of x, or what you are solving for.

$$x \text{ cm} =$$

    b. On the right side of the equation, place the available information related to the measurement or abbreviation that was placed on the left side. In this example that is *cm*. This information is placed in the equation as a common fraction; match the appropriate abbreviation or measurement. Thus the abbreviation that matches the x quantity must be placed in the numerator. We also know that there are 2.5 cm in each inch. This information is the denominator of our fraction.

$$x \text{ cm} = \frac{2.5 \text{ cm}}{1 \text{ inch}}$$

c. Next, find the information that matches the measurement or abbreviation used in the denominator of the fraction you created. In this example *inch* is in the denominator and the length we are given is 18 inches. Therefore the full equation is

$$x \text{ cm} = \frac{2.5 \text{ cm}}{1 \text{ inch}} \times \frac{18 \text{ inches}}{1}$$

d. Now cancel out the like abbreviations on the right side of the equation. If you have set up the problem correctly, the remaining measurement or abbreviation should match that used on the left side of the equation. You are now ready to solve for x.

$$x \text{ cm} = \frac{2.5 \text{ cm}}{1 \text{ inch}} \times \frac{18 \text{ inches}}{1}$$

$$x = \frac{2.5 \times 18}{1 \times 1} = \frac{45}{1}$$

$$x = 45 \text{ cm}$$

The answer to the problem is 45 cm.

HOUSEHOLD CONVERSIONS: PROPORTION METHOD

EXAMPLE 1: 1½ cups equals how many milliliters?

   a. 1 cup : 240 mL ::

   b. 1 cup : 240 mL :: _____ cups : _____ mL

    1 cup : 240 mL :: 1½ cups : x mL

   c. 1 : 240 :: 1½ : x

   d. $x = \dfrac{240}{1} \times \dfrac{3}{2}$

    $x = \dfrac{720}{2} = 360 \text{ mL}$

   e. 1½ cups = 360 mL

EXAMPLE 2: 35 kg equals how many pounds?

   a. 1 kg : 2.2 lb ::

   b. 1 kg : 2.2 lb :: _____ kg : _____ lb

    1 kg : 2.2 lb :: 35 kg : x lb

   c. 1 : 2.2 :: 35 : x

   d. $1x = 2.2 \times 35$

    $x = 77$

   e. 35 kg = 77 lb

EXAMPLE 3: 18 inches equals how many centimeters?

    a. 2.5 cm : 1 inch : :

    b. 2.5 cm : 1 inch : : _____ cm : _____ inch

       2.5 cm : 1 inch : : x cm : 18 inches

    c. 2.5 : 1 : : x : 18

    d. $x = 2.5 \times 18$

       $x = 45$ cm

    e. 18 inches = 45 cm

Memorize the tables of metric and household measurements. Study the material on using dimensional analysis or proportions for the calculation of problems relating to the metric and household systems of measure. Complete the following work sheet, which provides for extensive practice in the manipulation of measurements within the metric and household systems. Check your answers. If you have difficulties, go back and review the necessary material. When you feel ready to evaluate your learning, take the first posttest. Check your answers. An acceptable score as indicated on the posttest signifies that you are ready for the next chapter. An unacceptable score signifies a need for further study before taking the second posttest.

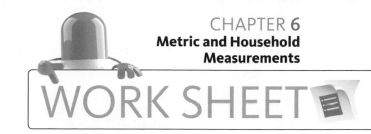

WORK SHEET

DIRECTIONS: Change to equivalents within the metric system. Solve the problems and show your work.

1. 230 mcg = _____ g **2.** 5 mg = _____ mcg **3.** 2.5 g = _____ mcg

4. 4000 mcg = _____ mg **5.** 0.33 g = _____ mg **6.** 6 kg = _____ g

7. 725 mL = _____ L **8.** 2000 mcg = _____ g **9.** 3 cm = _____ mm

10. 620 g = _____ kg **11.** 0.036 mg = _____ mcg **12.** 460 mL = _____ L

13. 0.66 mg = _____ mcg **14.** 0.5 g = _____ mcg **15.** 18 inches = _____ cm

16. 350,000 mcg = _____ g **17.** 25 mg = _____ g **18.** 1.46 L = _____ mL

19. 2.5 kg = _____ g **20.** 12 mg = _____ mcg **21.** 3.4 kg – _____ g

22. 920 mcg = _____ g **23.** 25 mm = _____ cm **24.** 300 mcg = _____ mg

25. 0.16 L = _____ mL   **26.** 0.01 g = _____ mg   **27.** 500 mcg = _____ mg

28. 360 mg = _____ g   **29.** 1.7 L = _____ mL   **30.** 0.45 g = _____ mg

31. 240 mL = _____ L   **32.** 10 mcg = _____ mg

DIRECTIONS: Change the following measurements into the approximate equivalents within the metric or household system, as indicated. Solve the problems and show your work.

33. 3 inches = _____ cm   **34.** 2¼ cups = _____ mL   **35.** 2 tsp = _____ mL

36. 3 Tbsp = _____ mL   **37.** 1½ cups = _____ mL   **38.** 8 kg = _____ lb

39. 3825 g = _____ lb   **40.** 7 inches = _____ cm   **41.** 3 lb = _____ kg

42. 12 kg = _____ lb   **43.** 1400 g = _____ lb   **44.** 2½ feet = _____ inches

45. 150 lb = _____ kg

ANSWERS ON PP. 128–129.

NAME _____

DATE _____

ACCEPTABLE SCORE **29**

YOUR SCORE _____

POSTTEST 1

DIRECTIONS: Change to equivalent measurements. Solve each problem and show your work.

1. 5000 mcg = _____ g

2. 10 mg = _____ mcg

3. 0.81 L = _____ mL

4. 3.5 mg = _____ g

5. 2¼ feet = _____ inches

6. 0.12 g = _____ mcg

7. 16 kg = _____ lb

8. 280 mL = _____ L

9. 0.4 kg = _____ g

10. 42 inches = _____ feet

11. 28 lb = _____ g

12. 4 inches = _____ cm

13. 500,000 mcg = _____ g

14. 37 mL = _____ L

15. 20 mL = _____ cc

16. 1⅓ cups = _____ mL

17. 2.5 g = _____ mg

18. 350 mg = _____ g

19. 6700 g = _____ kg

20. 0.3 L = _____ mL

21. 4 mg = _____ mcg

22. 2600 g = _____ lb

23. 1½ tsp = _____ mL

24. 0.2 L = _____ mL

25. 533 mL = _____ L   **26.** 1.5 g = _____ mcg   **27.** 620 mg = _____ g

28. 2.3 kg = _____ g   **29.** 15 inches = _____ feet   **30.** 7 lb = _____ kg

ANSWERS ON PP. 129–130.

NAME _____

DATE _____

ACCEPTABLE SCORE __**29**__

YOUR SCORE _____

POSTTEST 2

DIRECTIONS: Change to equivalent measurements. Solve each problem and show your work.

1. 4000 mcg = _____ mg

2. 150 g = _____ kg

3. 2½ cups = _____ mL

4. 800 g = _____ lb

5. 44 kg = _____ lb

6. 760 mg = _____ g

7. 0.55 L = _____ mL

8. 35 mm = _____ cm

9. 4 Tbsp = _____ mL

10. 2⅛ lb = _____ g

11. 0.1 L = _____ mL

12. 32 mg = _____ mcg

13. 618 mL = _____ L

14. 100,000 mcg = _____ g

15. 28 inches = _____ feet

16. 714 mL = _____ L

17. 350 mg = _____ g

18. 250,000 mcg = _____ g

19. 0.87 g = _____ mg

20. 7 mg = _____ mcg

21. 37 mcg = _____ mg

22. 1.4 L = _____ mL

23. 0.78 g = _____ mg

24. 225 mcg = _____ mg

25. 4500 g = _____ kg   **26.** 0.2 L = _____ mL   **27.** 3⅓ feet = _____ inches

28. 420 mg = _____ g   **29.** 2.6 g = _____ mcg   **30.** 73 lb = _____ kg

ANSWERS ON PP. 130–131.

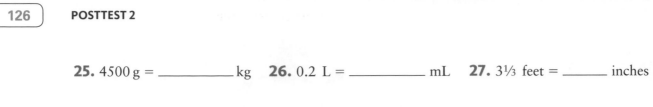

evolve   For additional information, refer to the Introducing Drug Measures
section of *Drug Calculations Companion,* Version 5, on Evolve.

ANSWERS

CHAPTER 6 Metric and Household Measurements—Pretest, pp. 109–110

1. 0.8 g	11. 100 mL	21. 0.06 g
2. 3000 mcg	12. 116.6 lb or 116⅗ lb	22. 250 mcg
3. 0.255 g	13. 5 mcg	23. 250 mL
4. 46,000 mcg	14. 800 g	24. 20.45 kg
5. 3 mg	15. 0.25 mg	25. 0.01 g
6. 680 mg	16. 300 mL	26. 1200 g
7. 0.326 L	17. 10,000 g	27. 25 mL
8. 72.6 lb or 72⅗ lb	18. 630 mL	28. 710 mg
9. 2100 mg	19. 0.733 kg	29. 0.48 L
10. 3 kg	20. 1,250,000 mcg	30. 1⁴³⁄₁₀₀ lb or 1.43 lb

Dimensional Analysis—Pretest, pp. 109–110

1. $x\ g = \dfrac{1\ g}{1,000,000\ mcg} \times \dfrac{800,000\ mcg}{1} = 0.8\ g$

2. $x\ mcg = \dfrac{1000\ mcg}{1\ mg} \times \dfrac{3\ mg}{1} = 3000\ mcg$

3. $x\ g = \dfrac{1\ g}{1000\ mg} \times \dfrac{225\ mg}{1} = 0.255\ g$

4. $x\ mcg = \dfrac{1000\ mcg}{1\ mg} \times \dfrac{46\ mg}{1} = 46,000\ mcg$

5. $x\ mg = \dfrac{1\ mg}{1000\ mcg} \times \dfrac{3000\ mcg}{1} = 3\ mg$

6. $x\ mg = \dfrac{1000\ mg}{1\ g} \times \dfrac{0.68\ g}{1} = 680\ mg$

7. $x\ L = \dfrac{1\ L}{1000\ mL} \times \dfrac{326\ mL}{1} = 0.326\ L$

8. $x\ lb = \dfrac{2.2\ lb}{1\ kg} \times \dfrac{33\ kg}{1} = 72.6\ lb$

9. $x\ mg = \dfrac{1000\ mg}{1\ g} \times \dfrac{2.1\ g}{1} = 2100\ mg$

10. $x\ kg = \dfrac{1\ kg}{1000\ g} \times \dfrac{3000\ g}{1} = 3\ kg$

11. $x\ mL = \dfrac{1000\ mL}{1\ L} \times \dfrac{0.1\ L}{1} = 100\ mL$

12. $x\ lb = \dfrac{2.2\ lb}{1\ kg} \times \dfrac{53\ kg}{1} = 116.6\ lb$

13. $x\ mcg = \dfrac{1000\ mcg}{1\ mg} \times \dfrac{0.005\ mg}{1} = 5\ mcg$

14. $x\ g = \dfrac{1000\ g}{1\ kg} \times \dfrac{0.8\ kg}{1} = 800\ g$

15. $x\ mg = \dfrac{1\ mg}{1000\ mcg} \times \dfrac{250\ mcg}{1} = 0.25\ mg$

16. $x\ mL = \dfrac{240\ mL}{1\ cup} \times \dfrac{1.25\ cups}{1} = 300\ mL$

17. $x\ g = \dfrac{1000\ g}{2.2\ lb} \times \dfrac{22\ lb}{1} = 10,000\ g$

18. $x\ mL = \dfrac{1000\ mL}{1\ L} \times \dfrac{0.63\ L}{1} = 630\ mL$

19. $x\ kg = \dfrac{1\ kg}{1000\ g} \times \dfrac{733\ g}{1} = 0.733\ kg$

20. $x\ mcg = \dfrac{1,000,000\ mcg}{1\ g} \times \dfrac{1.25\ g}{1} = 1,250,000\ mcg$

21. $x\ g = \dfrac{1\ g}{1000\ mg} \times \dfrac{60\ mg}{1} = 0.06\ g$

22. $x\ mcg = \dfrac{1000\ mcg}{1\ mg} \times \dfrac{0.25\ mg}{1} = 250\ mcg$

23. $x\ mL = \dfrac{1000\ mL}{1\ L} \times \dfrac{0.25\ L}{1} = 250\ mL$

24. $x\ kg = \dfrac{1\ kg}{2.2\ lb} \times \dfrac{45\ lb}{1} = 20.45\ kg$

25. $x\ g = \dfrac{1\ g}{1,000,000\ mcg} \times \dfrac{10,000\ mcg}{1} = 0.01\ g$

26. $x\ g = \dfrac{1000\ g}{1\ kg} \times \dfrac{1.2\ kg}{1} = 1200\ g$

ANSWERS

27. $x \text{ mL} = \dfrac{15 \text{ mL}}{1 \text{ Tbsp}} \times \dfrac{1\frac{2}{3} \text{ Tbsp}}{1} = 25 \text{ mL}$

29. $x \text{ L} = \dfrac{1 \text{ L}}{1000 \text{ mL}} \times \dfrac{480 \text{ mL}}{1} = 0.48 \text{ L}$

28. $x \text{ mg} = \dfrac{1000 \text{ mg}}{1 \text{ g}} \times \dfrac{0.71 \text{ g}}{1} = 710 \text{ mg}$

30. $x \text{ lb} = \dfrac{2.2 \text{ lb}}{1000 \text{ g}} \times \dfrac{650 \text{ g}}{1} = 1.43 \text{ lb}$

CHAPTER 6 Metric and Household Measurements—Work Sheet, pp. 121–122

1. 0.00023 g	16. 0.35 g	31. 0.24 L
2. 5000 mcg	17. 0.025 g	32. 0.01 mg
3. 2,500,000 mcg	18. 1460 mL	33. 7.5 cm
4. 4 mg	19. 2500 g	34. 540 mL
5. 330 mg	20. 12,000 mcg	35. 10 mL
6. 6000 g	21. 3400 g	36. 45 mL
7. 0.725 L	22. 0.00092 g	37. 360 mL
8. 0.002 g	23. 2.5 cm	38. $17\frac{3}{5}$ lb or 17.6 lb
9. 30 mm	24. 0.3 mg	39. 8.415 lb, $8\frac{83}{200}$ lb, or 8.41 lb
10. 0.62 kg	25. 160 mL	40. 17.5 cm
11. 36 mcg	26. 10 mg	41. 1.36 kg
12. 0.46 L	27. 0.5 mg	42. $26\frac{2}{5}$ lb or 26.4 lb
13. 660 mcg	28. 0.36 g	43. $3\frac{2}{25}$ lb or 3.08 lb
14. 500,000 mcg	29. 1700 mL	44. 30 inches
15. 45 cm	30. 450 mg	45. 68.18 kg

Dimensional Analysis—Work Sheet, pp. 121–122

1. $x \text{ g} = \dfrac{1 \text{ g}}{1,000,000 \text{ mcg}} \times \dfrac{230 \text{ mcg}}{1}$
$= 0.00023 \text{ g}$

2. $x \text{ mcg} = \dfrac{1000 \text{ mcg}}{1 \text{ mg}} \times \dfrac{5 \text{ mg}}{1} = 5000 \text{ mcg}$

3. $x \text{ mcg} = \dfrac{1,000,000 \text{ mcg}}{1 \text{ g}} \times \dfrac{2.5 \text{ g}}{1}$
$= 2,500,000 \text{ mcg}$

4. $x \text{ mg} = \dfrac{1 \text{ mg}}{1000 \text{ mcg}} \times \dfrac{4000 \text{ mcg}}{1} = 4 \text{ mg}$

5. $x \text{ mg} = \dfrac{1000 \text{ mg}}{1 \text{ g}} \times \dfrac{0.33 \text{ g}}{1} = 330 \text{ mg}$

6. $x \text{ g} = \dfrac{1000 \text{ g}}{1 \text{ kg}} \times \dfrac{6 \text{ kg}}{1} = 6000 \text{ g}$

7. $x \text{ L} = \dfrac{1 \text{ L}}{1000 \text{ mL}} \times \dfrac{725 \text{ mL}}{1} = 0.725 \text{ L}$

8. $x \text{ g} = \dfrac{1 \text{ g}}{1,000,000 \text{ mcg}} \times \dfrac{2,000 \text{ mcg}}{1}$
$= 0.002 \text{ g}$

9. $x \text{ mm} = \dfrac{10 \text{ mm}}{1 \text{ cm}} \times \dfrac{3 \text{ cm}}{1} = 30 \text{ mm}$

10. $x \text{ kg} = \dfrac{1 \text{ kg}}{1000 \text{ g}} \times \dfrac{620 \text{ g}}{1} = 0.62 \text{ kg}$

11. $x \text{ mcg} = \dfrac{1000 \text{ mcg}}{1 \text{ mg}} \times \dfrac{0.036 \text{ mg}}{1} = 36 \text{ mcg}$

12. $x \text{ L} = \dfrac{1 \text{ L}}{1000 \text{ mL}} \times \dfrac{460 \text{ mL}}{1} = 0.46 \text{ L}$

13. $x \text{ mcg} = \dfrac{1000 \text{ mcg}}{1 \text{ mg}} \times \dfrac{0.66 \text{ mg}}{1} = 660 \text{ mcg}$

14. $x \text{ mcg} = \dfrac{1,000,000 \text{ mcg}}{1 \text{ g}} \times \dfrac{0.5 \text{ g}}{1}$
$= 500,000 \text{ mcg}$

15. $x \text{ cm} = \dfrac{2.5 \text{ cm}}{1 \text{ in}} \times \dfrac{18 \text{ in}}{1} = 45 \text{ cm}$

16. $x \text{ g} = \dfrac{1 \text{ g}}{1,000,000 \text{ mcg}} \times \dfrac{350,000 \text{ mcg}}{1}$
$= 0.35 \text{ g}$

17. $x \text{ g} = \dfrac{1 \text{ g}}{1000 \text{ mg}} \times \dfrac{25 \text{ mg}}{1} = 0.025 \text{ g}$

18. $x \text{ mL} = \dfrac{1000 \text{ mL}}{1 \text{ L}} \times \dfrac{1.46 \text{ L}}{1} = 1460 \text{ mL}$

ANSWERS

19. $x \text{ g} = \dfrac{1000 \text{ g}}{1 \text{ kg}} \times \dfrac{2.5 \text{ kg}}{1} = 2500 \text{ g}$

20. $x \text{ mcg} = \dfrac{1000 \text{ mcg}}{1 \text{ mg}} \times \dfrac{12 \text{ mg}}{1}$
$= 12{,}000 \text{ mcg}$

21. $x \text{ g} = \dfrac{1000 \text{ g}}{1 \text{ kg}} \times \dfrac{3.4 \text{ kg}}{1} = 3400 \text{ g}$

22. $x \text{ g} = \dfrac{1 \text{ g}}{1{,}000{,}000 \text{ mcg}} \times \dfrac{920 \text{ mcg}}{1}$
$= 0.00092 \text{ g}$

23. $x \text{ cm} = \dfrac{1 \text{ cm}}{10 \text{ mm}} \times \dfrac{25 \text{ mm}}{1} = 2.5 \text{ cm}$

24. $x \text{ mg} = \dfrac{1 \text{ mg}}{1000 \text{ mcg}} \times \dfrac{300 \text{ mcg}}{1} = 0.3 \text{ mg}$

25. $x \text{ mL} = \dfrac{1000 \text{ mL}}{1 \text{ L}} \times \dfrac{0.16 \text{ L}}{1} = 160 \text{ mL}$

26. $x \text{ mg} = \dfrac{1000 \text{ mg}}{1 \text{ g}} \times \dfrac{0.01 \text{ g}}{1} = 10 \text{ mg}$

27. $x \text{ mg} = \dfrac{1 \text{ mg}}{1000 \text{ mcg}} \times \dfrac{500 \text{ mcg}}{1} = 0.5 \text{ mg}$

28. $x \text{ g} = \dfrac{1 \text{ g}}{1000 \text{ mg}} \times \dfrac{360 \text{ mg}}{1} = 0.36 \text{ g}$

29. $x \text{ mL} = \dfrac{1000 \text{ mL}}{1 \text{ L}} \times \dfrac{1.7 \text{ L}}{1} = 1700 \text{ mL}$

30. $x \text{ mg} = \dfrac{1000 \text{ mg}}{1 \text{ g}} \times \dfrac{0.45 \text{ g}}{1} = 450 \text{ mg}$

31. $x \text{ L} = \dfrac{1 \text{ L}}{1000 \text{ mL}} \times \dfrac{240 \text{ mL}}{1} = 0.24 \text{ L}$

32. $x \text{ mg} = \dfrac{1 \text{ mg}}{1000 \text{ mcg}} \times \dfrac{10 \text{ mcg}}{1} = 0.01 \text{ mg}$

33. $x \text{ cm} = \dfrac{2.5 \text{ cm}}{1 \text{ in}} \times \dfrac{3 \text{ in}}{1} - 7.5 \text{ cm}$

34. $x \text{ mL} = \dfrac{240 \text{ mL}}{1 \text{ cup}} \times \dfrac{2.25 \text{ cups}}{1} = 540 \text{ mL}$

35. $x \text{ mL} = \dfrac{5 \text{ mL}}{1 \text{ tsp}} \times \dfrac{2 \text{ tsp}}{1} = 10 \text{ mL}$

36. $x \text{ mL} = \dfrac{15 \text{ mL}}{1 \text{ Tbsp}} \times \dfrac{3 \text{ Tbsp}}{1} = 45 \text{ mL}$

37. $x \text{ mL} = \dfrac{240 \text{ mL}}{1 \text{ cup}} \times \dfrac{1.5 \text{ cups}}{1} = 360 \text{ mL}$

38. $x \text{ lb} = \dfrac{2.2 \text{ lb}}{1 \text{ kg}} \times \dfrac{8 \text{ kg}}{1} = 17.6 \text{ lb}$

39. $x \text{ lb} = \dfrac{2.2 \text{ lb}}{1000 \text{ g}} \times \dfrac{3825 \text{ g}}{1} = 8.415 \text{ lb}$

40. $x \text{ cm} = \dfrac{2.5 \text{ cm}}{1 \text{ in}} \times \dfrac{7 \text{ in}}{1} = 17.5 \text{ cm}$

41. $x \text{ kg} = \dfrac{1 \text{ kg}}{2.2 \text{ lb}} \times \dfrac{3 \text{ lb}}{1} = 1.36 \text{ kg}$

42. $x \text{ lb} = \dfrac{2.2 \text{ lb}}{1 \text{ kg}} \times \dfrac{12 \text{ kg}}{1} = 26.4 \text{ lb}$

43. $x \text{ lb} = \dfrac{2.2 \text{ g}}{1000 \text{ g}} \times \dfrac{1400 \text{ g}}{1} = 3.08 \text{ lb}$

44. $x \text{ inches} = \dfrac{12 \text{ inches}}{1 \text{ foot}} \times \dfrac{2\frac{1}{2} \text{ feet}}{1}$
$= 30 \text{ inches}$

45. $x \text{ kg} = \dfrac{1 \text{ kg}}{2.2 \text{ lb}} \times \dfrac{150 \text{ lb}}{1} = 68.18 \text{ kg}$

CHAPTER 6 Metric and Household Measurements—Posttest 1, pp. 123–124

1. 0.005 g
2. 10,000 mcg
3. 810 mL
4. 0.035 g
5. 27 inches
6. 120,000 mcg
7. 35⅕ lb or 35.2 lb
8. 0.28 L
9. 400 g
10. 3½ feet
11. 12,727.27 g
12. 10 cm
13. 0.5 g
14. 0.037 L
15. 20 cc
16. 320 mL
17. 2500 mg
18. 0.35 g
19. 6.7 kg
20. 300 mL
21. 4000 mcg
22. 5¹⁸⁄₂₅ lb or 5.72 lb
23. 7.5 mL
24. 200 mL
25. 0.533 L
26. 1,500,000 mcg
27. 0.62 g
28. 2300 g
29. 1¼ feet
30. 3.18 kg

Dimensional Analysis—Posttest 1, pp. 123–124

1. $x \text{ g} = \dfrac{1 \text{ g}}{1,000,000 \text{ mcg}} \times \dfrac{5000 \text{ mcg}}{1}$
$= 0.005 \text{ g}$

2. $x \text{ mcg} = \dfrac{1000 \text{ mcg}}{1 \text{ mg}} \times \dfrac{10 \text{ mg}}{1}$
$= 10,000 \text{ mcg}$

3. $x \text{ mL} = \dfrac{1000 \text{ mL}}{1 \text{ L}} \times \dfrac{0.81 \text{ L}}{1} = 810 \text{ mL}$

4. $x \text{ g} = \dfrac{1 \text{ g}}{1000 \text{ mg}} \times \dfrac{35 \text{ mg}}{1} = 0.035 \text{ g}$

5. $x \text{ inches} = \dfrac{12 \text{ inches}}{1 \text{ foot}} \times \dfrac{2\frac{1}{4} \text{ feet}}{1}$
$= 27 \text{ inches}$

6. $x \text{ mcg} = \dfrac{1,000,000 \text{ mcg}}{1 \text{ g}} \times \dfrac{0.12 \text{ g}}{1}$
$= 120,000 \text{ mcg}$

7. $x \text{ lb} = \dfrac{2.2 \text{ lb}}{1 \text{ kg}} \times \dfrac{16 \text{ kg}}{1} = 35.2 \text{ lb}$

8. $x \text{ L} = \dfrac{1 \text{ L}}{1000 \text{ mL}} \times \dfrac{280 \text{ mL}}{1} = 0.28 \text{ L}$

9. $x \text{ g} = \dfrac{1000 \text{ g}}{1 \text{ kg}} \times \dfrac{0.4 \text{ kg}}{1} = 400 \text{ g}$

10. $x \text{ feet} = \dfrac{1 \text{ foot}}{12 \text{ inches}} \times \dfrac{42 \text{ inches}}{1} = 3.5 \text{ feet}$

11. $x \text{ g} = \dfrac{1000 \text{ g}}{2.2 \text{ lb}} \times \dfrac{28 \text{ lb}}{1} = 12,727.27 \text{ g}$

12. $x \text{ cm} = \dfrac{2.5 \text{ cm}}{1 \text{ inch}} \times \dfrac{4 \text{ inches}}{1} = 10 \text{ cm}$

13. $x \text{ g} = \dfrac{1 \text{ g}}{1,000,000 \text{ mcg}} \times \dfrac{500,000 \text{ mcg}}{1}$
$= 0.5 \text{ g}$

14. $x \text{ L} = \dfrac{1 \text{ L}}{1000 \text{ mL}} \times \dfrac{37 \text{ mL}}{1} = 0.037 \text{ L}$

15. $x \text{ cc} = \dfrac{1 \text{ cc}}{1 \text{ mL}} \times \dfrac{20 \text{ mL}}{1} = 20 \text{ cc}$

16. $x \text{ mL} = \dfrac{240 \text{ mL}}{1 \text{ cup}} \times \dfrac{1\frac{1}{3} \text{ cups}}{1} = 320 \text{ mL}$

17. $x \text{ mg} = \dfrac{1000 \text{ mg}}{1 \text{ g}} \times \dfrac{2.5 \text{ g}}{1} = 2500 \text{ mg}$

18. $x \text{ g} = \dfrac{1 \text{ g}}{1000 \text{ mg}} \times \dfrac{350 \text{ mg}}{1} = 0.35 \text{ g}$

19. $x \text{ kg} = \dfrac{1 \text{ kg}}{1000 \text{ g}} \times \dfrac{6700 \text{ g}}{1} = 6.7 \text{ kg}$

20. $x \text{ mL} = \dfrac{1000 \text{ mL}}{1 \text{ L}} \times \dfrac{0.3 \text{ L}}{1} = 300 \text{ mL}$

21. $x \text{ mcg} = \dfrac{1000 \text{ mcg}}{1 \text{ mg}} \times \dfrac{4 \text{ mg}}{1} = 4000 \text{ mcg}$

22. $x \text{ lb} = \dfrac{2.2 \text{ lb}}{1000 \text{ g}} \times \dfrac{2600 \text{ g}}{1} = 5.72 \text{ lb}$

23. $x \text{ mL} = \dfrac{5 \text{ mL}}{1 \text{ tsp}} \times \dfrac{1\frac{1}{2} \text{ tsp}}{1} = 7.5 \text{ mL}$

24. $x \text{ mL} = \dfrac{1000 \text{ mL}}{1 \text{ L}} \times \dfrac{0.2 \text{ L}}{1} = 2000 \text{ mL}$

25. $x \text{ L} = \dfrac{1 \text{ L}}{1000 \text{ mL}} \times \dfrac{533 \text{ mL}}{1} = 0.533 \text{ L}$

26. $x \text{ mcg} = \dfrac{1,000,000 \text{ mcg}}{1 \text{ g}} \times \dfrac{1.5 \text{ g}}{1}$
$= 1,500,000 \text{ mcg}$

27. $x \text{ g} = \dfrac{1 \text{ g}}{1000 \text{ mg}} \times \dfrac{620 \text{ mg}}{1} = 0.62 \text{ g}$

28. $x \text{ g} = \dfrac{1000 \text{ g}}{1 \text{ kg}} \times \dfrac{2.3 \text{ kg}}{1} = 2300 \text{ g}$

29. $x \text{ feet} = \dfrac{1 \text{ foot}}{12 \text{ inches}} \times \dfrac{15 \text{ inches}}{1} = 1.25 \text{ feet}$

30. $x \text{ kg} = \dfrac{1 \text{ kg}}{2.2 \text{ lb}} \times \dfrac{7 \text{ lb}}{1} = 3.18 \text{ kg}$

CHAPTER 6 Metric and Household Measurements—Posttest 2, pp. 125–126

1. 4 mg
2. 0.15 kg
3. 600 mL
4. $1\frac{19}{25}$ lb or 1.76 lb
5. $96\frac{4}{5}$ lb or 96.8 lb
6. 0.76 g
7. 550 mL
8. 3.5 cm
9. 60 mL
10. 965.909 g
11. 100 mL
12. 32,000 mcg
13. 0.618 L
14. 0.1 g
15. $2\frac{1}{3}$ feet
16. 0.714 L
17. 0.35 g
18. 0.25 g
19. 870 mg
20. 7000 mcg
21. 0.037 mg

ANSWERS

22. 1400 mL   **25.** 4.5 kg   **28.** 0.42 g
23. 780 mg   **26.** 200 mL   **29.** 2,600,000 mcg
24. 0.225 mg   **27.** 40 inches   **30.** 33.18 kg

Dimensional Analysis—Posttest 2, pp. 125–126

1. $x \text{ mg} = \dfrac{1 \text{ mg}}{1000 \text{ mcg}} \times \dfrac{4000 \text{ mcg}}{1} = 4 \text{ mg}$

2. $x \text{ kg} = \dfrac{1 \text{ kg}}{1000 \text{ mcg}} \times \dfrac{150 \text{ g}}{1} = 0.15 \text{ kg}$

3. $x \text{ mL} = \dfrac{240 \text{ mL}}{1 \text{ cup}} \times \dfrac{1\frac{1}{2} \text{ cups}}{1} = 600 \text{ mL}$

4. $x \text{ lb} = \dfrac{2.2 \text{ lb}}{1000 \text{ g}} \times \dfrac{800 \text{ g}}{1} = 1.76 \text{ lb}$

5. $x \text{ lb} = \dfrac{2.2 \text{ lb}}{1 \text{ kg}} \times \dfrac{44 \text{ kg}}{1} = 96.8 \text{ lb}$

6. $x \text{ g} = \dfrac{1 \text{ g}}{1000 \text{ mg}} \times \dfrac{760 \text{ mg}}{1} = 0.76 \text{ g}$

7. $x \text{ mL} = \dfrac{1000 \text{ mL}}{1 \text{ L}} \times \dfrac{0.55 \text{ L}}{1} = 550 \text{ mL}$

8. $x \text{ cm} = \dfrac{1 \text{ cm}}{10 \text{ mm}} \times \dfrac{35 \text{ mm}}{1} = 3.5 \text{ cm}$

9. $x \text{ mL} = \dfrac{15 \text{ mL}}{1 \text{ Tbsp}} \times \dfrac{4 \text{ Tbsp}}{1} = 60 \text{ mL}$

10. $x \text{ g} = \dfrac{1000 \text{ g}}{2.2 \text{ lb}} \times \dfrac{2\frac{1}{8} \text{ lb}}{1} = 965.909 \text{ g}$

11. $x \text{ mL} = \dfrac{1000 \text{ mL}}{1 \text{ L}} \times \dfrac{0.1 \text{ L}}{1} = 100 \text{ mL}$

12. $x \text{ mcg} = \dfrac{1000 \text{ mcg}}{1 \text{ mg}} \times \dfrac{32 \text{ mg}}{1}$
$= 32{,}000 \text{ mcg}$

13. $x \text{ L} = \dfrac{1 \text{ L}}{1000 \text{ mL}} \times \dfrac{618 \text{ mL}}{1} = 0.618 \text{ L}$

14. $x \text{ g} = \dfrac{1 \text{ g}}{1{,}000{,}000 \text{ mcg}} \times \dfrac{100{,}000 \text{ mcg}}{1}$
$= 0.1 \text{ g}$

15. $x \text{ feet} = \dfrac{1 \text{ foot}}{12 \text{ inches}} \times \dfrac{28 \text{ inches}}{1}$
$= 2.33 \text{ feet}$

16. $x \text{ L} = \dfrac{1 \text{ L}}{1000 \text{ mL}} \times \dfrac{714 \text{ mL}}{1} = 0.714 \text{ L}$

17. $x \text{ g} = \dfrac{1 \text{ g}}{1000 \text{ mg}} \times \dfrac{350 \text{ mg}}{1} = 0.35 \text{ g}$

18. $x \text{ g} = \dfrac{1 \text{ g}}{1{,}000{,}000 \text{ mcg}} \times \dfrac{250{,}000 \text{ mcg}}{1}$
$= 0.25 \text{ g}$

19. $x \text{ mg} = \dfrac{1000 \text{ mg}}{1 \text{ g}} \times \dfrac{0.87 \text{ g}}{1} = 870 \text{ mg}$

20. $x \text{ mcg} = \dfrac{1000 \text{ mcg}}{1 \text{ mg}} \times \dfrac{7 \text{ mg}}{1} = 7000 \text{ mcg}$

21. $x \text{ mg} = \dfrac{1 \text{ mg}}{1000 \text{ mcg}} \times \dfrac{37 \text{ mcg}}{1} = 0.037 \text{ mg}$

22. $x \text{ mL} = \dfrac{1000 \text{ mL}}{1 \text{ L}} \times \dfrac{1.4 \text{ L}}{1} = 1400 \text{ mL}$

23. $x \text{ mg} = \dfrac{1000 \text{ mg}}{1 \text{ g}} \times \dfrac{0.78 \text{ g}}{1} = 780 \text{ mg}$

24. $x \text{ mg} = \dfrac{1 \text{ mg}}{1000 \text{ mcg}} \times \dfrac{225 \text{ mcg}}{1} = 0.225 \text{ mg}$

25. $x \text{ kg} = \dfrac{1 \text{ kg}}{1000 \text{ g}} \times \dfrac{4500 \text{ g}}{1} = 4.5 \text{ kg}$

26. $x \text{ mL} = \dfrac{1000 \text{ mL}}{1 \text{ L}} \times \dfrac{0.2 \text{ L}}{1} = 200 \text{ mL}$

27. $x \text{ inches} = \dfrac{12 \text{ inches}}{1 \text{ foot}} \times \dfrac{3\frac{1}{3} \text{ feet}}{1}$
$= 40 \text{ inches}$

28. $x \text{ g} = \dfrac{1 \text{ g}}{1000 \text{ mg}} \times \dfrac{420 \text{ mg}}{1} = 0.42 \text{ g}$

29. $x \text{ mcg} = \dfrac{1{,}000{,}000 \text{ mcg}}{1 \text{ g}} \times \dfrac{2.6 \text{ g}}{1}$
$= 2{,}600{,}000 \text{ mcg}$

30. $x \text{ kg} = \dfrac{1 \text{ kg}}{2.2 \text{ lb}} \times \dfrac{73 \text{ lb}}{1} = 33.18 \text{ kg}$

ANSWERS

NAME _____

DATE _____

ACCEPTABLE SCORE __14__

YOUR SCORE _____

PRETEST

DIRECTIONS: Change to approximate equivalents as indicated. Solve the problems by using proportions. Show your work. (Round weights and temperatures to nearest tenth.)

1. 110 lb = _____ kg

2. 480 mL = _____ cups

3. 36 kg = _____ lb

4. 90 mL = _____ fl oz

5. 3 cups = _____ mL

6. 8.2 kg = _____ lb

7. 600 mL = _____ cups

8. 2 cups = _____ mL

9. 7 fl oz = _____ mL

10. 360 mL = _____ fl oz

11. 85 lb = _____ kg

12. 1½ fl oz = _____ mL

13. 98.8° F = _____ ° C

14. 41° C = _____ ° F

15. 97.6° F = _____ ° C

16. 38.5° C = _____ ° F

17. 20 cm = _____ inches

18. 50 inches = _____ cm

ANSWERS ON P. 147.

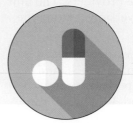

Calculations Used in Patient Assessments

LEARNING OBJECTIVES

Upon completion of the materials provided in this chapter, you will be able to perform computations accurately by mastering the following mathematical concepts:

1 Recalling equivalent apothecary and metric measures
2 Computing equivalents between the apothecary and metric systems by using dimensional analysis to calculate intake and output (I&O), weights, and lengths.
3 Converting from the Fahrenheit scale to the Celsius scale
4 Converting from the Celsius scale to the Fahrenheit scale

In addition to the calculation of drug dosages, nurses calculate aspects of a patient's assessment: intake and output (I&O), weight, lengths, and temperature. The nurse should know the approximate equivalents between the metric and apothecary systems for the calculation of I&O, weight, and lengths. A patient's temperature may require the conversion between the Celsius and Fahrenheit systems. This chapter is devoted to the common calculations that may be used in patient assessments.

APPROXIMATE EQUIVALENTS BETWEEN THE MEASUREMENT SYSTEMS

A list of the most commonly used equivalents among household, apothecary, and metric systems of measure is provided in Box 7-1. Memorize these equivalents. Sometimes a nurse will have to convert from one system to the other. This can be done by using a proportion or dimensional analysis.

BOX 7-1 HOUSEHOLD/APOTHECARY/METRIC EQUIVALENTS

Household Measure	=	Apothecary Measure	=	Metric Measure
		1 fluid ounce (fl oz)	=	30 milliliters (mL)
		6 fluid ounces (fl oz)	=	180 milliliters (mL)
1 standard measuring cup	=	8 fluid ounces (fl oz)	=	240 milliliters (mL)
		2.2 pounds (lb)	=	1000 grams (g) or 1 kilogram (kg)
		1 inch	=	2.5 cm

CALCULATING INTAKE AND OUTPUT

Intake and output (I&O) is an important assessment performed by health care providers. The unit of measure for I&O calculation is typically milliliters, which may require conversions among the household, apothecary, and metric measurement systems.

EXAMPLE 1: (no conversions): A patient consumes 240 mL of orange juice and 240 mL of milk for breakfast, 360 mL of coffee and 90 mL of gelatin for lunch, and 120 mL of apple juice and 240 mL of water for dinner. The patient voided four times during the shift for 300 mL, 200 mL, 400 mL, and 300 mL of urine. Calculate the I&O from 6 AM to 6 PM.

Solution:

Intake	Output
240 mL	300 mL
240 mL	200 mL
360 mL	400 mL
90 mL	300 mL
120 mL	1200 mL
240 mL	
1290 mL	

Therefore 1290 mL would be recorded for the intake and 1200 mL would be recorded for the output during the 6 AM to 6 PM shift.

EXAMPLE 2: (with conversions): A patient consumes 1 cup of coffee and 6 oz of milk for breakfast, 2 cups of coffee and 2 oz of gelatin for lunch, and ½ cup water and 4 oz of ice cream for dinner. The patient voided four times during the shift for 240 mL, 280 mL, 480 mL, and 360 mL of urine. Calculate the I&O from 6 AM to 6 PM.

Solution using dimensional analysis method:

1 cup coffee   1 cup = 240 mL (no conversion needed)

6 oz milk $x \text{ mL} = \dfrac{30 \text{ mL}}{1 \text{ oz}} \times \dfrac{6 \text{ oz}}{1} = 180 \text{ mL}$

2 cups coffee $x \text{ mL} = \dfrac{240 \text{ mL}}{1 \text{ cup}} \times \dfrac{2 \text{ cups}}{1} = 480 \text{ mL}$

2 oz gelatin $x \text{ mL} = \dfrac{30 \text{ mL}}{1 \text{ oz}} \times \dfrac{2 \text{ oz}}{1} = 60 \text{ mL}$

½ cup water $x \text{ mL} = \dfrac{240 \text{ mL}}{1 \text{ cup}} \times \dfrac{0.5 \text{ cup}}{1} = 120 \text{ mL}$

4 oz ice cream $x \text{ mL} = \dfrac{30 \text{ mL}}{1 \text{ oz}} \times \dfrac{4 \text{ oz}}{1} = 120 \text{ mL}$

Solution using proportion method:

1 cup coffee	1 cup = 240 mL (no conversion needed)
6 oz milk	1 oz : 30 mL :: 6 oz : x mL $x = 180$ mL
2 cups coffee	1 cup : 240 mL :: 2 cups : x mL $x = 480$ mL
2 oz gelatin	1 oz : 30 mL :: 2 oz : x mL $x = 60$ mL
½ cup water	1 cup : 240 mL :: ½ cup : x mL $x = 120$ mL
4 oz ice cream	1 oz : 30 mL :: 4 oz : x mL $x = 120$ mL

Intake			Output
1 cup coffee	=	240 mL	240 mL
6 oz milk	=	180 mL	280 mL
2 cups coffee	=	480 mL	480 mL
2 oz gelatin	=	60 mL	360 mL
½ cup water	=	120 mL	1360 mL
4 oz ice cream	=	120 mL	
		1200 mL	

Therefore 1200 mL would be recorded for the intake and 1360 mL would be recorded for the output during the 6 AM to 6 PM shift.

EXAMPLE 3: (complex I&O): A patient has intravenous (IV) fluids of 0.9% normal saline infusing at 100 mL/h at 6 AM. After morning labs are reviewed, the IV fluids are decreased to 50 mL/h at 10 AM. The IV fluids are held for 2 hours while 1 unit of packed red blood cells (300 mL) is infused from 1 PM to 3 PM. The patient consumes 4 oz of orange juice for breakfast, 240 mL of milk for lunch, and 120 mL of coffee with dinner. At 1 PM, the patient has 200 mL of emesis. At 6 PM, the patient's Foley catheter is emptied of 1200 mL and a surgical drain is emptied of 50 mL. Calculate the I&O from 6 AM to 6 PM.

Solution using an I&O sheet:

	6-7	7-8	8-9	9-10	10-11	11-12	12-1	1-2	2-3	3-4	4-5	5-6	Total
Intake:													
Oral			120				240					120	480
IV	100	100	100	100	50	50	50	off	off	50	50	50	700
Blood								150	150				300
Shift Total:													1480
Output:													
Urine												1200	1200
Drains												50	50
Emesis								200					200
Shift Total:													1450

Therefore 1480 mL would be recorded for the intake and 1450 mL would be recorded for the output during the 6 AM to 6 PM shift. Note that all values entered into the I&O sheet are in milliliters.

CALCULATING PATIENT WEIGHT

EXAMPLE 1: 5.5 lb equals how many kilograms?

Dimensional Analysis Method

$$x \text{ kg} = \frac{1 \text{ kg}}{2.2 \text{ lb}}$$

$$x \text{ kg} = \frac{1 \text{ kg}}{2.2 \text{ lb}} \times \frac{5.5 \text{ lb}}{1}$$

$$x \text{ kg} = \frac{1 \text{ kg}}{2.2 \text{ lb}} \times \frac{5.5 \text{ lb}}{1} = 2.5 \text{ kg}$$

Proportion Method

$$1 \text{ kg} : 2.2 \text{ lb} : x \text{ kg} : 5.5 \text{ lb}$$

$$2.2x = 5.5$$

$$x = \frac{5.5}{2.2} = 2.5 \text{ kg}$$

EXAMPLE 2: 28 kg equals how many pounds?

Dimensional Analysis Method

$$x \text{ lb} = \frac{2.2 \text{ lb}}{1 \text{ kg}}$$

$$x \text{ lb} = \frac{2.2 \text{ lb}}{1 \text{ kg}} \times \frac{28 \text{ kg}}{1}$$

$$x \text{ lb} = \frac{2.2 \text{ lb}}{1 \text{ kg}} \times \frac{28 \text{ kg}}{1} = 61.6 \text{ lb}$$

Proportion Method

$$1 \text{ kg} : 2.2 \text{ lb} :: 28 \text{ kg} : x \text{ lb}$$

$$x = 2.2 \times 28$$

$$x = 61.6 \text{ lb}$$

CALCULATING PATIENT LENGTHS

EXAMPLE 1: 62 inches equals how many centimeters?

Dimensional Analysis Method

$$x \text{ cm} = \frac{2.5 \text{ cm}}{1 \text{ inch}}$$

$$x \text{ cm} = \frac{2.5 \text{ cm}}{1 \text{ inch}} \times \frac{62 \text{ inches}}{1}$$

$$x \text{ cm} = \frac{2.5 \text{ cm}}{1 \text{ inch}} \times \frac{62 \text{ inches}}{1} = 155 \text{ cm}$$

Proportion Method

$$1 \text{ inch} : 2.5 \text{ cm} :: 62 \text{ inches} : x \text{ cm}$$

$$x = 2.5 \times 62$$

$$x = 155 \text{ cm}$$

EXAMPLE 2: 10 cm equals how many inches?

Dimensional Analysis Method

$$x \text{ in} = \frac{1 \text{ inch}}{2.5 \text{ cm}}$$

$$x \text{ in} = \frac{1 \text{ inch}}{2.5 \text{ cm}} \times \frac{10 \text{ cm}}{1}$$

$$x \text{ in} = \frac{1 \text{ inch}}{2.5 \text{ cm}} \times \frac{10 \text{ cm}}{1} = 4 \text{ inches}$$

Proportion Method

$$2.5 \text{ cm} : 1 \text{ inch} :: 10 \text{ cm} : x \text{ inches}$$

$$2.5x = 10$$

$$x = \frac{10}{2.5} = 4 \text{ inches}$$

APPROXIMATE EQUIVALENTS BETWEEN CELSIUS AND FAHRENHEIT MEASUREMENTS

Hospitals and health care centers use the metric system of measurement, including thermometers calibrated in the Celsius scale. It may be necessary for the nurse to convert the Celsius, or centigrade, scale to the Fahrenheit scale for patient or family information. Because not everyone concerned with patient care uses the same scale, it is also important for the nurse to be able to convert the Fahrenheit scale to the Celsius scale.

Most hospitals now use digital thermometers rather than mercury thermometers. The following thermometers are included for illustration purposes only. Digital thermometers are available in the Fahrenheit or Celsius scale. Patients frequently ask for conversion charts at the time of discharge so that they can understand the readings if they are allowed to take their hospital thermometers home. The conversion charts are helpful for the nurse as well. However, the nurse should be able to convert from one scale to the other if necessary.

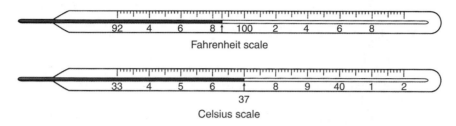

For conversion from one scale to another, the following proportion may be used:

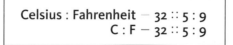

Celsius : Fahrenheit − 32 :: 5 : 9
C : F − 32 :: 5 : 9

C or F will be the unknown.
Extend the decimal to hundredths; round to tenths.
Another means of converting Celsius and Fahrenheit temperatures to equivalents is given in Box 7-2.

BOX 7-2 CONVERTING CELSIUS AND FAHRENHEIT TEMPERATURES

Fahrenheit to Celsius	Celsius to Fahrenheit
Subtract 32	Multiply by 1.8
Divide by 1.8	Add 32

The following examples illustrate each method. (Round temperatures to nearest tenth.)

EXAMPLE 1: 100.6° F equals _____ ° C.

a. C : F − 32 :: 5 : 9

b. C : 100.6 − 32 :: 5 : 9

c. 9C = (100.6 − 32) × 5

d. 9C = 68.6 × 5

e. 9C = 343

f. $C = \dfrac{343}{9}$

g. C = 38.11

h. 100.6° F = 38.1° C.

a. 100.6 − 32 − 68.6

b. 68.6 ÷ 1.8 = 38.111,
or 38.1° C

EXAMPLE 2: 37.6° C equals _____ ° F.

a. $C : F - 32 :: 5 : 9$

b. $37.6 : F - 32 :: 5 : 9$

c. $5(F - 32) = 9 \times 37.6$

d. $5F - 160 = 338.4$

e. $5F - 160 + 160 = 338.4 + 160$

f. $5F = 498.4$

g. $F = \dfrac{498.4}{5}$

h. $F = 99.68$

i. $37.6° \, C = 99.7° \, F.$

a. $37.6 \times 1.8 = 67.68$

b. $67.68 + 32 = 99.68,$ or 99.7° F

Memorize the table of approximate equivalents for the household, apothecary, and metric systems of measure. Study the material on the calculations of I&O, lengths, weight, and temperature conversions. Complete the following work sheet, which provides for extensive practice. Check your answers. If you have difficulties, go back and review the necessary material. When you feel ready to evaluate your learning, take the first posttest. Check your answers. An acceptable score as indicated on the posttest signifies that you are ready for the next chapter. An unacceptable score signifies a need for further study before you take the second posttest.

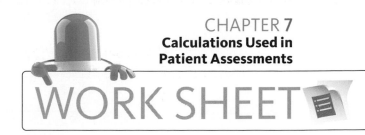

WORK SHEET

DIRECTIONS: Change to approximate equivalents as indicated. Solve the problems by using a proportion. Show your work.

1. 22 lb = _____ kg

2. 3 cups = _____ mL

3. 210 mL = _____ fl oz

4. 10 kg = _____ lb

5. 1740 mL = _____ fl oz

6. ½ fl oz = _____ mL

7. 4.2 inches = _____ cm

8. 6 fl oz = _____ mL

9. 3600 mL = _____ fl oz

10. 360 mL = _____ cups

11. 3.3 kg = _____ lb

12. 6 lb = _____ kg

13. 30 cm = _____ inches

14. 5 lb – _____ kg

15. 2400 mL – _____ cups

16. 2 cups = _____ mL

17. 365 kg = _____ lb

18. 4 fl oz = _____ mL

19. 12 lb = _____ g

20. 75 lb = _____ kg

21. 6 cups = _____ mL

22. 4500 g = _____ kg

23. 25 kg = _____ lb

24. 99.6° F = _____ ° C

25. 101.8° F = _____ ° C

26. 40.4° C = _____ ° F

27. 36.8° C = _____ ° F

28. 39.2° C = _____ ° F   **29.** 98.4° F = _____ ° C   **30.** 41.2° C = _____ ° F

31. 103.6° F = _____ ° C   **32.** 102.2° F = _____ ° C   **33.** 100.4° F = _____ ° C

34. A patient consumes 180 mL of apple juice and 120 mL of milk for breakfast, 240 mL of coffee and 120 mL of gelatin for lunch, and 120 mL of ice cream and 240 mL of tea for dinner. The patient voided four times during the shift for 340 mL, 220 mL, 440 mL, and 300 mL of urine. Calculate the I&O from 6 AM to 6 PM.

35. A patient consumes 2 cups of tea and 8 oz of milk for breakfast, 1 cup of coffee and 6 oz of gelatin for lunch, and ½ cup of broth and 4 oz of ice cream for dinner. The patient voided five times during the shift for 120 mL, 200 mL, 240 mL, 400 mL, and 320 mL of urine. Calculate the I&O from 6 AM to 6 PM.

36. A patient has intravenous (IV) fluids of D5 ½ NS with 20 mEq KCl infusing at 100 mL/h at 6 AM. An order is received to increase the IV fluids to 125 mL/h at 11 AM. The IV fluids are held for 2 hours while vancomycin 1 g in 250 mL of 0.9% NS is infused from 3 PM to 5 PM. The patient consumes 6 oz of broth and 3 oz of gelatin for breakfast, 240 mL of milk for lunch, and 120 mL of coffee with dinner. At 2 PM, the patient has 200 mL removed during a thoracentesis. At 6 PM, the patient's Foley catheter is emptied of 1100 mL and 150 mL is emptied from a surgical drain. Calculate the I&O from 6 AM to 6 PM using the following I&O sheet.

	6-7	7-8	8-9	9-10	10-11	11-12	12-1	1-2	2-3	3-4	4-5	5-6	**Total**
Intake:													
Oral													
IV													
IV Meds													
Shift Total:													
Output:													
Urine													
Drains													
Thora.													
Shift Total:													

ANSWERS ON P. 147.

NAME _____

DATE _____

ACCEPTABLE SCORE ___**16**___

YOUR SCORE _____

POSTTEST 1

DIRECTIONS: Change to approximate equivalents as indicated. Solve the problems by using proportions. Show your work.

1. 3 fl oz = _____ mL

2. 1½ cups = _____ mL

3. 7½ lb = _____ g

4. 17 fl oz = _____ mL

5. 20 lb = _____ kg

6. 900 mL = _____ fl oz

7. 60 mL = _____ fl oz

8. 5 fl oz = _____ mL

9. 32 kg = _____ lb

10. 50 inches = _____ cm

11. 60 cm = _____ inches

12. 40.8° C = _____ ° F

13. 104.2° F = _____ ° C

14. 37.2° C = _____ ° F

15. 99.4° F = _____ ___ ° C

16. A patient is nothing by mouth (NPO) and is receiving D5 ½ NS with 20 mEq KCl at 125 mL/h. The patient voided three times during the shift for 320 mL, 480 mL, and 320 mL of urine. Calculate the I&O from 6 AM to 6 PM.

17. A patient receives 8 oz of Pulmocare every 6 hours followed by 4 oz of water per gastrostomy tube on an 8-2-8-2 schedule. The patient consumes 2 oz of ice pop one time. The patient's Foley catheter is emptied of 800 mL of urine at 6 PM. Calculate the I&O from 6 AM to 6 PM.

ANSWERS

CHAPTER 9 Interpretation of the Physician's Orders—Posttest 1, p. 171

1.	1430	**6.**	0345	**11.**	11:15 PM	**16.**	4:30 PM
2.	1030	**7.**	2130	**12.**	4:40 AM	**17.**	7:00 PM
3.	1700	**8.**	0400	**13.**	5:45 PM	**18.**	10:30 PM
4.	2400, or 0000	**9.**	1830	**14.**	9:20 AM	**19.**	7:50 AM
5.	0800	**10.**	2215	**15.**	6:45 PM	**20.**	1:15 AM

CHAPTER 9 Interpretation of the Physician's Orders—Posttest 2, p. 173

¹1/12/19	Cefuroxime						
	1 g dose	IV route	q8 h interval	08	16	24	
²1/12/19	Lasix						
	40 mg dose	po route	twice daily interval		09	21	
³1/12/19	Slow-K						
	10 mEq dose	po route	twice daily interval		09	21	

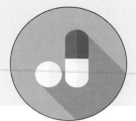

CHAPTER **10**

Reading Medication Labels

LEARNING OBJECTIVES

Upon completion of the materials provided in this chapter, you will be able to identify the following parts of each drug label:

1 Trade name of the medication
2 Generic name of the medication
3 Strength of the medication dosage
4 Form in which the medication is provided
5 Route of administration
6 Total amount or volume of the medication provided in the container
7 Directions for mixing or preparation of the medication if required

The safe administration of medications to patients begins with the nurse accurately reading and interpreting the drug label. Thus it is important for the nurse to be familiar and comfortable with the information that is found on the drug label.

PARTS OF A DRUG LABEL

1. TRADE NAME. The trade name (also known as the brand or proprietary name) is usually capitalized and written in bold print. It is the first name written on the label. The trade name is always followed by the ® registration symbol. Different manufacturers market the same medication under different trade names.

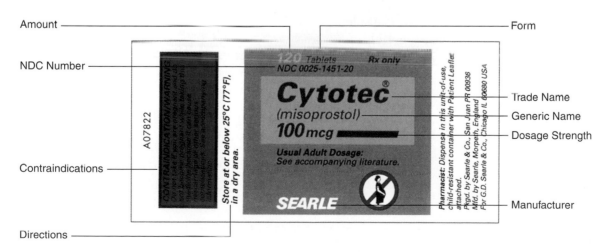

2. GENERIC NAME. The generic name is the official name of the drug. Each drug has only *one* generic name. This name appears directly under the trade name, usually in smaller or different type letters. Physicians may order a patient's medication by generic or trade name. Nurses need to be familiar with both names and cross-check references as needed. Occasionally, only the generic name will appear on the label.

3. DOSAGE STRENGTH. The strength indicates the amount or weight of the medication that is supplied in the specific unit of measure. This amount may be per capsule, tablet, or milliliter, for example.

4. FORM. The form indicates how the drug is supplied. Examples of various forms are tablets, capsules, liquids, suppositories, and ointments.

5. ROUTE. The label will indicate how the drug is to be administered. The route can be oral, topical, injection (subcutaneous, intradermal, intramuscular), or intravenous.

6. AMOUNT. The total amount or volume of the medication may be indicated. Some examples are 250 mL of oral suspension and a bottle that contains 50 capsules.

7. DIRECTIONS. Some medications must be mixed before use. The amounts and types of diluent required will be listed along with the resulting strengths of the medication. This information may also be found on package inserts.

Other information may be found on drug labels: the name of the manufacturer, expiration date, special instructions for storage, a National Drug Code (NDC) number, and contraindications.

EXAMPLES FOR PRACTICE IN READING DRUG LABELS

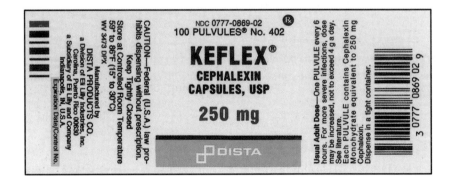

1. Trade name ....Keflex
2. Generic name ....cephalexin
3. Dosage strength ....250 mg
4. Form.......................................Capsules
5. Amount...................................100
6. Directions ....Keep tightly closed. Store at controlled room temperature 59° to 86° F (15° to 30° C).
7. NDC number 0777-0869-02
8. Manufacturer..........................DISTA
9. Expiration date ....(Yellow highlight)

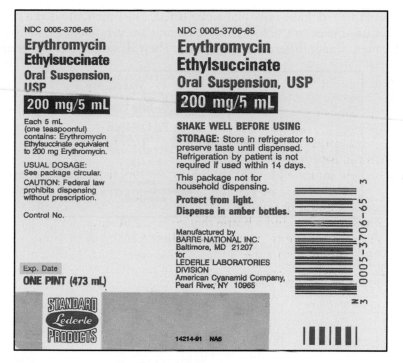

1. Trade name ....Erythromycin
2. Generic name ....erythromycin ethylsuccinate
3. Dosage strength......................200 mg/5 mL
4. Form ....Suspension
5. Route ....Oral
6. Amount.................................1 pint (473 mL)
7. Directions.............................Shake well before using. Storage: Store in refrigerator to preserve taste until dispensed. Refrigeration by patient is not required if used within 14 days. Protect from light. Dispense in amber bottles.
8. NDC number 0005-3706-65
9. Manufacturer ....Barre-National Inc., Lederle Laboratories Division
10. Expiration date ....(Yellow highlight)

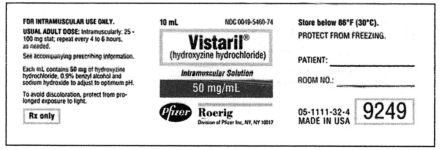

1. Trade name ....Vistaril
2. Generic name ....hydroxyzine hydrochloride
3. Dosage strength ....50 mg/mL
4. Form......................................Intramuscular solution
5. Route ....Intramuscular injection
6. Amount..................................Total amount of 10 mL in vial
7. Directions ....Storage: Store below 86° F (30° C). Protect from freezing. To avoid discoloration, protect from prolonged exposure to light.
8. NDC number 0049-5460-74
9. Manufacturer..........................Pfizer Roerig

Occasionally, a drug label will have only one name listed. The one name is the generic name. These are drugs that have been in use for many years and are very well known. The drug companies do not market them under different trade names. They all simply use the generic name.

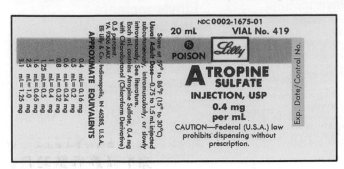

1. Trade name .... None
2. Generic name .... atropine sulfate
3. Dosage strength .... 0.4 mg per mL
4. Form .... Liquid
5. Route .... Injection
6. Amount .... 20 mL
7. NDC number 0002-1675-01
8. Expiration date .... (Yellow highlight)
9. Manufacturer .... Lilly
10. Caution .... Federal (U.S.A.) law prohibits dispensing without prescription.

Study the material and examples for practice in reading drug labels. When you feel ready to evaluate your learning, take the first posttest. Check your answers. An acceptable score as indicated on the posttest signifies that you are ready for the next chapter. An unacceptable score signifies a need for further study before you take the second posttest.

hw ✓ 6/4

NAME _____

DATE _____

ACCEPTABLE SCORE __19__

YOUR SCORE _____

DIRECTIONS: Identify the requested parts of each of the following medication labels.

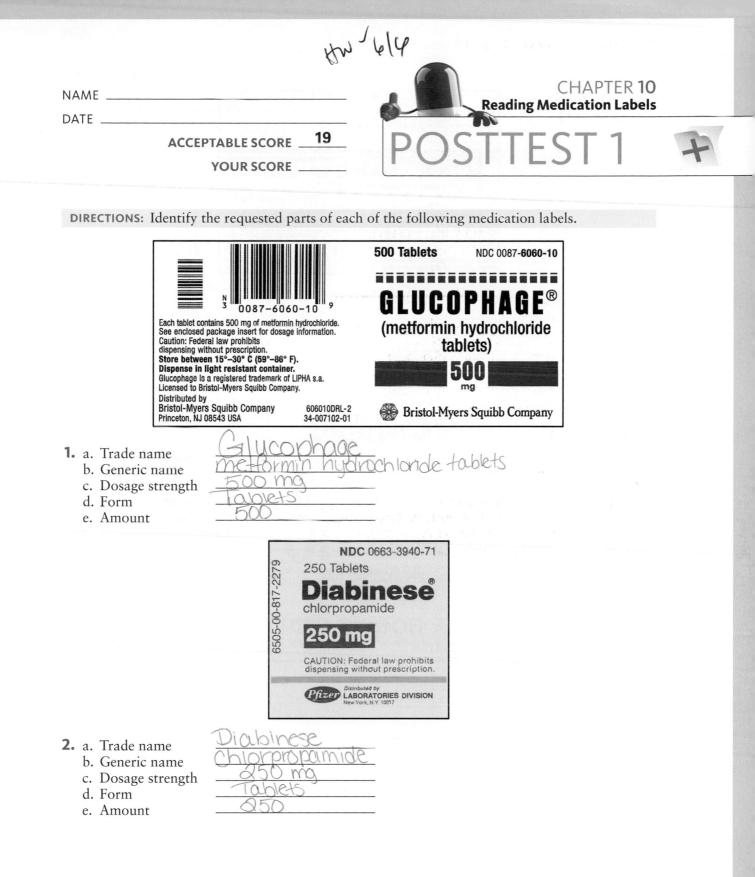

1. a. Trade name _Glucophage_
   b. Generic name _metformin hydrochloride tablets_
   c. Dosage strength _500 mg_
   d. Form _Tablets_
   e. Amount _500_

2. a. Trade name _Diabinese_
   b. Generic name _Chlorpropamide_
   c. Dosage strength _250 mg_
   d. Form _Tablets_
   e. Amount _250_

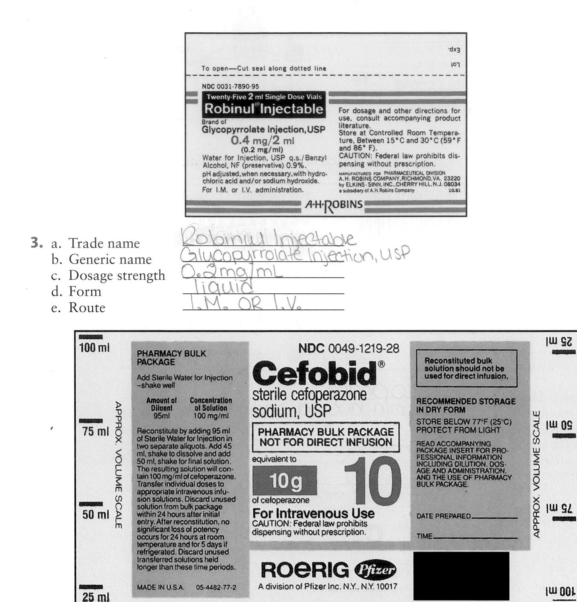

3. a. Trade name   Robinul Injectable
    b. Generic name   Glucopyrrolate Injection, USP
    c. Dosage strength   0.2mg/mL
    d. Form   liquid
    e. Route   I.M. OR I.V.

4. a. Trade name   Cefobid
    b. Generic name   Sterile cefoperazone sodium, USP
    c. Dosage strength   10g
    d. Form   phdliquid >liquid
    e. Route   I.V.

ANSWERS ON P. 183.

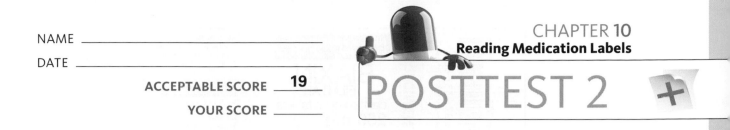

NAME _____

DATE _____

ACCEPTABLE SCORE __19__

YOUR SCORE _____

CHAPTER 10
Reading Medication Labels

POSTTEST 2

DIRECTIONS: Identify the requested parts of each of the following medication labels.

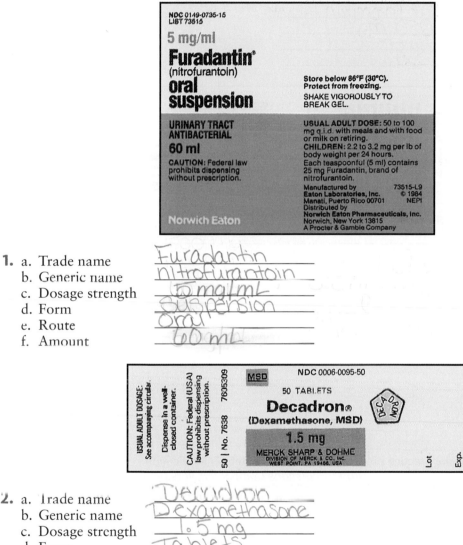

1. a. Trade name   *Furadantin*
   b. Generic name   *nitrofurantoin*
   c. Dosage strength *5 mg/mL*
   d. Form   *suspension*
   e. Route   *oral*
   f. Amount   *60 mL*

2. a. Trade name   *Decadron*
   b. Generic name   *Dexamethasone*
   c. Dosage strength *1.5 mg*
   d. Form   *Tablets*

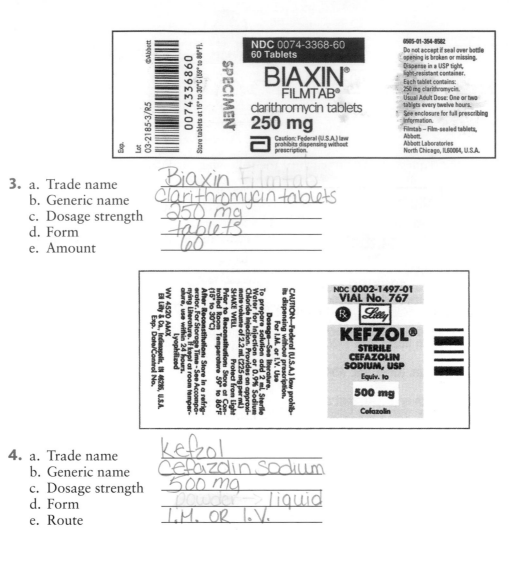

3. a. Trade name   ~~Biaxin Filmtab~~
   b. Generic name   ~~Clarithromycin tablets~~
   c. Dosage strength   ~~250 mg~~
   d. Form   ~~tablets~~
   e. Amount   ~~60~~

4. a. Trade name   ~~Kefzol~~
   b. Generic name   ~~Cefazolin sodium~~
   c. Dosage strength   ~~500 mg~~
   d. Form   ~~powder → liquid~~
   e. Route   ~~I.M. or I.V.~~

ANSWERS ON P. 183.

evolve   For additional practice problems, refer to the Safety in Medication
Administration section of *Drug Calculations Companion,* Version 5,
on Evolve.

ANSWERS

CHAPTER 10 Reading Medication Labels—Posttest 1, pp. 179–180

1. a. Glucophage
   b. metformin hydrochloride
   c. 500 mg
   d. tablets
   e. 500 tablets

2. a. Diabinese
   b. chlorpropamide
   c. 250 mg
   d. tablets
   e. 250 tablets

3. a. Robinul
   b. glycopyrrolate
   c. 0.4 mg/2 mL or 0.2 mg/mL
   d. milliliters, liquid
   e. IM or IV

4. a. Cefobid
   b. cefoperazone sodium
   c. 10 g
   d. milliliters, powder reconstituted into liquid
   e. IV

CHAPTER 10 Reading Medication Labels—Posttest 2, pp. 181–182

1. a. Furadantin
   b. nitrofurantoin
   c. 5 mg/mL
   d. suspension
   e. oral
   f. 60 mL

2. a. Decadron
   b. dexamethasone
   c. 1.5 mg
   d. tablets

3. a. Biaxin
   b. clarithromycin
   c. 250 mg
   d. tablet
   e. 60 tablets

4. a. Kefzol
   b. cefazolin sodium
   c. 225 mg/mL
   d. milliliters, powder reconstituted into liquid
   e. IM or IV

PART FOUR

CALCULATION of DRUG DOSAGES

Oral Dosages

1 Using the dimensional analysis method to solve problems of oral dosages involving tablets, capsules, liquid medications, and those measured in milliequivalents

2 Converting all measures within the problem to equivalent measures in one system of measurement if required

3 Using a proportion to solve problems of oral dosages involving tablets, capsules, liquid medications, and those measured in milliequivalents

4 Using the stated formula as an alternative method of solving problems of oral dosages involving tablets, capsules, liquid medications, and those measured in milliequivalents

Oral drugs are preferred for administration of medications because they are easy to take and convenient for the patient. Oral medications are absorbed through the gastrointestinal tract; therefore the skin is not interrupted. Oral medications may be more economical because the production cost is usually lower than for other forms of medication.

Oral medications are absorbed primarily in the small intestine. Because of the differences in absorption factors, they might not be as effective as other forms of medication. Some oral medications are irritating to the alimentary canal and must be given with meals or a snack. Others may be harmful to the teeth and should be taken through a straw or feeding tube.

Oral medications are supplied in a variety of forms (Figure 11-1). The most common form is a tablet. Tablets come in many colors, sizes, and shapes. A tablet is produced from a drug powder. The tablet may be grooved for ease in administering only a fraction of the whole tablet. Some tablets are scored into halves, and others are divided into fourths (Figure 11-2).

Many physicians order medications that allow their patients to cut the tablets in half at home. With the rising cost of medications, this strategy helps to decrease the cost for the patient and encourages compliance in taking the medication.

If a patient has difficulty swallowing pills, some pills may be crushed using a mortar and pestle or a device that is specifically made for crushing pills (Figure 11-3). Before crushing any medication in pill form, verify that the medication can be crushed. Some medications, such as those that are enteric coated or sustained or extended release, should not be crushed.

! ● ALERT

Before crushing, verify from the pharmacist that the medication may be crushed and the instructions for crushing.

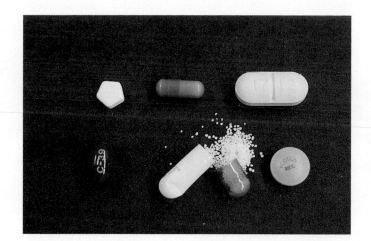

FIGURE 11-1   Forms of solid oral medication. *Top row:* Uniquely shaped tablet, capsule, scored tablet. *Bottom row:* Gelatin-coated liquid, extended-release capsule, and enteric-coated tablet. (From Potter PA, Perry AG, Stockert PA, Hall AM: *Fundamentals of nursing,* ed 8, St Louis, 2013, Mosby.)

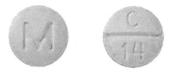

FIGURE 11-2   Scored medication tablet. (From *Mosby's drug consult 2007,* St Louis, 2007, Mosby.)

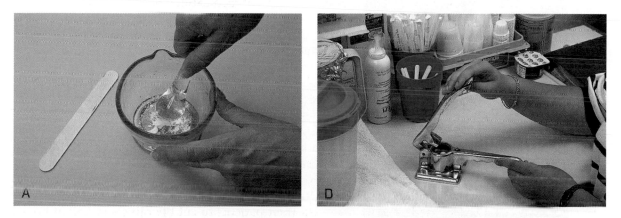

FIGURE 11-3   **A,** Mortar and pestle. **B,** Pill crusher. (From Perry AG, Potter PA, Elkin MK: *Nursing interventions and clinical skills,* ed 5, St Louis, 2012, Mosby.)

Oral medications may also be supplied in capsule form. A capsule is a hard or soft gelatin that houses a powder, liquid, or granular form of a specific medicine(s). Capsules are produced in a variety of sizes and colors (Figure 11-4). Capsules cannot be divided or crushed.

Oral medications may also be administered in liquid form such as an elixir or an oral suspension. Oral liquid medications can be measured with a medication cup, oral syringe (syringe without the needle attached), or dropper (Figures 11-5 to 11-7).

Table 11-1 describes the forms of a variety of medications.

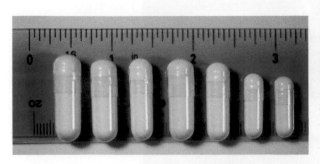

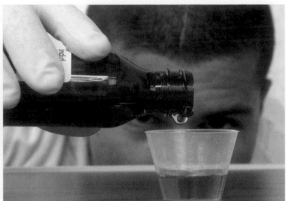

FIGURE 11-4   Various sizes and numbers of gelatin capsules (actual size). (From Clayton BD, Willihnganz M: *Basic pharmacology for nurses,* ed 16, St Louis, 2013, Mosby.)

FIGURE 11-5   Oral liquid medication measured with a medication cup. (From Potter PA, Perry AG, Stokert PA, Hall AM: *Fundamentals of Nursing,* ed 8, St Louis, 2013, Mosby.)

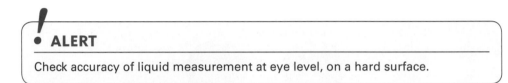

! **ALERT**

Check accuracy of liquid measurement at eye level, on a hard surface.

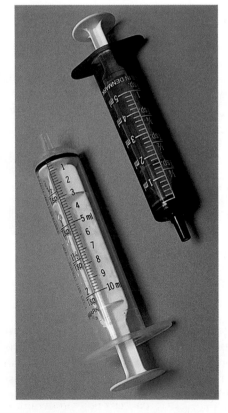

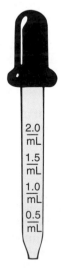

FIGURE 11-6   Plastic oral syringe. (From Clayton BD, Willihnganz M: *Basic pharmacology for nurses,* ed 16, St Louis, 2013, Mosby.)

FIGURE 11-7   Medicine dropper. (From Clayton BD, Willihnganz M: *Basic pharmacology for nurses,* ed 16, St Louis, 2013, Mosby.)

TABLE 11-1 FORMS OF MEDICATION

Medication Forms Commonly Prepared for Administration by Oral Route

Solid Forms	Description
Caplet	Shaped like capsule and coated for ease of swallowing
Capsule	Medication encased in a gelatin shell
Tablet	Powdered medication compressed into hard disk or cylinder; in addition to primary medication, contains binders (adhesive to allow powder to stick together), disintegrators (to promote tablet dissolution), lubricants (for ease of manufacturing), and fillers (for convenient tablet size)
Enteric-coated tablet	Coated tablet that does not dissolve in stomach; coatings dissolve in intestine, where medication is absorbed
Pill	Contains one or more medications, shaped into globules, ovoids, or oblong shapes; rarely used (have been replaced by tablets)

Liquid Forms	Description
Elixir	Clear fluid containing water and/or alcohol; often sweetened
Extract	Syrup or dried form of pharmacologically active medication, usually made by evaporating solution
Aqueous solution	Substance dissolved in water and syrups
Aqueous suspension	Finely divided drug particles dispersed in liquid medium; when left standing, particles settle to bottom of container; shake before use
Syrup	Medication dissolved in a concentrated sugar solution
Tincture	Alcohol extract from plant or vegetable

Solid Forms	Description

Other Oral Forms and Terms Associated with Oral Preparations

Troche (lozenge)	Flat, round tablets that dissolve in mouth to release medication; not meant for ingestion; should not be swallowed
Aerosol	Aqueous medication sprayed and absorbed in mouth and upper airway; not meant for ingestion
Sustained release	Tablet or capsule that contains small particles of a medication coated with material that requires a varying amount of time to dissolve

Medication Forms Commonly Prepared for Administration by Topical Route

Ointment (salve or cream)	Semisolid, externally applied preparation, usually containing one or more medications
Liniment	Usually contains alcohol, oil, or soapy emollient; applied to skin
Lotion	Liquid suspension that usually protects, cools, or cleanses skin
Paste	Thick ointment; absorbed through skin more slowly than ointment; often used for skin protection
Transdermal disk or patch	Medicated disk or patch absorbed through skin slowly over long period (e.g., 24 hours, 1 week)

Medication Forms Commonly Prepared for Administration by Parenteral Route

Solution	Sterile preparation that contains water with one or more dissolved compounds
Powder	Sterile particles of medication that are dissolved in a sterile liquid (e.g., water, normal saline) before administration

Medication Forms Commonly Prepared for Instillation into Body Cavities

Solution	Substance dissolved in water or other liquid
Intraocular disk	Small, flexible oval (similar to contact lens) consisting of two soft, outer layers and a middle layer containing medication; slowly releases medication when moistened by ocular fluid
Suppository	Solid dosage form mixed with gelatin and shaped to form pellet for insertion into body cavity (rectum or vagina); melts when it reaches body temperature, releasing medication for absorption

Modified from Potter PA, Perry AG: *Fundamentals of nursing,* ed 7, St Louis, 2009, Mosby.

Oral Dosages Involving Capsules and Tablets: Dimensional Analysis Method

Dimensional analysis is another method for setting up problems to calculate drug dosages. The advantage of dimensional analysis is that only one equation is needed. This is true even if the information supplied indicates a need to convert to like units before setting up the proportion to perform the actual calculation of the amount of medication to be given to the patient.

EXAMPLE 1: The order states Augmentin 500 mg po daily. The drug is supplied in 250-mg tablets. How many tablets will the nurse administer?

a. On the left side of the equation, place the name or abbreviation of the drug form of x, or what you are solving for.

$$x \text{ tablet} =$$

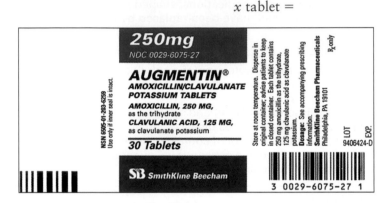

b. On the right side of the equation, place the available information related to the measurement or abbreviation that was placed on the left side. In this example that is *tablet*. This information is placed in the equation as a common fraction; match the appropriate abbreviation or measurement. Thus the abbreviation that matches the x quantity must be placed in the numerator. We also know from the problem that each tablet contains 250 mg of Augmentin. This information is the denominator of our fraction.

$$x \text{ tablet} = \frac{1 \text{ tablet}}{250 \text{ mg}}$$

c. Next, find the information that matches the measurement or abbreviation used in the denominator of the fraction you created. In this example mg is in the denominator and our order is for 500 mg. Therefore the full equation is

$$x \text{ tablet} = \frac{1 \text{ tablet}}{250 \text{ mg}} \times \frac{500 \text{ mg}}{1}$$

d. Now cancel out the like abbreviations on the right side of the equation. If you have set up the problem correctly, the remaining measurement or abbreviation should match that used on the left side of the equation. You are now ready to solve for x.

$$x \text{ tablet} = \frac{1 \text{ tablet}}{250 \text{ mg}} \times \frac{500 \text{ mg}}{1}$$

$$x = \frac{500}{250}$$

$$x = 2 \text{ tablets}$$

The answer to the problem is 2 tablets.

EXAMPLE 2: The physician orders aspirin 975 mg po four times a day. Aspirin 325-mg tablets are available. How many tablets will the nurse administer? _____

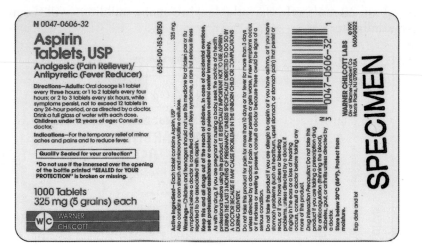

a. On the left side of the equation, place the name or abbreviation of the drug form of x, or what you are solving for.

$$x \text{ tablet} =$$

b. On the right side of the equation, place the available information related to the measurement or abbreviation that was placed on the left side. In this example that is *tablet*. This information is placed in the equation as a common fraction; match the appropriate abbreviation or measurement. Thus the abbreviation that matches the x quantity must be placed in the numerator. We also know from the problem that each tablet contains 325 mg of aspirin. This information is the denominator of our fraction.

$$x \text{ tablet} = \frac{1 \text{ tablet}}{325 \text{ mg}}$$

c. Next, find the information that matches the measurement or abbreviation used in the denominator of the fraction you created. In this example *mg* is in the denominator and our order is for 975 mg. Therefore the full equation is

$$x \text{ tablet} = \frac{1 \text{ tablet}}{325 \text{ mg}} \times \frac{975 \text{ mg}}{1}$$

d. Now cancel out the like abbreviations on the right side of the equation. If you have set up the problem correctly, the remaining measurement or abbreviation should match that used on the left side of the equation. You are now ready to solve for x.

$$x \text{ tablet} = \frac{1 \text{ tablet}}{\frac{325 \text{ mg}}{1}} \times \frac{\overset{3}{\cancel{975}} \text{ mg}}{1}$$

$$x = \frac{975}{325} = \frac{3}{1}$$

$$x = 3 \text{ tablets}$$

The answer to the problem is 3 tablets.

Oral Dosages Involving Liquids: Dimensional Analysis Method

EXAMPLE 1: The physician orders phenobarbital 45 mg po two times a day. Phenobarbital elixir, 20 mg/5 mL, is available. How many milliliters will the nurse administer? _____

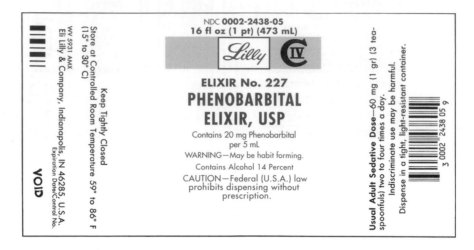

a. On the left side of the equation, place the name or abbreviation of the drug form of x, or what you are solving for.

$$x \text{ mL} =$$

b. On the right side of the equation, place the available information related to the measurement or abbreviation that was placed on the left side. In this example, that is *mL*. This information is placed in the equation as a common fraction; match the appropriate abbreviation or measurement. Thus the abbreviation that matches the x quantity must be placed in the numerator. We also know from the problem that each 5 *mL* contains 20 mg of phenobarbital elixir. This information is the denominator of our fraction.

$$x \text{ mL} = \frac{5 \text{ mL}}{20 \text{ mg}}$$

c. Next, find the information that matches the measurement or abbreviation used in the denominator of the fraction you created. In this example *mg* is in the denominator and our order is for 45 mg. Therefore the full equation is

$$x \text{ mL} = \frac{5 \text{ mL}}{20 \text{ mg}} \times \frac{45 \text{ mg}}{1}$$

d. Now cancel out the like abbreviations on the right side of the equation. If you have set up the problem correctly, the remaining measurement or abbreviation should match that used on the left side of the equation. You are now ready to solve for x.

$$x \text{ mL} = \frac{5 \text{ mL}}{\underset{4}{\cancel{20} \ \cancel{\text{mg}}}} \times \frac{\overset{9}{\cancel{45} \ \cancel{\text{mg}}}}{1}$$

$$x = \frac{5 \times 9}{4 \times 1} = \frac{45}{4}$$

$$x = 11.25 \text{ mL}$$

The answer to the problem is 11.25 mL.

EXAMPLE 2: The physician orders Thorazine 20 mg po q 4 h. The drug is available in 120-mL bottles of Thorazine syrup containing 10 mg/5 mL. How many milliliters will the nurse administer? _____

  a. On the left side of the equation, place the name or abbreviation of the drug form of x, or what you are solving for.

$$x \text{ mL} =$$

  b. On the right side of the equation, place the available information related to the measurement or abbreviation that was placed on the left side. In this example that is mL. This information is placed in the equation as a common fraction; match the appropriate abbreviation or measurement. Thus the abbreviation that matches the x quantity must be placed in the numerator. We also know from the problem that each 5 mL contains 10 mg of Thorazine. This information is the denominator of our fraction.

$$x \text{ mL} = \frac{5 \text{ mL}}{10 \text{ mg}}$$

  c. Next, find the information that matches the measurement or abbreviation used in the denominator of the fraction you created. In this example mg is in the denominator and our order is for 20 mg. Therefore the full equation is

$$x \text{ mL} = \frac{5 \text{ mL}}{10 \text{ mg}} \times \frac{20 \text{ mg}}{1}$$

  d. Now cancel out the like abbreviation on the right side of the equation. If you have set up the problem correctly, the remaining measurement or abbreviation should match that used on the left side of the equation. You are now ready to solve for x.

$$x \text{ mL} = \frac{5 \text{ mL}}{\cancel{10} \text{ mg} \atop 1} \times \frac{\overset{2}{\cancel{20}} \text{ mg}}{1}$$

$$x = \frac{5 \times 2}{1} = \frac{10}{1}$$

$$x = 10 \text{ mL}$$

The answer to the problem is 10 mL.

Oral Dosages Involving Milliequivalents: Dimensional Analysis Method

EXAMPLE: The physician orders potassium chloride (KCl) 60 mEq three times a day with meals. KCl 40 mEq/30 mL is available. How many milliliters will the nurse administer? _____

A **milliequivalent** is the number of grams of a solute contained in 1 mL of a normal solution. The milliequivalent is used in a drug dosage proportion, the same as a form of measurement in the metric system.

  a. On the left side of the equation, place the name or abbreviation of the drug form of x, or what you are solving for.

$$x \text{ mL} =$$

  b. On the right side of the equation, place the available information related to the measurement or abbreviation that was placed on the left side. In this example that is mL. This information is placed in the equation as a common fraction; match the appropriate abbreviation or measurement. Thus the abbreviation that matches the x quantity must be placed in the numerator. We also know from the problem that each 30 mL contains 40 mEq of potassium chloride (KCI). This information is the denominator of our fraction.

$$x \text{ mL} = \frac{30 \text{ mL}}{40 \text{ mEq}}$$

c. Next, find the information that matches the measurement or abbreviation used in the denominator of the fraction you created. In this example *mEq* is in the denominator and our order is for 60 mEq. Therefore the full equation is

$$x \text{ mL} = \frac{30 \text{ mL}}{40 \text{ mEq}} \times \frac{60 \text{ mEq}}{1}$$

d. Now cancel out the like abbreviations on the right side of the equation. If you have set up the problem correctly, the remaining measurement or abbreviation should match that used on the left side of the equation. You are now ready to solve for x.

$$x \text{ mL} = \frac{30 \text{ mL}}{\overset{}{\underset{2}{40} \text{ mEq}}} \times \frac{\overset{3}{60} \text{ mEq}}{1}$$

$$x = \frac{30 \times 3}{2 \times 1} = \frac{90}{2}$$

$$x = 45 \text{ mL}$$

The answer to the problem is 45 mL.

Oral Dosages Involving Capsules and Tablets: Proportion Method

Sometimes the physician's order is in one strength of measurement, and the drug is supplied in another strength of measurement. It is therefore necessary to convert one of the measurements so that they are both in the same strength of measurement. After this is done, another proportion will be written to calculate the actual drug dosage.

EXAMPLE 1: The physician orders ampicillin 0.5 g po four times a day. The drug is supplied in 250-mg capsules. How many capsules will the nurse administer? _____

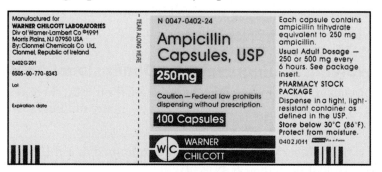

The physician's order is in grams and the drug is supplied in milligrams. The order and the supplied drug must be in the same strength of measurement because only two different abbreviations can be used in each proportion. Therefore first convert 0.5 g to milligrams.

$$1000 \text{ mg} : 1 \text{ g} :: x \text{ mg} : 0.5 \text{ g}$$

$$1000 : 1 :: x : 0.5$$

$$1x = 1000 \times 0.5$$

$$x = 500 \text{ mg}$$

$$0.5 \text{ g} = 500 \text{ mg}$$

Now that the order and the supplied drug are in the same strength of measurement, a proportion may be written to calculate the amount of the drug to be given.

    a. 250 mg : 1 capsule ::

    b. 250 mg : 1 capsule :: _____ mg : _____ capsule

    250 mg : 1 capsule :: 500 mg : x capsule

    c. 250 : 1 :: 500 : x

    d. $250x = 1 \times 500$

$$250x = 500$$

$$x = \frac{500}{250}$$

$$x = 2$$

    e. x = 2 capsules. Therefore to give 0.5 g of the medication, the nurse will administer 2 capsules.

How many capsules will be given in 1 day? _____

The drug is to be given four times a day.

    a. 2 capsules : 1 dose ::

    b. 2 capsules : 1 dose :: _____ capsules : _____ dose

    2 capsules : 1 dose :: x capsules : 4 doses

    c. 2 : 1 :: x : 4

    d. $1x = 2 \times 4$

      $x = 8$

    e. 8 capsules will be given each day.

EXAMPLE 2: The physician orders aspirin 975 mg po four times a day. Aspirin 325-mg tablets are available. How many tablets will the nurse administer? _____

    a. On the left side of the proportion place what you know or have available. In this example, each tablet contains 325 mg. So the left side of the proportion is

1 tablet : 325 mg ::

    b. The right side of the proportion is determined by the physician's order and the abbreviations used on the left side of the proportion. Only *two* different abbreviations may be used in a single proportion. The abbreviations must be in the same position on the right as they are on the left.

1 tablet : 325 mg :: _____ tablet : _____ mg

In the example, the physician has ordered 975 mg.

1 tablet : 325 mg :: _____ tablet : 975 mg

We need to find the number of tablets to be given, so we use the symbol x to represent the unknown. Therefore the full proportion is

1 tablet : 325 mg :: x tablet : 975 mg

c. Rewrite the proportion without using the abbreviations.

1 : 325 :: x : 975

d. Solve for x.

$$325x = 1 \times 975$$

$$325x = 975$$

$$x = \frac{975}{325}$$

$$x = 3$$

e. Label your answer as determined by the abbreviation placed next to x in the original proportion.

975 mg = 3 tablets

Oral Dosages Involving Liquids: Proportion Method

EXAMPLE 1: The physician orders phenobarbital 45 mg po two times a day. Phenobarbital elixir, 20 mg/5 mL, is available. How many milliliters will the nurse administer? _____

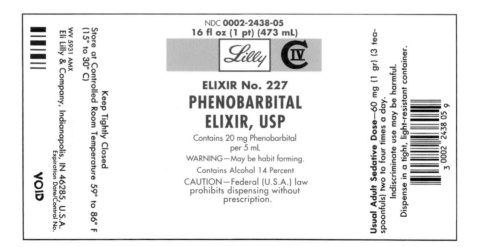

A proportion can be written to calculate the actual amount of the drug to be administered.

a. 20 mg : 5 mL ::

b. 20 mg : 5 mL :: _____ mg : _____ mL
20 mg : 5 mL :: 45 mg : x mL

c. 20 : 5 :: 45 : x

d. $20x = 5 \times 45$

$$20x = 225$$

$$x = \frac{225}{20}$$

$$x = 11.25$$

e. $x = 11.25$ mL. Therefore 11.25 mL is the amount of each individual dose twice a day.

EXAMPLE 2: The physician orders Thorazine 20 mg po q 4 h. The drug is available in 120-mL bottles of Thorazine syrup containing 10 mg/5 mL. How many milliliters will the nurse administer? _____ How many doses are available in 120 mL? _____

1. **a.** 10 mg : 5 mL ::
   b. 10 mg : 5 mL :: _____ mg : _____ mL
      10 mg : 5 mL :: 20 mg : x mL
   c. 10 : 5 :: 20 : x
   d. $10x = 5 \times 20$

   $10x = 100$

   $$x = \frac{100}{10}$$

   $x = 10$

   e. $x = 10$ mL. Therefore 10 mL is the amount of each individual dose q 4 h.

A proportion can be written to calculate the number of doses in a 120-mL bottle.

   a. 10 mL : 1 dose ::
   b. 10 mL : 1 dose :: _____ mL : _____ dose
      10 mL : 1 dose :: 120 mL : x dose
   c. 10 : 1 :: 120 : x
   d. $10x = 120$

   $$x = \frac{120}{10}$$

   $x = 12$

   e. $x = 12$ doses. Therefore each 120-mL bottle contains 12 doses.

Oral Dosages Involving Milliequivalents: Proportion Method

EXAMPLE: The physician orders potassium chloride (KCl) 60 mEq three times a day with meals. KCl 40 mEq/30 mL is available. How many milliliters will the nurse administer? _____

A **milliequivalent** is the number of grams of a solute contained in 1 mL of a normal solution. The milliequivalent is used in a drug dosage proportion, the same as a form of measurement in the apothecary or metric system.

   a. 40 mEq : 30 mL ::
   b. 40 mEq : 30 mL :: _____ mEq : _____ mL
      40 mEq : 30 mL :: 60 mEq : x mL
   c. 40 : 30 :: 60 : x
   d. $40x = 30 \times 60$

   $40x = 1800$

   $$x = \frac{1800}{40}$$

   $x = 45$

   e. $x = 45$ mL. Therefore to give 60 mEq of the medication, the nurse will administer 45 mL.

Alternative Formula Method of Oral Drug Dosage Calculation

A formula has been used for many years in the calculation of drug dosages by nurses. The formula method may be the method that some students learned first in an earlier nursing role (e.g., for a nurse who was a licensed practical nurse or who is returning to work in the area of direct patient care). If this is the case and the student accurately uses the formula method, we do not recommend changing to dimensional analysis or the proportion method. Remember, choose the method that you feel is best for you and consistently use the chosen method. We do not recommend switching back and forth between the formula method and the proportion method. When you use the formula method, the *desired and available amounts must be in the same units of measurement.*

$$\text{Formula:} \quad \frac{D}{A} \times Q = x$$

D represents the **desired** amount of the medication that has been ordered by the physician.

A represents the strength of the medication that is **available.**

Q represents the **quantity** or amount of the medication that contains the available strength.

> **! ALERT**
>
> When the medication is a solid such as a tablet, capsule, or caplet, the quantity will always be 1. If the medication is in liquid form, the number will vary. Remember from the math review, the denominator of a whole number is always one: $\frac{1}{1}$, $\frac{2}{1}$, $\frac{3}{1}$, etc.

x represents the dose that is unknown.

This formula can be read as:

Desired over (or divided by) available multiplied by the quantity available equals *x*, or the amount to be given to the patient.

Oral Dosages Involving Capsules and Tablets: Alternative Formula

If the physician's order is in one strength of measurement and the drug is supplied in another strength of measurement, it will still be necessary to convert one of the measurements so that both are expressed in the same system. After this is done, the formula may be used to calculate the drug dose to be administered.

EXAMPLE 1: The physician orders ampicillin 0.5 g po four times a day. The drug is supplied in 250-mg capsules. How many capsules will the nurse administer? _____

The physician's order is expressed in grams and the drug is supplied in milligrams. Therefore convert the order to milligrams as outlined in Chapter 6.

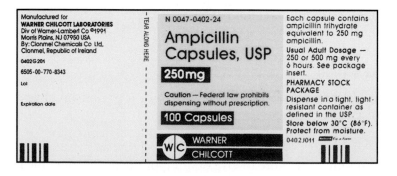

$$1000 \text{ mg} : 1 \text{ g} :: x \text{ mg} : 0.5 \text{ g}$$
$$1000 : 1 :: x : 0.5$$
$$x = 1000 \times 0.5$$
$$x = 500 \text{ mg}$$

Now the numbers may be filled into the formula $\dfrac{D}{A} \times Q = x$

a. The desired amount of ampicillin is 500 mg. The available amount or strength of ampicillin supplied is 250 mg.

$$\frac{500}{250}$$

b. The quantity available is in capsule form, or 1.

$$\frac{500 \text{ mg}}{250 \text{ mg}} = \frac{1}{1}$$

c. Rewrite the problem with the abbreviations canceled.

$$\frac{500 \cancel{\text{ mg}}}{250 \cancel{\text{ mg}}} = \frac{1}{1}$$

d. Solve for x.

$$x = \frac{500 \times 1}{250 \times 1}$$

$$x = \frac{500}{250}$$

$$x = 2$$

e. Label your answer as determined by the quantity.

$$500 \text{ mg} = 2 \text{ capsules}$$

EXAMPLE 2: The physician orders aspirin 975 mg po four times a day. Aspirin is available in 325-mg tablets. How many tablets will the nurse administer? _____

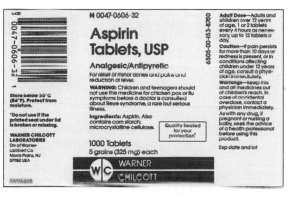

$$\frac{D}{A} \times Q = x$$

a. The desired amount of aspirin is 975 mg. The available amount or strength of the aspirin supplied is 325 mg.

$$\frac{975 \text{ mg}}{325 \text{ mg}}$$

b. The quantity of the medication for 325 mg is 1 tablet.

$$\frac{975 \text{ mg}}{325 \text{ mg}} = \frac{1}{1}$$

c. Rewrite the problem with the abbreviations canceled.

$$\frac{975 \cancel{\text{ mg}}}{325 \cancel{\text{ mg}}} = \frac{1}{1}$$

d. Solve for x.

$$x = \frac{975}{325} \times \frac{1}{1}$$

$$x = \frac{975 \times 1}{325 \times 1}$$

$$x = \frac{975}{325}$$

$$x = 3$$

e. Label your answer as determined by the quantity.

$$975 \text{ mg} = 3 \text{ tablets}$$

Oral Dosages Involving Liquids: Alternative Formula

EXAMPLE: The physician orders phenobarbital 45 mg po two times a day. Phenobarbital elixir, 20 mg/5 mL, is available. How many milliliters will the nurse administer? _____

The numbers may be filled into the formula $\dfrac{D}{A} \times Q = x$.

a. The desired amount is 45 mg. The available amount or strength of phenobarbital is 20 mg.

$$\frac{45 \text{ mg}}{20 \text{ mg}}$$

b. The quantity available is 5 mL.

$$\frac{45 \text{ mg}}{20 \text{ mg}} \times \frac{5 \text{ mL}}{1 \text{ mL}}$$

c. Rewrite the problem with the abbreviations canceled.

$$\frac{45 \cancel{\text{mg}}}{20 \cancel{\text{mg}}} \times \frac{5 \cancel{\text{mL}}}{1 \cancel{\text{mL}}}$$

d. Solve for x.

$$x = \frac{45}{20} \times \frac{5}{1}$$

$$x = \frac{45}{\underset{4}{\cancel{20}}} \times \frac{\overset{1}{\cancel{5}}}{1}$$

$$x = \frac{45 \times 1}{4 \times 1}$$

$$x = \frac{45}{4}$$

$$x = 11.25$$

e. Label your answer as determined by the quantity.

$$45 \text{ mg} = 11.25 \text{ mL}$$

Complete the following work sheet, which provides for extensive practice in the calculation of oral dosage problems. Check your answers. It is sometimes impossible to administer the exact amount ordered. All capsules and tablets that are not scored are impossible to divide accurately. If you have difficulties, go back and review the necessary material. When you feel ready to evaluate your learning, take the first posttest. Check your answers. An acceptable score as indicated on the posttest signifies that you are ready for the next chapter. An unacceptable score signifies a need for further study before taking the second posttest.

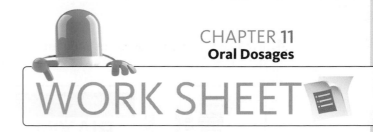

WORK SHEET

DIRECTIONS: The medication order is listed at the beginning of each problem. Calculate the oral doses. Show your work. Shade each medicine cup or oral syringe when provided to indicate the correct dose.

1. The physician orders Minipress 2 mg po two times a day for Mr. Shaw's high blood pressure. How many capsules will the nurse administer per dose? _____

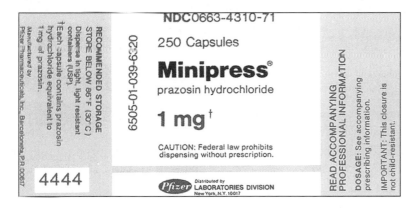

2. Mrs. Taylor has a long history of seizures. Elixir of phenobarbital 30 mg po q 12 h is ordered. How many milliliters will the nurse administer per dose? _____

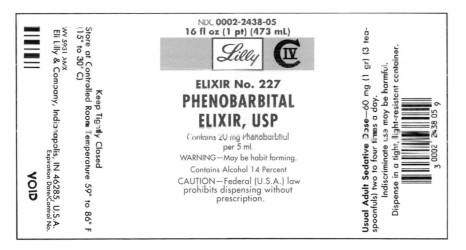

3. The physician orders Crystodigin 0.2 mg po two times a day for 4 days, then 0.15 mg po two times a day. You have Crystodigin 0.05-mg tablets available. How many tablets will you give for each dose the first 4 days? _____ How many tablets will you give for each dose thereafter? _____

4. Mr. Davis has a diagnosis of acute maxillary sinusitis. His physician orders Biaxin 500 mg q 12 h × 10 days. How many tablets will the nurse administer per dose? _____

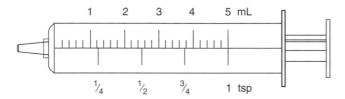

5. Mrs. Rios complains of nausea. Compazine 2.5 mg po three times a day is ordered. The stock supply is Compazine syrup 5 mg/5 mL. How many milliliters will the nurse administer per dose? _____

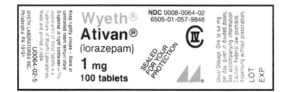

6. The physician orders Ativan 2 mg at bedtime. How many tablets will the nurse administer per dose? _____

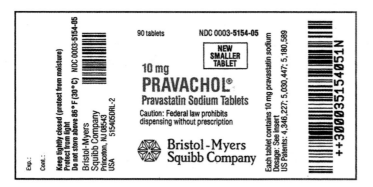

7. The physician orders Pravachol 20 mg po at bedtime. How many tablets will the nurse administer per dose? _____

8. Mandelamine 1 g po four times a day is scheduled for Mr. Eaton to treat his urinary tract infection. You have 0.5-g tablets available. How many tablets will you administer per dose? _____

9. The physician orders Prozac 40 mg po daily in AM. How many milliliters will the nurse administer per dose? _____

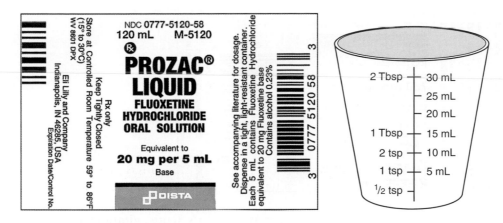

10. Mr. Chang has Parkinson's disease and is to receive Cogentin 1 mg po at 1900. How many tablets will the nurse administer per dose? _____

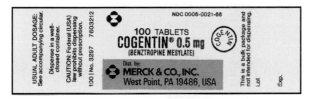

11. Mrs. Martin receives Motrin 800 mg po three times a day for arthritis pain. The drug is supplied in 400-mg tablets. How many tablets will the nurse administer per dose? _____

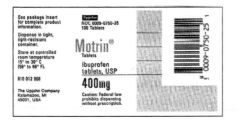

12. The physician orders lithium carbonate 0.6 g po two times a day. The drug is supplied in 300-mg scored tablets. How many tablets will the nurse administer per dose? _____ How many milligrams will be given each day? _____

13. Your patient is taking minoxidil 30 mg daily for hypertension. How many tablets will you administer per dose? _____

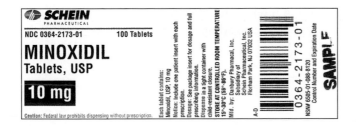

14. Mr. Hill is to receive Cipro 0.75 g q 12 h for a knee infection. How many tablets will the nurse administer per dose? _____

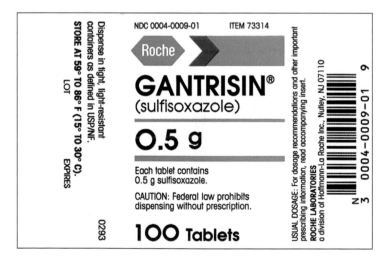

15. The physician orders Geodon 80 mg bid to treat Mrs. Basey's acute agitation. You have 40-mg capsules available. How many capsules will you administer per dose? _____

16. The physician orders Gantrisin 4 g po STAT, then 2 g q 6 h. How many tablets will be given for the STAT dose? _____ How many tablets will be given for each of the 2-g doses? _____

17. The physician orders acyclovir 800 mg po q 4 h while the patient is awake. Acyclovir 400-mg tablets are available. How many tablets will the nurse administer per dose? _____

18. The physician orders Gaviscon 30 mL po four times a day. Gaviscon is supplied in 360-mL bottles. How many mLs will be given in 1 day? _____

19. Ms. Vega complains of a rash on her abdomen, and the physician orders Benadryl 30 mg po three times a day. How many milliliters will the nurse administer per dose? _____

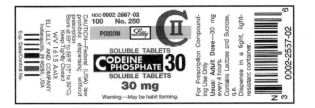

20. Mr. Gifford has had a lumbar laminectomy and requires pain medication. The patient has an order for codeine 60 mg po q 3 h prn. How many tablets will the nurse administer per dose? _____

21. The physician orders Amoxil suspension 5.5 mL (125 mg/5 mL strength) po q 6 h for your patient who had a tonsillectomy. How many milligrams will you administer every 6 hours? _____

22. Mr. Sawyer is admitted with congestive heart failure. His orders require Lasix 80 mg po daily. How many tablets will the nurse administer per dose? _____

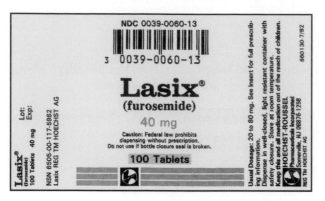

23. The physician orders nitroglycerin 0.4 mg sublingual prn for angina. The patient should take no more than three tablets in 15 minutes. Mr. Cane took two tablets 5 minutes apart. How many milligrams did he receive? _____

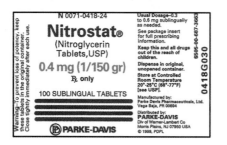

24. Mr. Koehler has rheumatoid arthritis and has Decadron 1.5 mg po q 12 h ordered. You have Decadron elixir 0.5 mg/5 mL. How many milliliters will you administer per dose? _____ How many ounces will you administer per dose? _____

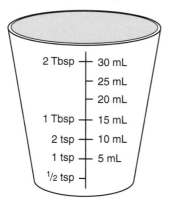

25. Your adult patient has acute bronchitis and has cefaclor 500 mg po q 12 h ordered. How many milliliters will you administer per dose? _____

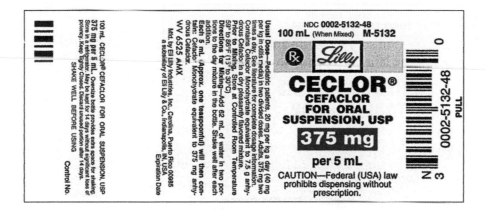

26. Mrs. Turner is admitted with hypertension. Apresoline 25 mg po four times a day is ordered. You have 50-mg scored tablets available. How many tablets will you administer per dose? _____

27. Your patient complains of indigestion during meals. Mylanta 30 mL po pc four times a day is ordered. Mylanta is supplied in a 360-mL bottle. There are _____ doses in one 360-mL bottle.

28. The physician orders Halcion 0.25 mg po at bedtime. How many tablets will the nurse administer per dose? _____

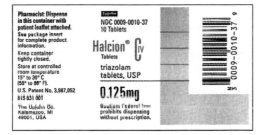

29. Mr. Bates has a history of seizure activity. Phenobarbital 15 mg po q 3 h is ordered. How many tablets will the nurse administer per dose? _____

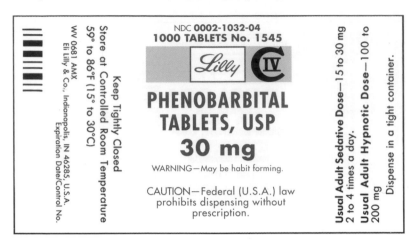

30. Mrs. Ortega has chronic sinusitis. Her physician orders amoxicillin 125 mg po q 8 h. How many milliliters will the nurse administer per dose? _____

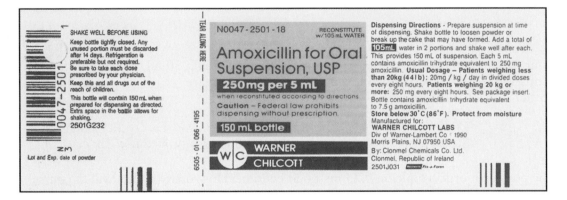

31. The physician prescribes Tenormin 25 mg po q 4 h for Mr. Hutton's high blood pressure. You have Tenormin 50-mg scored tablets available. How many tablets will you administer per dose? _____

32. The physician orders quinidine 0.6 g po q 4 h. Quinidine is supplied in 200-mg tablets. How many tablets will you give for one dose? _____ How many tablets will you give in 24 hours? _____

33. Mrs. Farmer has Phenergan 12.5 mg po three times a day ordered for relief of nausea. The drug is available in syrup containing 6.25 mg/5 mL. How many milliliters will the nurse administer per dose? _____

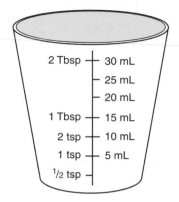

34. Your patient has Cipro 750 mg po q 12 h ordered for a severe respiratory tract infection. You have Cipro oral suspension 500 mg/5 mL available. How many milliliters will you administer per dose? _____

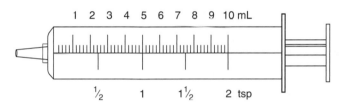

35. Mr. Golden, recovering from a left great toe amputation, has Colace elixir 100 mg po at bedtime ordered for constipation. How many milliliters will the nurse administer per dose? _____

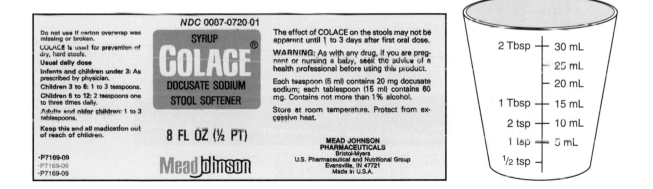

36. Mr. Malito is to receive Procanbid 1 g po now. How many tablets will you administer per dose? _____

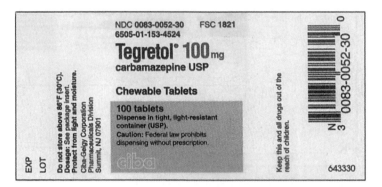

37. Mr. Mikal was admitted for treatment of leukemia and receives Deltasone 7.5 mg po three times a day as part of his chemotherapy. The drug is available in 2.5-mg tablets. How many tablets will the nurse administer per dose? _____

38. The physician orders Tegretol 0.2 g po three times a day for Mr. Pine's epilepsy. How many tablets will the nurse administer per dose? _____

39. Lortab 5/500 po now is ordered for Mrs. Lindl for pain. How many tablets will she receive per dose? _____ How much acetaminophen is in each tablet? _____

40. Mrs. Cross was admitted with a myasthenia crisis. Decadron 0.5 mg po q 12 h is ordered. How many tablets will the nurse administer per dose? _____

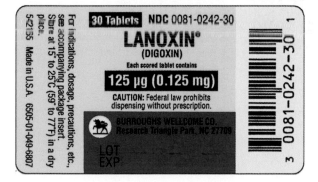

41. Mr. Cook requires medication for nausea. Compazine 10 mg po q 4 h prn is ordered. You have Compazine 5-mg tablets available. How many tablets will you administer per dose? _____

42. Mr. Pace receives Atarax 100 mg po at bedtime prn to relieve anxiety. You have 50-mg tablets available. How many tablets will you administer per dose? _____

43. The physician orders Rifadin 600 mg po 1 hour before dinner daily. How many capsules will the nurse administer per dose? _____

NDC 0068-0508-30

300 mg   MARION MERRELL DOW INC.

RIFADIN®
(rifampin capsules)

300 mg

30 Capsules

Each capsule contains: rifampin.............................300 mg
Usual Dose: See accompanying product information.
CAUTION: Federal law prohibits dispensing without prescription.
Keep tightly closed. Store in a dry place. Avoid excessive heat.
Dispense in tight, light-resistant container with child-resistant closure.

© 1993 Marion Merrell Dow Inc.

Merrell Dow Pharmaceuticals Inc.
Subsidiary of Marion Merrell Dow Inc.
Kansas City, MO 64114   H 3 6 4 C

44. Mr. Day receives Lanoxin 0.25 mg po daily for atrial fibrillation. How many tablets will the nurse administer per dose? _____

30 Tablets NDC 0081-0242-30

LANOXIN®
(DIGOXIN)

Each scored tablet contains

125 μg (0.125 mg)

CAUTION: Federal law prohibits dispensing without prescription.

BURROUGHS WELLCOME CO.
Research Triangle Park, NC 27709

45. Mr. Payne receives Keflex 500 mg po four times a day before his dental extraction. How many capsules will the nurse administer in each dose? _____ How many capsules will the nurse administer for 1 day? _____

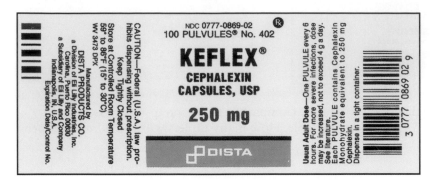

46. Mr. Tune is experiencing gastroesophageal reflux. The physician orders Nexium 40 mg po daily for 3 days. How many capsules will the nurse administer per dose? _____

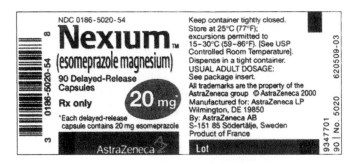

47. Mrs. Graves receives phenobarbital tablets 90 mg po q 3 h prn for seizure activity. How many tablets will the nurse administer per dose? _____

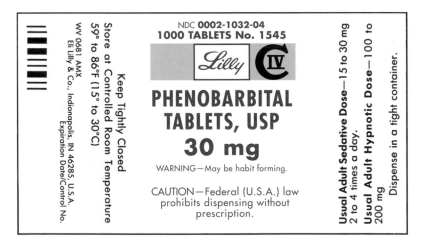

48. Mr. Vee is enrolled in a smoking-cessation program. He is to begin with Wellbutrin 150 mg po daily for 3 days. How many tablets will the nurse administer per dose? _____

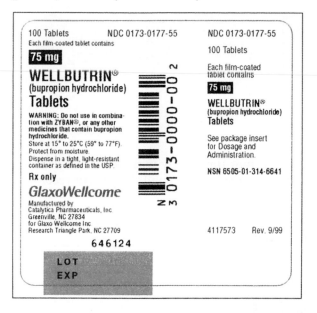

49. Mr. Sahl, recovering from a coronary artery bypass graft, receives aspirin 650 mg po twice a day. How many tablets will the nurse administer per dose? _____

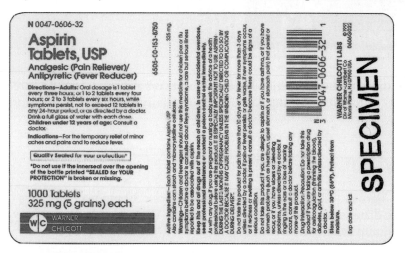

50. Mr. Dale receives Zantac 150 mg two times a day as part of his treatment for esophagitis. How many milliliters will the nurse administer per dose? _____

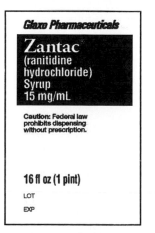

51. Mrs. Line has erythromycin 500 mg po q 6 h prescribed for treatment of her strep throat. How many tablets will you administer per dose? _____

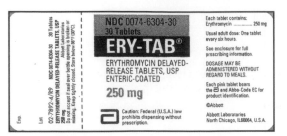

52. The physician has prescribed Cytotec 0.2 mg po four times daily with meals and at bedtime for a patient with a history of gastric ulcers. How many tablets will the patient receive for each dose? _____

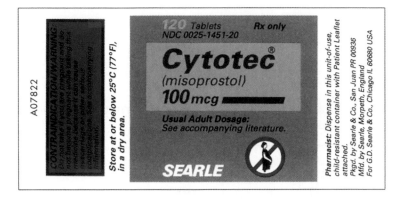

53. Mr. Romero, admitted with chronic obstructive lung disease, takes Bentyl 20 mg po three times a day ac. The drug is available in 10-mg capsules. How many capsules will the nurse administer per dose? _____

54. Mrs. Tyth has pruritic dermatosis. The physician prescribes Atarax 30 mg po two times daily as part of her therapy. The drug is supplied in syrup containing 10 mg/5 mL. How many milliliters will the nurse administer per dose? _____

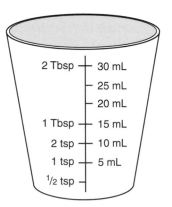

55. Mrs. Gale, admitted for alcohol abuse, has an order for ascorbic acid 0.75 g po daily while hospitalized. You have 250-mg tablets available. How many tablets will you administer per dose? _____

56. Your patient who is receiving chemotherapy has an order for Zofran 8 mg po ½ hour before chemotherapy for relief of nausea. The drug is supplied in 4-mg tablets. How many tablets will the nurse administer per dose? _____

57. Mr. Nade, hospitalized for a radical neck dissection, has Vistaril 15 mg po four times a day ordered to suppress nausea. You have Vistaril 25 mg/5 mL available. How many milliliters will you administer per dose? _____

58. Mrs. Snell requires Lopressor 100 mg po two times daily. How many tablets will the nurse administer per dose? _____

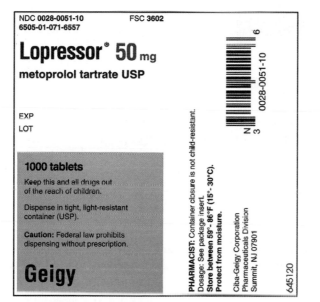

59. Your patient with type 2 adult-onset diabetes mellitus receives metformin hydrochloride 1 g po twice daily. How many tablets will the nurse administer per dose? _____

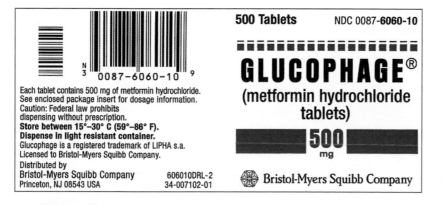

60. Mr. Aden requires Chloromycetin 250 mg po q 6 h for treatment of a *Salmonella* infection. You have Chloromycetin 150 mg/5 mL available. How many milliliters will you administer per dose? _____

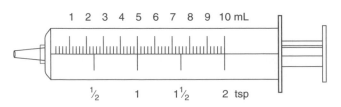

61. Mr. Scheottle receives Vibramycin 100 mg po q 12 h for treatment of inclusion conjunctivitis. How many milliliters will the nurse administer per dose? _____

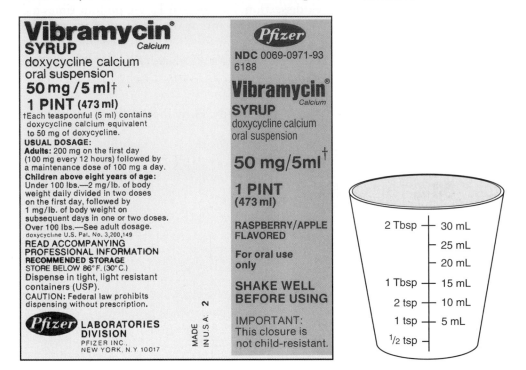

62. Your patient, admitted for cardiac catheterization, receives HydroDIURIL 25 mg po two times a day for hypertension. You have 50-mg scored tablets available. How many tablets will you administer per dose? _____

63. Tylenol 240 mg po q 4 h is ordered for a temperature of 38.9° C. You have Tylenol 80-mg chewable tablets available. How many tablets will be required for each dose? _____

64. The physician prescribes Lanoxin elixir 90 mcg po two times a day for your patient with atrial fibrillation. How many milliliters will you administer per dose? _____

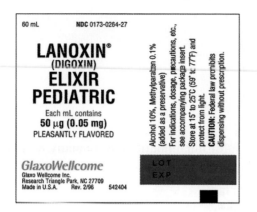

65. Mr. Ceney, admitted for contact dermatitis, receives elixir of Benadryl 10 mL po q 6 h prn for relief of itching. The drug is supplied as 12.5 mg/5 mL. This dose delivers _____ mg.

66. The physician orders Indocin 50 mg po twice a day. How many capsules will the nurse administer per dose? _____

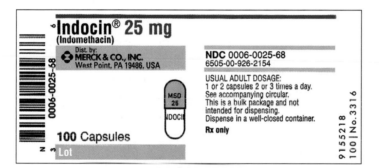

67. Your patient receives Dilantin 90 mg po three times a day for past seizure activity. How many capsules will you administer per dose? _____

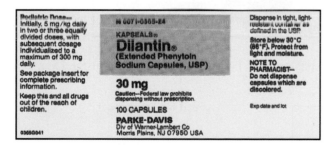

68. The physician orders Lipitor 40 mg po daily. You have available 10-mg, 20-mg, and 40-mg tablets. Which tablet would be most appropriate? _____ How many tablets will you administer per dose? _____

69. Your patient, admitted with a small-bowel obstruction, has KCl 10 mEq po daily ordered for his low potassium level. The drug is available as a liquid in KCl 20 mEq/15 mL. How many milliliters will you administer per dose? _____

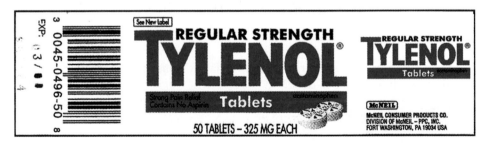

70. Mr. Brown receives dexamethasone 1.5 mg po q 12 h for inflammation. How many tablets will the nurse administer per dose? _____

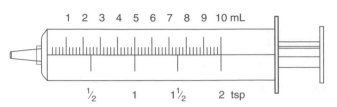

71. Mrs. Roget has been receiving digoxin 0.5 mg po daily for her cardiac dysrhythmia. The drug is available in 0.25-mg tablets. How many tablets will the nurse administer per dose? _____

72. Acetaminophen 650 mg po q 4 h is prescribed for a temperature of more than 38.5° C × 24 h. How many tablets will the nurse administer every 4 hours? _____

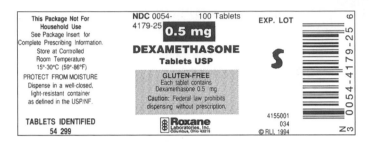

73. The physician prescribes Decadron 0.5 mg po q 12 h for your patient's keratitis. How many tablets will you administer per dose? _____

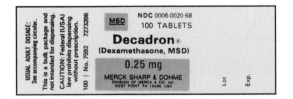

74. The physician orders Keflex 375 mg po q 6 h for Mr. Pein after his thyroidectomy. How many milliliters will the nurse administer per dose? _____

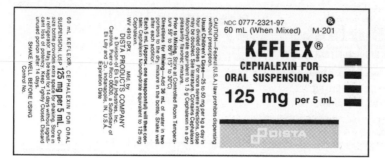

75. Mrs. Fare receives codeine 30 mg po q 3 h prn for pain relief after knee replacement surgery. How many tablets will you administer? _____

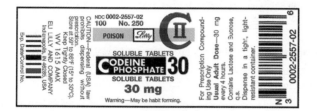

76. The physician orders Crystodigin 0.3 mg po daily. You have Crystodigin in 0.05-mg, 0.15-mg, and 0.2-mg tablets. The best way to administer this drug is to give _____ tablets of _____ mg each.

77. Mr. Zeman has prednisone 7.5 mg po daily ordered for exfoliative dermatitis. Prednisone is supplied in 5-mg scored tablets. How many tablets will the nurse administer per dose? _____

78. Your patient who has had a partial craniotomy has Ceclor suspension 250 mg po four times a day ordered. How many milliliters will you administer per dose? _____

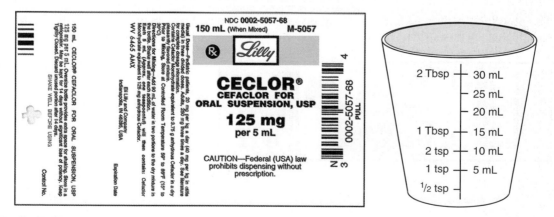

79. Your patient, who has undergone a coronary artery bypass graft, receives Surfak 250 mg po daily as a stool softener. How many capsules will you administer per dose? _____

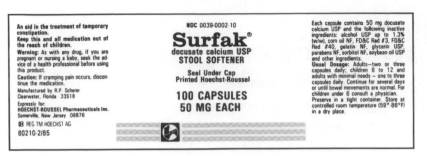

80. The physician orders 20 mEq KCl elixir po three times a day. Elixir of KCl 15 mEq/11.25 mL is available. How many milliliters will you administer per dose? _____

81. Your patient with epilepsy receives phenobarbital 55 mg po two times a day. How many milliliters will you administer per dose? _____

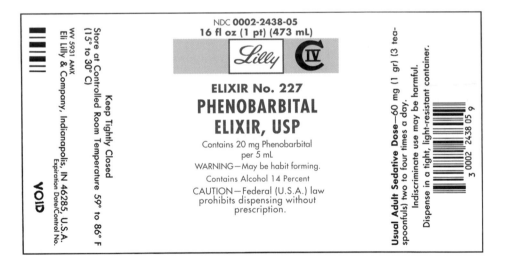

82. The physician orders Aldomet 250 mg po two times a day. How many tablets will the nurse administer per dose? _____

83. Mrs. Richardson, a patient who had a thyroidectomy, receives Synthroid 0.05 mg po daily in the morning. How many tablets will the nurse administer per dose? _____

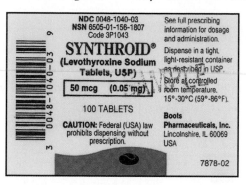

84. The physician orders Theo-Dur 0.2 g po q 8 h. Theo-Dur is supplied in 100-mg, 200-mg, and 300-mg sustained-action tablets. Give _____ tablets of _____ mg. How many milligrams will be given per day? _____

85. Your patient who had a valve repair begins receiving Coumadin 15 mg po STAT. Coumadin 5-mg scored tablets are available. How many tablets will you administer per dose? _____

86. Your patient, who has an ulcer, receives cimetidine 800 mg po at bedtime. How many tablets will you administer each night? _____

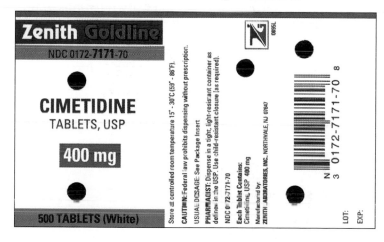

87. Your patient receives Keflex 0.5 g po four times a day. You have Keflex 250-mg capsules available. How many capsules will you administer? _____

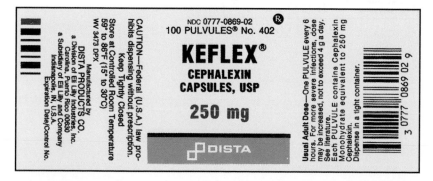

88. The physician orders imipramine 50 mg po once in the morning and once at bedtime. The drug is supplied in 25-mg tablets. How many tablets will the nurse administer per dose? _____

89. Your patient with depression receives Prozac 30 mg po twice a day. How many pills will you administer per dose? _____

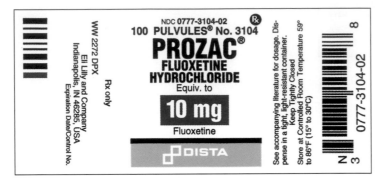

90. A patient receives Lasix 6 mg po twice a day with meals. Lasix is available in an oral solution of 10 mg/mL. How many milliliters will be given per dose? _____

91. Mrs. Adams receives Cleocin 150 mg po q 6 h for her upper respiratory tract infection. Cleocin is supplied in 75-mg capsules. How many capsules will the nurse administer per dose? _____

92. Your patient receives Dilantin 200 mg po three times a day for seizures. How many capsules will you administer per dose? _____

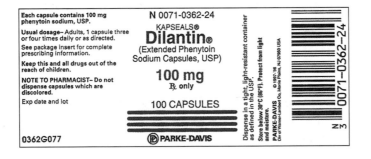

93. The physician orders Coumadin 10 mg po at 1800 today. How many tablets will the nurse administer per dose? _____

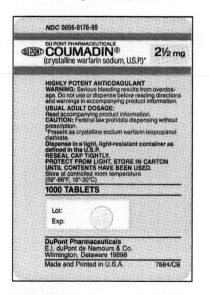

94. Your patient with diabetes receives Diabinese 0.25 g po daily in the morning. How many tablets will you administer per dose? _____

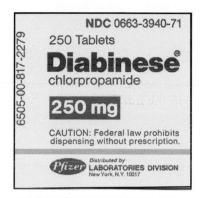

95. The physician prescribes Apresoline 25 mg po two times a day for Mr. Yu's hypertension. You have Apresoline scored tablets 10 mg available. How many tablets will you administer per dose? _____

96. The physician orders Flexeril 30 mg po at bedtime. Flexeril 10-mg tablets are available. How many tablets will the nurse administer per dose? _____

97. Your patient has begun receiving prednisone 15 mg po daily for asthma. Prednisone is available in 5-mg tablets. How many tablets will you administer per dose? _____

98. Mr. Gray, who has undergone cervical diskectomy, receives Restoril 0.015 g po at bedtime for insomnia. How many capsules will the nurse administer per dose? _____

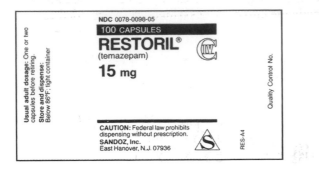

99. A patient receives KCl elixir 30 mEq po three times a day with juice. KCl 6.7 mEq/5 mL is available. How many milliliters will the nurse administer per dose? _____

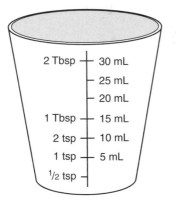

100. Mrs. Endres receives furosemide 20 mg po q 8 h for congestive heart failure. How many tablets will the nurse administer per dose? _____

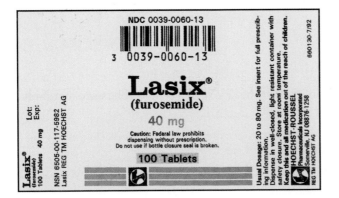

ANSWERS ON PP. 238–242 AND 244–260.

NAME _____

DATE _____

ACCEPTABLE SCORE __24__

YOUR SCORE _____

_hw ✓ 6/13_

POSTTEST 1

DIRECTIONS: The medication order is listed at the beginning of each problem. Calculate the oral doses. Show your work. Shade each medicine cup or oral syringe when provided to indicate the correct dose.

1. The physician orders aspirin 975 mg po four times a day for a patient who had a mitral valve repair. How many tablets will the nurse administer per dose? __3 tablets__

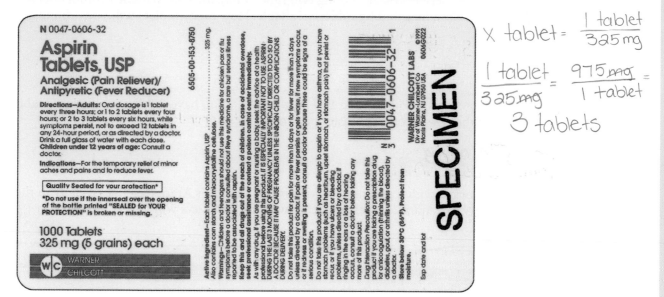

$$X \text{ tablet} = \frac{1 \text{ tablet}}{325 \text{ mg}}$$

$$\frac{1 \text{ tablet}}{325 \text{ mg}} = \frac{975 \text{ mg}}{1 \text{ tablet}} =$$

3 tablets

2. Mr. Clay receives tetracycline 0.5 g po four times a day for a gastrointestinal infection. How many capsules will the nurse administer per dose? __1 capsules__

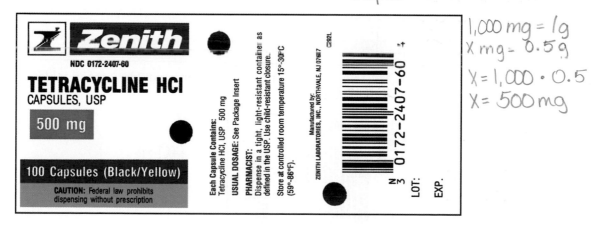

1,000 mg = 1 g
X mg = 0.5 g
X = 1,000 • 0.5
X = 500 mg

3. The physician orders ampicillin 1 g po q 6 h for treatment of shigellosis. How many capsules will the nurse administer per dose? ___4 capsules___

Handwritten:
$$1{,}000\ mg = 1g$$
$$X\ mg = 1g$$
$$X = 1{,}000 \cdot 1$$
$$X = \frac{1{,}000\ mg}{250\ mg} = 4\ capsules$$

Medication label:

Manufactured for
WARNER CHILCOTT LABORATORIES
Div of Warner-Lambert Co ©1991
Morris Plains, NJ 07950 USA
By: Clonmel Chemicals Co Ltd.
Clonmel, Republic of Ireland
0402G201
6505-00-770-8343
Lot
Expiration date

— TEAR ALONG HERE —

N 0047-0402-24

Ampicillin Capsules, USP

250mg

Caution — Federal law prohibits dispensing without prescription.

100 Capsules

WC WARNER CHILCOTT

Each capsule contains ampicillin trihydrate equivalent to 250 mg ampicillin.
Usual Adult Dosage — 250 or 500 mg every 6 hours. See package insert.
PHARMACY STOCK PACKAGE
Dispense in a tight, light-resistant container as defined in the USP.
Store below 30°C (86°F). Protect from moisture.
0402J011

4. The physician prescribes Allegra 60 mg two times a day for your patient's complaints of allergic rhinitis. You have 0.03-g tablets available. How many tablets will you administer per dose? ___2 tablets___

Handwritten:
$$1000\ mg = 1g$$
$$X\ mg = 0.03g$$
$$1000 \cdot 0.03 = 30 \cdot 2 = 60$$

5. The physician orders levothyroxine 100 mcg po daily. You have 0.05-mg tablets available. How many tablets will you administer per dose? ___2 tablets___

Handwritten:
$$1{,}000\ mcg = 1mg$$
$$X\ mcg = 0.05\ mg$$
$$1{,}000 \cdot 0.05 = 50 \cdot 2 = 100\ mcg$$

6. Mr. Shen, admitted with a psychoneurotic disorder, receives Atarax 25 mg po daily in the morning. You have Atarax 10 mg/5 mL. How many milliliters will you administer per dose? ___12.5 mL___

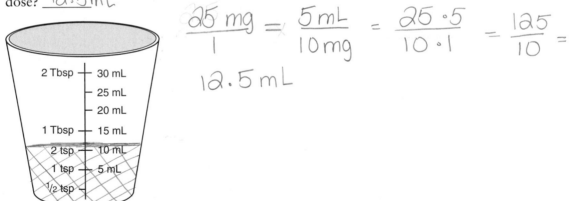

Handwritten:
$$\frac{25\ mg}{1} = \frac{5\ mL}{10\ mg} = \frac{25 \cdot 5}{10 \cdot 1} = \frac{125}{10} =$$
$$12.5\ mL$$

7. Your cardiac patient has Cardizem 60 mg four times a day ordered. How many tablets will you administer per dose? ___2 tablets___

Handwritten:
$$\frac{120\ mg}{60\ mg} = 2\ tablets$$

Medication label:

NDC 0088-1792-47   6505-01-259-2914

120 mg **Hoechst Marion Roussel**

CARDIZEM®
(diltiazem HCl)

120 mg

100 Tablets

Each tablet contains: diltiazem hydrochloride... (equivalent to 110.3 mg as diltiazem). Dosage and Administration: Read package insert for prescribing information. Warning: Federal law prohibits dispensing without prescription. Pharmacist: Dispense in tight, light-resistant container as defined in USP. Important: This package is not child resistant. Store at controlled room temperature 59–86°F (15–30°C). Keep out of reach of children.

© 1996, Hoechst Marion Roussel, Inc.
Hoechst Marion Roussel, Inc.
Kansas City, MO 64137 USA

EXP.: B6   50007212

0088-1792-47

8. The physician prescribes codeine 30 mg po q 3 h prn for pain relief for your patient with a total hip replacement. How many tablets will you administer per dose? 1 tablet

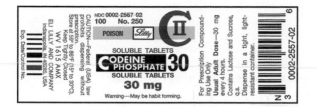

9. Your patient receives Vistaril 50 mg po three times a day for preoperative anxiety. Vistaril oral suspension 25 mg/5 mL is available. How many milliliters will you administer per dose? 10 mL

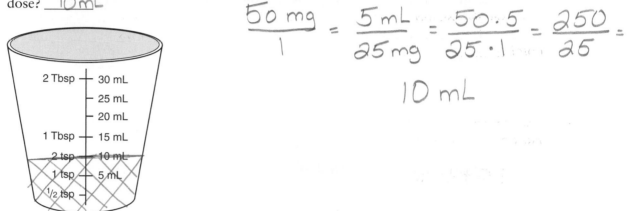

$$\frac{50\ mg}{1} = \frac{5\ mL}{25\ mg} = \frac{50 \cdot 5}{25 \cdot 1} = \frac{250}{25} = $$

$$10\ mL$$

10. The physician orders Prozac liquid 30 mg po twice a day. How many milliliters will you administer per dose? 7.5 mL

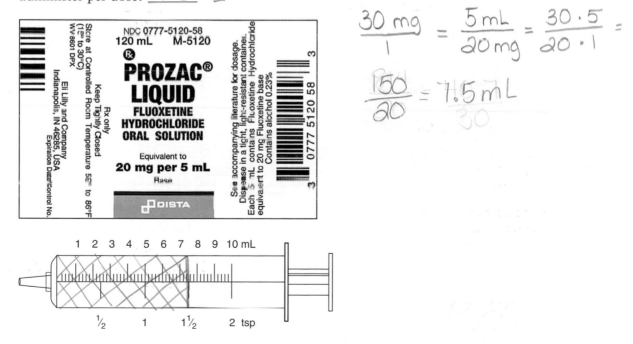

$$\frac{30\ mg}{1} = \frac{5\ mL}{20\ mg} = \frac{30 \cdot 5}{20 \cdot 1} = $$

$$\frac{150}{20} = 7.5\ mL$$

11. Your patient receives Crystodigin 0.1 mg po daily for an atrial arrhythmia. Crystodigin tablets 0.2 mg are available. How many tablets will you administer per dose? <u>0.5 tablets</u>

$$\frac{0.1 \text{ mg}}{0.2 \text{ mg}} = 0.5$$

12. The physician prescribes KCl 20 mEq po twice a day for hypokalemia. KCl liquid is supplied 30 mEq/22.5 mL. How many milliliters will the nurse administer per dose? <u>15 mL</u>

$$\frac{20 \text{ mEq}}{1} = \frac{22.5 \text{ mL}}{30 \text{ mEq}} = \frac{20 \cdot 22.5}{30 \cdot 1} = \frac{450}{30} = 15 \text{ mL}$$

13. The physician orders Lipitor 40 mg po daily. How many tablets will you give per dose? <u>2 tablets</u>

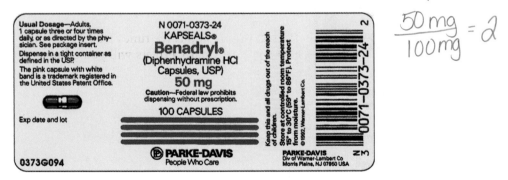

$$\frac{20 \text{ mg}}{40 \text{ mg}} = 2$$

14. Your patient with a lumbar laminectomy has Benadryl 100 mg po at bedtime prn ordered for insomnia. How many capsules will you administer per dose? <u>2 capsules</u>

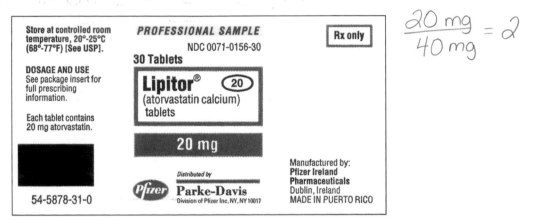

$$\frac{50 \text{ mg}}{100 \text{ mg}} = 2$$

15. Your patient has Lasix 38 mg po q 12 h ordered for hypercalcemia. You have Lasix 10 mg/mL. How many milliliters will you administer per dose? <u>3.8 mL</u>

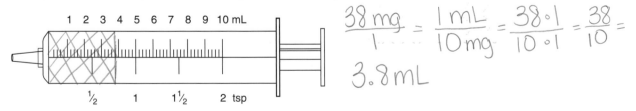

$$\frac{38 \text{ mg}}{1} = \frac{1 \text{ mL}}{10 \text{ mg}} = \frac{38 \cdot 1}{10 \cdot 1} = \frac{38}{10} =$$

3.8 mL

16. Mrs. Cook receives Keflex 100 mg po q 6 h for a sinus infection. How many milliliters will the nurse administer per dose? __4 mL__

$$\frac{5mL}{125mg} = \frac{100mg}{1} = \frac{500}{125} = 4mL$$

NDC 0777-2321-97
60 mL (When Mixed)   M-201 ®

KEFLEX®
CEPHALEXIN FOR
ORAL SUSPENSION, USP
125 mg per 5 mL

DISTA

17. The physician orders Mevacor 30 mg po daily to be given with the evening meal. You have 10-mg tablets available. How many tablets will you administer per dose? __3 tablets__

18. Mr. Jones receives Inderal 80 mg po two times a day for a dysrhythmia. You have Inderal 40-mg scored tablets. How many tablets will you administer per dose? __2 tablets__

19. The physician prescribes Apresoline 20 mg po three times a day for your patient's hypertension. You have 10-mg tablets available. How many tablets will you administer per dose? __2 tablets__

20. Your patient with epilepsy receives phenobarbital 90 mg po three times a day. How many tablets will you administer in each dose? __1.5__ How many tablets will you administer in 1 day? __4.5 tablets__

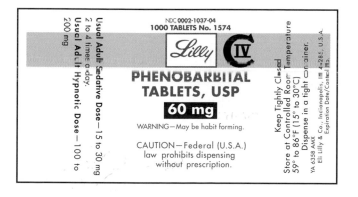

NDC 0002-1037-04
1000 TABLETS No. 1574

Lilly C IV

**PHENOBARBITAL
TABLETS, USP**
60 mg

WARNING—May be habit forming.

CAUTION—Federal (U.S.A.)
law prohibits dispensing
without prescription.

Usual Adult Sedative Dose—15 to 30 mg
2 to 4 times a day.
Usual Adult Hypnotic Dose—100 to
200 mg

Keep Tightly Closed
Store at Controlled Room Temperature
59° to 86°F (15° to 30°C)
Dispense in a tight container.

YA 6358 AMX
Eli Lilly & Co., Indianapolis, IN 46285, U.S.A.
Expiration Date/Control No.

21. Mrs. Luther has alprazolam 0.5 mg po three times a day prescribed for her panic disorder. You have 0.25-mg tablets available. How many tablets will you administer per dose? *2 tablets*

22. Mr. Barry has Ambien 10 mg po at bedtime ordered for insomnia. How many tablets will the nurse administer per dose? *2 tablets*

A07757-3

Store at controlled room temperature 20°-25°C (68°-77°F).

Usual Adult Dosage: One or two tablets at bedtime as directed. See complete prescribing information.

100 Tablets
NDC 0025-5401-31   Rx only

Ambien **CIV**
(zolpidem tartrate)

5mg

Pharmacist: Dispense in a tight, light-resistant, child-resistant container.

SEARLE

Mfd. and distr. by G.D. Searle & Co. Chicago IL 60680 USA
by agreement with Lorex Pharmaceuticals Skokie IL.
Ambien is a registered trademark of Sanofi-Synthelabo, Inc.

3 0025-5401-31 8

23. Mrs. Torres has metoprolol 150 mg po twice daily ordered for hypertension. You have metoprolol 100-mg scored tablets available. How many tablets will you administer per dose? *1.5 tablets*

24. The physician orders Zocor 30 mg po daily in the evening. How many tablets will you administer per dose? *3 tablets*

5   **Zocor® 10 mg**
(Simvastatin)

Dist. by:
MERCK & CO., INC.
West Point, PA 19486, USA

Store between 5 - 30°C (41 - 86°F).

60 Tablets

Lot

0006-0735-61

N3   Exp.

Zocor® 10 mg
(Simvastatin)

NDC 0006-0735-61
6505-01-354-4545

USUAL ADULT DOSAGE:
See accompanying circular.
Rx only

60 Tablets

Lot

Exp.

LIFT HERE

9098605
60 | No. 3589

25. Mr. Bond has Allegra 60 mg po twice a day ordered. Allegra 30-mg tablets are available. How many tablets will you administer per dose? *2 tablets*

ANSWERS ON PP. 242–244 AND 260–264.

NAME _____

DATE _____

ACCEPTABLE SCORE __24__

YOUR SCORE _____

CHAPTER **11**
Oral Dosages

POSTTEST 2

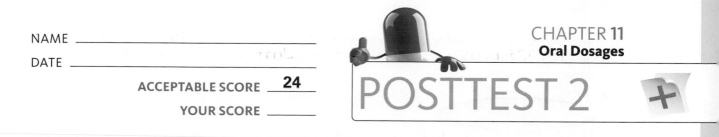

DIRECTIONS: The medication order is listed at the beginning of each problem. Calculate the oral doses. Show your work. Shade each medicine cup or oral syringe when provided to indicate correct dose.

1. Your patient receives Feldene 20 mg po daily for gouty arthritis. Feldene 10-mg capsules are available. How many capsules will you administer per dose? _____

2. The physician orders Zofran 8 mg po before chemotherapy. How many milliliters will the nurse administer per dose? _____

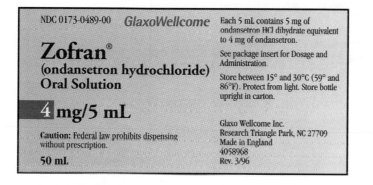

NDC 0173-0489-00   *GlaxoWellcome*

Zofran®
(ondansetron hydrochloride)
Oral Solution

4 mg/5 mL

Caution: Federal law prohibits dispensing without prescription.

50 mL

Each 5 mL contains 5 mg of ondansetron HCl dihydrate equivalent to 4 mg of ondansetron.

See package insert for Dosage and Administration.

Store between 15° and 30°C (59° and 86°F). Protect from light. Store bottle upright in carton.

Glaxo Wellcome Inc.
Research Triangle Park, NC 27709
Made in England
4058968
Rev. 3/96

3. Mr. Theson receives Vistaril 60 mg po q 6 h for relief of nausea after his acoustic neuroma revision. Vistaril oral suspension, 25 mg/5 mL, is supplied. How many milliliters will the nurse administer? _____

4. The physician orders Glucotrol 15 mg daily. Glucotrol 10 mg scored tablets are available. How many tablets will the nurse administer per dose? _____

5. Your patient who is being treated for congestive heart failure requires KCl 5 mEq po two times a day for hypokalemia. KCl 20 mEq/30 mL is available. How many milliliters will you administer per dose? _____

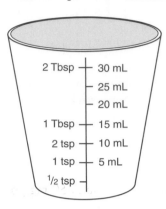

6. Your patient who has had a tonsillectomy receives Keflex 250 mg po four times a day. How many capsules will you administer per dose? _____

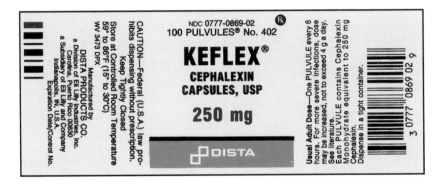

7. Mrs. Pace receives prednisone 7.5 mg po four times a day for asthma. Prednisone is supplied as 2.5-mg tablets. How many tablets will the nurse administer per dose? _____

8. Your patient receives Lanoxin 0.05 mg po daily for cardiac arrhythmia. How many milliliters will you administer per dose? _____

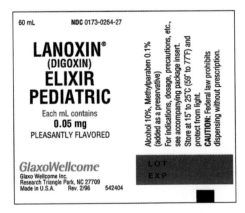

9. The physician orders Macrodantin 0.1 g po four times a day. How many capsules will the nurse administer per dose? _____

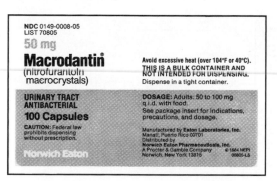

10. Your patient who had a bilateral turbinate reduction receives acetaminophen 650 mg po q 4 h for pain relief. Acetaminophen is supplied in 325-mg tablets. How many tablets will you administer per dose? _____

11. The physician prescribes Dilantin 100 mg po twice a day for seizure activity in your patient with epilepsy. Dilantin 50-mg Infatabs are available. How many tablets will you administer per dose? _____

12. Mr. Bales requires Pen V K 250 mg po q 6 h for bacterial endocarditis. Pen-V K solution 125 mg/5 mL is available. How many milliliters will the nurse administer per dose? _____

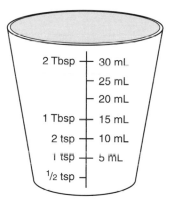

13. The physician orders Deltasone 20 mg po four times a day. Deltasone is supplied in 2.5-mg, 5-mg, and 50-mg tablets. The nurse will give _____ tablets of _____ mg.

14. Mr. Cy, who has had mitral valve repair, receives Lanoxin 0.25 mg po daily. How many tablets will the nurse administer per dose? _____

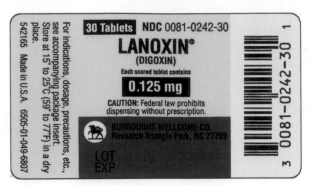

15. Colace syrup 25 mg po three times a day prn for constipation is ordered for your patient after an ethmoidectomy. How many milliliters will you administer per dose? _____

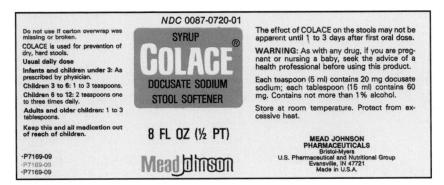

16. Mr. Tate, who suffers from chronic gout, has Zyloprim 0.15 g po daily in the mornings. How many tablets will he receive per dose? _____

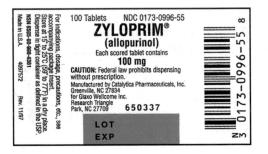

17. Your patient with hypertension has verapamil 80 mg po three times a day ordered. You have 40-mg tablets. How many tablets will you administer per dose? _____

18. The physician orders Zyprexa 15 mg po daily for bipolar mania. How many tablets will the nurse administer per dose? _____

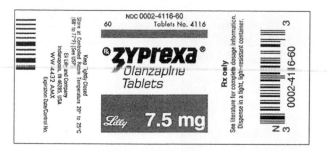

19. Your patient was admitted with seizure activity. The physician orders phenobarbital 30 mg po q 8 h. How many tablets will you administer per dose?

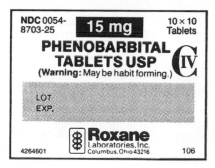

20. The physician orders Flagyl 750 mg po three times a day for 5 days for a yeast infection. Flagyl is supplied in 250-mg tablets. How many tablets will the nurse administer per dose? _____

21. Mr. Luke's physician has ordered Norvasc 10 mg po daily for hypertension. Norvasc 5-mg tablets are available. How many tablets will you administer per dose? _____

22. Mrs. Martin is prescribed Tofranil-PM 0.225 g po at bedtime for depression. How many capsules will you administer per dose? _____

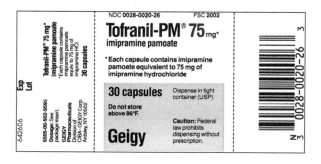

23. The physician orders Vibramycin 100 mg po daily. You have Vibramycin syrup 50 mg/5 mL. How many milliliters will you administer per dose? _____

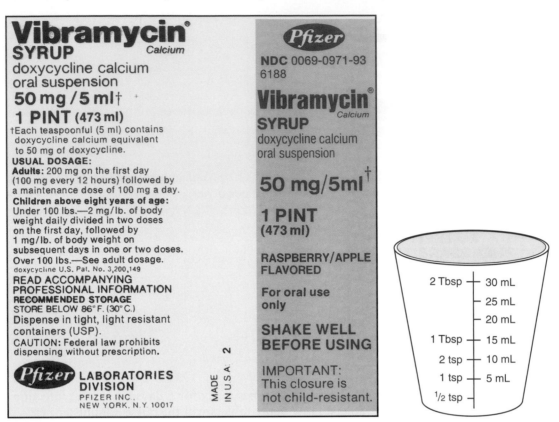

24. Vasotec 5 mg po twice a day is ordered for Mr. Butter's congestive heart failure. How many tablets will the nurse administer per dose? _____

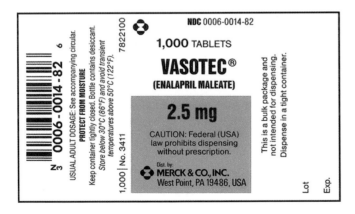

25. Ms. Wang is to receive Zithromax oral suspension 1 g po now. How many milliliters will you administer per dose? _____

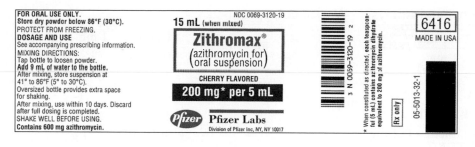

ANSWERS ON PP. 243–244 AND 265–268.

evolve   For additional practice problems, refer to the Basic Calculations section of *Drug Calculations Companion,* Version 5, on Evolve.

ANSWERS

CHAPTER 11 Dimensional Analysis—Worksheet, pp. 201–224

1. $x \text{ capsules} = \dfrac{1 \text{ capsule}}{1 \text{ mg}} \times \dfrac{2 \text{ mg}}{1} = 2 \text{ capsules}$

2. $x \text{ mL} = \dfrac{5 \text{ mL}}{20 \text{ mg}} \times \dfrac{30 \text{ mg}}{1} = 7.5 \text{ mL}$

3. $x \text{ tablets} = \dfrac{1 \text{ tablet}}{0.05 \text{ mg}} \times \dfrac{0.2 \text{ mg}}{1} = 4 \text{ tablets}$

   $x \text{ tablets} = \dfrac{1 \text{ tablet}}{0.05 \text{ mg}} \times \dfrac{0.15 \text{ mg}}{1} = 3 \text{ tablets}$

4. $x \text{ tablets} = \dfrac{1 \text{ tablet}}{250 \text{ mg}} \times \dfrac{500 \text{ mg}}{1} = 2 \text{ tablets}$

5. $x \text{ mL} = \dfrac{5 \text{ mL}}{5 \text{ mg}} \times \dfrac{2.5 \text{ mg}}{1} = 2.5 \text{ mL}$

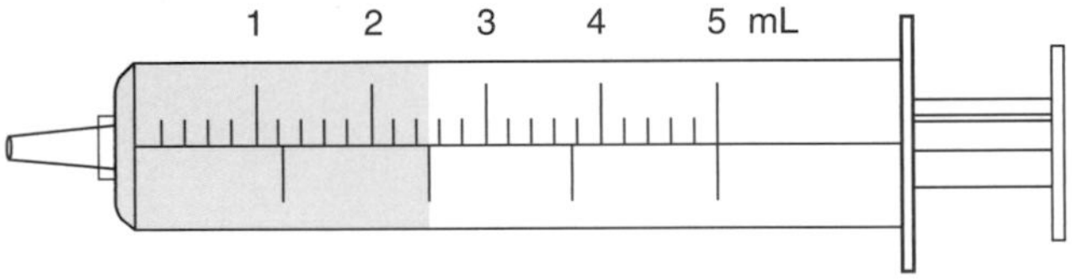

6. $x \text{ tablets} = \dfrac{1 \text{ tablet}}{1 \text{ mg}} \times \dfrac{2 \text{ mg}}{1} = 2 \text{ tablets}$

7. $x \text{ tablets} = \dfrac{1 \text{ tablet}}{10 \text{ mg}} \times \dfrac{20 \text{ mg}}{1} = 2 \text{ tablets}$

8. $x \text{ tablets} = \dfrac{1 \text{ tablet}}{0.5 \text{ g}} \times \dfrac{1 \text{ g}}{1} = 2 \text{ tablets}$

9. $x \text{ mL} = \dfrac{5 \text{ mL}}{20 \text{ mg}} \times \dfrac{40 \text{ mg}}{1} = 10 \text{ mL}$

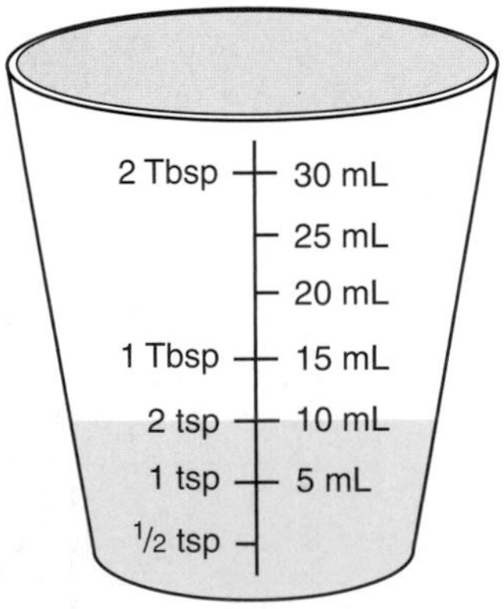

10. $x \text{ tablets} = \dfrac{1 \text{ tablet}}{0.5 \text{ mg}} \times \dfrac{1 \text{ mg}}{1} = 2 \text{ tablets}$

11. $x \text{ tablets} = \dfrac{1 \text{ tablet}}{400 \text{ mg}} \times \dfrac{800 \text{ mg}}{1} = 2 \text{ tablets}$

12. $x \text{ tablets} = \dfrac{1 \text{ tablet}}{300 \text{ mg}} \times \dfrac{1000 \text{ mg}}{1 \text{ g}} \times \dfrac{0.6 \text{ g}}{1} = 2 \text{ tablets}$

    $x \text{ mg} = \dfrac{300 \text{ mg}}{1 \text{ tablet}} \times \dfrac{2 \text{ tablets}}{1 \text{ dose}} \times \dfrac{2 \text{ doses}}{1 \text{ day}} = 1200 \text{ mg}$

13. $x \text{ tablets} = \dfrac{1 \text{ tablet}}{10 \text{ mg}} \times \dfrac{30 \text{ mg}}{1} = 3 \text{ tablets}$

14. $x \text{ tablets} = \dfrac{1 \text{ tablet}}{750 \text{ mg}} \times \dfrac{1000 \text{ mg}}{1 \text{ g}} \times \dfrac{0.75 \text{ g}}{1} = 1 \text{ tablet}$

15. $x \text{ capsules} = \dfrac{1 \text{ capsule}}{40 \text{ mg}} \times \dfrac{80 \text{ mg}}{1} = 2 \text{ capsules}$

16. $x \text{ tablets} = \dfrac{1 \text{ tablet}}{0.5 \text{ g}} \times \dfrac{4 \text{ g}}{1} = 8 \text{ tablets}$

    $x \text{ tablets} = \dfrac{1 \text{ tablet}}{0.5 \text{ g}} \times \dfrac{2 \text{ g}}{1} = 4 \text{ tablets}$

17. $x \text{ tablets} = \dfrac{1 \text{ tablet}}{400 \text{ mg}} \times \dfrac{800 \text{ mg}}{1} = 2 \text{ tablets}$

18. $x = \dfrac{30 \text{ mL}}{\text{Dose}} \times \dfrac{4 \text{ doses}}{1} = 120 \text{ mL}$

19. $x \text{ mL} = \dfrac{5 \text{ mL}}{12.5 \text{ mg}} \times \dfrac{30 \text{ mg}}{1} = 12 \text{ mL}$

20. $x \text{ tablets} = \dfrac{1 \text{ tablet}}{30 \text{ mg}} \times \dfrac{60 \text{ mg}}{1} = 2 \text{ tablets}$

21. $x \text{ mg} = \dfrac{125 \text{ mg}}{5 \text{ mL}} \times \dfrac{5.5 \text{ mL}}{1} = 137.5 \text{ mg}$

22. $x \text{ tablets} = \dfrac{1 \text{ tablet}}{40 \text{ mg}} \times \dfrac{80 \text{ mg}}{1} = 2 \text{ tablets}$

23. $x \text{ mg} = \dfrac{0.4 \text{ mg}}{1 \text{ tablet}} \times \dfrac{2 \text{ tablets}}{1} = 0.8 \text{ mg}$

24. $x \text{ mL} = \dfrac{5 \text{ mL}}{0.5 \text{ mg}} \times \dfrac{1.5 \text{ mg}}{1} = 15 \text{ mL}$

$x \text{ oz} = \dfrac{1 \text{ oz}}{30 \text{ mL}} \times \dfrac{15 \text{ mL}}{1} = 0.5 \text{ oz}$

33. $x \text{ mL} = \dfrac{5 \text{ mL}}{6.25 \text{ mg}} \times \dfrac{12.5 \text{ mg}}{1} = 10 \text{ mL}$

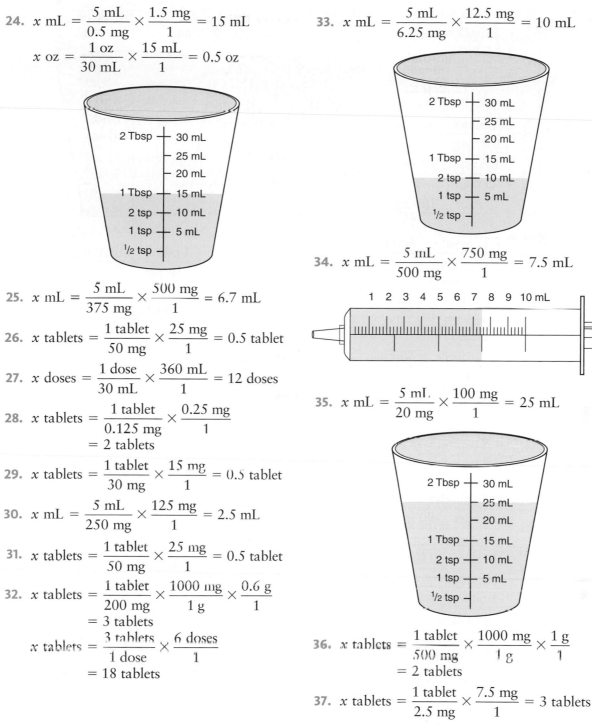

25. $x \text{ mL} = \dfrac{5 \text{ mL}}{375 \text{ mg}} \times \dfrac{500 \text{ mg}}{1} = 6.7 \text{ mL}$

26. $x \text{ tablets} = \dfrac{1 \text{ tablet}}{50 \text{ mg}} \times \dfrac{25 \text{ mg}}{1} = 0.5 \text{ tablet}$

27. $x \text{ doses} = \dfrac{1 \text{ dose}}{30 \text{ mL}} \times \dfrac{360 \text{ mL}}{1} = 12 \text{ doses}$

28. $x \text{ tablets} = \dfrac{1 \text{ tablet}}{0.125 \text{ mg}} \times \dfrac{0.25 \text{ mg}}{1} = 2 \text{ tablets}$

29. $x \text{ tablets} = \dfrac{1 \text{ tablet}}{30 \text{ mg}} \times \dfrac{15 \text{ mg}}{1} = 0.5 \text{ tablet}$

30. $x \text{ mL} = \dfrac{5 \text{ mL}}{250 \text{ mg}} \times \dfrac{125 \text{ mg}}{1} = 2.5 \text{ mL}$

31. $x \text{ tablets} = \dfrac{1 \text{ tablet}}{50 \text{ mg}} \times \dfrac{25 \text{ mg}}{1} = 0.5 \text{ tablet}$

32. $x \text{ tablets} = \dfrac{1 \text{ tablet}}{200 \text{ mg}} \times \dfrac{1000 \text{ mg}}{1 \text{ g}} \times \dfrac{0.6 \text{ g}}{1} = 3 \text{ tablets}$

$x \text{ tablets} = \dfrac{3 \text{ tablets}}{1 \text{ dose}} \times \dfrac{6 \text{ doses}}{1} = 18 \text{ tablets}$

34. $x \text{ mL} = \dfrac{5 \text{ mL}}{500 \text{ mg}} \times \dfrac{750 \text{ mg}}{1} = 7.5 \text{ mL}$

35. $x \text{ mL} = \dfrac{5 \text{ mL}}{20 \text{ mg}} \times \dfrac{100 \text{ mg}}{1} = 25 \text{ mL}$

36. $x \text{ tablets} = \dfrac{1 \text{ tablet}}{500 \text{ mg}} \times \dfrac{1000 \text{ mg}}{1 \text{ g}} \times \dfrac{1 \text{ g}}{1} = 2 \text{ tablets}$

37. $x \text{ tablets} = \dfrac{1 \text{ tablet}}{2.5 \text{ mg}} \times \dfrac{7.5 \text{ mg}}{1} = 3 \text{ tablets}$

38. $x \text{ tablets} = \dfrac{1 \text{ tablet}}{100 \text{ mg}} \times \dfrac{1000 \text{ mg}}{1 \text{ g}} \times \dfrac{0.2 \text{ g}}{1} = 2 \text{ tablets}$

ANSWERS

39. $x \text{ tablets} = \dfrac{1 \text{ tablet}}{5 \text{ mg}/500 \text{ mg}} \times \dfrac{5 \text{ mg}/500 \text{ mg}}{1}$
$\qquad = 1 \text{ tablet}$

$\qquad x \text{ acetaminophen} = \dfrac{500 \text{ mg}}{1 \text{ tablet}} \times \dfrac{1 \text{ tablet}}{1}$
$\qquad\qquad = 500 \text{ mg acetaminophen}$

40. $x \text{ tablets} = \dfrac{1 \text{ tablet}}{0.25 \text{ mg}} \times \dfrac{0.5 \text{ mg}}{1} = 2 \text{ tablets}$

41. $x \text{ tablets} = \dfrac{1 \text{ tablet}}{5 \text{ mg}} \times \dfrac{10 \text{ mg}}{1} = 2 \text{ tablets}$

42. $x \text{ tablets} = \dfrac{1 \text{ tablet}}{50 \text{ mg}} \times \dfrac{100 \text{ mg}}{1} = 2 \text{ tablets}$

43. $x \text{ capsules} = \dfrac{1 \text{ capsule}}{300 \text{ mg}} \times \dfrac{600 \text{ mg}}{1}$
$\qquad = 2 \text{ capsules}$

44. $x \text{ tablets} = \dfrac{1 \text{ tablet}}{0.125 \text{ mg}} \times \dfrac{0.25 \text{ mg}}{1}$
$\qquad = 2 \text{ tablets}$

45. $x \text{ capsules} = \dfrac{1 \text{ capsule}}{250 \text{ mg}} \times \dfrac{500 \text{ mg}}{1}$
$\qquad = 2 \text{ capsules}$

$\qquad x \text{ capsules} = \dfrac{2 \text{ capsules}}{1 \text{ dose}} \times \dfrac{4 \text{ doses}}{1}$
$\qquad\qquad = 8 \text{ capsules}$

46. $x \text{ capsules} = \dfrac{1 \text{ capsule}}{20 \text{ mg}} \times \dfrac{40 \text{ mg}}{1}$
$\qquad = 2 \text{ capsules}$

47. $x \text{ tablets} = \dfrac{1 \text{ tablet}}{30 \text{ mg}} \times \dfrac{90 \text{ mg}}{1} = 3 \text{ tablets}$

48. $x \text{ tablets} = \dfrac{1 \text{ tablet}}{75 \text{ mg}} \times \dfrac{150 \text{ mg}}{1} = 2 \text{ tablets}$

49. $x \text{ tablets} = \dfrac{1 \text{ tablet}}{325 \text{ mg}} \times \dfrac{650 \text{ mg}}{1} = 2 \text{ tablets}$

50. $x \text{ mL} = \dfrac{1 \text{ mL}}{15 \text{ mg}} \times \dfrac{150 \text{ mg}}{1} = 10 \text{ mL}$

51. $x \text{ tablets} = \dfrac{1 \text{ tablet}}{250 \text{ mg}} \times \dfrac{500 \text{ mg}}{1} = 2 \text{ tablets}$

52. $x \text{ tablets} = \dfrac{1 \text{ tablet}}{0.1 \text{ mg}} \times \dfrac{0.2 \text{ mg}}{1} = 2 \text{ tablets}$

53. $x \text{ capsules} = \dfrac{1 \text{ capsule}}{10 \text{ mg}} \times \dfrac{20 \text{ mg}}{1}$
$\qquad = 2 \text{ capsules}$

54. $x \text{ mL} = \dfrac{5 \text{ mL}}{10 \text{ mg}} \times \dfrac{30 \text{ mg}}{1} = 15 \text{ mL}$

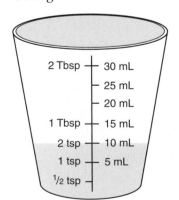

55. $x \text{ tablets} = \dfrac{1 \text{ tablet}}{250 \text{ mg}} \times \dfrac{1000 \text{ mg}}{1 \text{ g}} \times \dfrac{0.75 \text{ g}}{1}$
$\qquad = 3 \text{ tablets}$

56. $x \text{ tablets} = \dfrac{1 \text{ tablet}}{4 \text{ mg}} \times \dfrac{8 \text{ mg}}{1} = 2 \text{ tablets}$

57. $x \text{ mL} = \dfrac{5 \text{ mL}}{25 \text{ mg}} \times \dfrac{15 \text{ mg}}{1} = 3 \text{ mL}$

58. $x \text{ tablets} = \dfrac{1 \text{ tablet}}{50 \text{ mg}} \times \dfrac{100 \text{ mg}}{1} = 2 \text{ tablets}$

59. $x \text{ tablets} = \dfrac{1 \text{ tablet}}{500 \text{ mg}} \times \dfrac{1000 \text{ mg}}{1 \text{ g}} \times \dfrac{1 \text{ g}}{1}$
$\qquad = 2 \text{ tablets}$

60. $x \text{ mL} = \dfrac{5 \text{ mL}}{150 \text{ mg}} \times \dfrac{250 \text{ mg}}{1} = 8.33 \text{ mL}$

61. $x \text{ mL} = \dfrac{5 \text{ mL}}{50 \text{ mg}} \times \dfrac{100 \text{ mg}}{1} = 10 \text{ mL}$

ANSWERS

62. $x \text{ tablets} = \dfrac{1 \text{ tablet}}{50 \text{ mg}} \times \dfrac{25 \text{ mg}}{1} = 0.5 \text{ tablet}$

63. $x \text{ tablets} = \dfrac{1 \text{ tablet}}{80 \text{ mg}} \times \dfrac{240 \text{ mg}}{1} = 3 \text{ tablets}$

64. $x \text{ mL} = \dfrac{1 \text{ mL}}{0.05 \text{ mg}} \times \dfrac{1 \text{ mg}}{1000 \text{ mcg}} \times \dfrac{90 \text{ mcg}}{1}$
$= 1.8 \text{ mL}$

65. $x \text{ mg} = \dfrac{12.5 \text{ mg}}{5 \text{ mL}} \times \dfrac{10 \text{ mL}}{1} = 25 \text{ mg}$

66. $x \text{ capsules} = \dfrac{1 \text{ capsule}}{25 \text{ mg}} \times \dfrac{50 \text{ mg}}{1}$
$= 2 \text{ capsules}$

67. $x \text{ capsules} = \dfrac{1 \text{ capsule}}{30 \text{ mg}} \times \dfrac{90 \text{ mg}}{1}$
$= 3 \text{ capsules}$

68. 40-mg tablet
$x \text{ tablets} = \dfrac{1 \text{ tablet}}{40 \text{ mg}} \times \dfrac{40 \text{ mg}}{1} = 1 \text{ tablet}$

69. $x \text{ mL} = \dfrac{15 \text{ mL}}{20 \text{ mEq}} \times \dfrac{10 \text{ mEq}}{1} = 7.5 \text{ mL}$

70. $x \text{ tablets} = \dfrac{1 \text{ tablet}}{0.5 \text{ mg}} \times \dfrac{1.5 \text{ mg}}{1} = 3 \text{ tablets}$

71. $x \text{ tablets} = \dfrac{1 \text{ tablet}}{0.25 \text{ mg}} \times \dfrac{0.5 \text{ mg}}{1} = 2 \text{ tablets}$

72. $x \text{ tablets} = \dfrac{1 \text{ tablet}}{325 \text{ mg}} \times \dfrac{650 \text{ mg}}{1} = 2 \text{ tablets}$

73. $x \text{ tablets} = \dfrac{1 \text{ tablet}}{0.25 \text{ mg}} \times \dfrac{0.5 \text{ mg}}{1} = 2 \text{ tablets}$

74. $x \text{ mL} = \dfrac{5 \text{ mL}}{125 \text{ mg}} \times \dfrac{375 \text{ mg}}{1} = 15 \text{ mL}$

75. $x \text{ tablets} = \dfrac{1 \text{ tablet}}{30 \text{ mg}} \times \dfrac{30 \text{ mg}}{1} = 1 \text{ tablet}$

76. $x \text{ tablets} = \dfrac{1 \text{ tablet}}{0.15 \text{ mg}} \times \dfrac{0.3 \text{ mg}}{1}$
$= 2 \text{ tablets of } 0.15 \text{ mg}$

77. $x \text{ tablets} = \dfrac{1 \text{ tablet}}{5 \text{ mg}} \times \dfrac{7.5 \text{ mg}}{1}$
$= 1.5 \text{ tablets}$

78. $x \text{ mL} = \dfrac{5 \text{ mL}}{125 \text{ mg}} \times \dfrac{250 \text{ mg}}{1} = 10 \text{ mL}$

79. $x \text{ capsules} = \dfrac{1 \text{ capsule}}{50 \text{ mg}} \times \dfrac{250 \text{ mg}}{1}$
$= 5 \text{ capsules}$

80. $x \text{ mL} = \dfrac{11.25 \text{ mL}}{15 \text{ mEq}} \times \dfrac{20 \text{ mEq}}{1} = 15 \text{ mL}$

81. $x \text{ mL} = \dfrac{5 \text{ mL}}{20 \text{ mg}} \times \dfrac{55 \text{ mg}}{1} = 13.75 \text{ mL}$

82. $x \text{ tablets} = \dfrac{1 \text{ tablet}}{125 \text{ mg}} \times \dfrac{250 \text{ mg}}{1} = 2 \text{ tablets}$

83. $x \text{ tablets} = \dfrac{1 \text{ tablet}}{0.05 \text{ mg}} \times \dfrac{0.05 \text{ mg}}{1} = 1 \text{ tablet}$

84. $x \text{ mg} = \dfrac{1000 \text{ mg}}{1 \text{ g}} \times \dfrac{0.2 \text{ g}}{1}$
$= 1 \text{ tablet of } 200 \text{ mg}$
$x \text{ mg} = \dfrac{200 \text{ mg}}{1 \text{ dose}} \times \dfrac{3 \text{ doses}}{1} = 600 \text{ mg}$

85. $x \text{ tablets} = \dfrac{1 \text{ tablet}}{5 \text{ mg}} \times \dfrac{15 \text{ mg}}{1} = 3 \text{ tablets}$

86. $x \text{ tablets} = \dfrac{1 \text{ tablet}}{400 \text{ mg}} \times \dfrac{800 \text{ mg}}{1} = 2 \text{ tablets}$

87. $x \text{ capsules} = \dfrac{1 \text{ capsule}}{250 \text{ mg}} \times \dfrac{500 \text{ mg}}{1}$
$= 2 \text{ capsules}$

88. $x \text{ tablets} = \dfrac{1 \text{ tablet}}{25 \text{ mg}} \times \dfrac{50 \text{ mg}}{1} = 2 \text{ tablets}$

89. $x \text{ pills} = \dfrac{1 \text{ pill}}{10 \text{ mg}} \times \dfrac{30 \text{ mg}}{1} = 3 \text{ pills}$

90. $x \text{ mL} = \dfrac{1 \text{ mL}}{10 \text{ mg}} \times \dfrac{6 \text{ mg}}{1} = 0.6 \text{ mL}$

91. $x \text{ capsules} = \dfrac{1 \text{ capsule}}{75 \text{ mg}} \times \dfrac{150 \text{ mg}}{1}$
$= 2 \text{ capsules}$

ANSWERS

92. $x \text{ capsules} = \dfrac{1 \text{ capsule}}{100 \text{ mg}} \times \dfrac{200 \text{ mg}}{1}$
$= 2 \text{ capsules}$

93. $x \text{ tablets} = \dfrac{1 \text{ tablet}}{2.5 \text{ mg}} \times \dfrac{10 \text{ mg}}{1} = 4 \text{ tablets}$

94. $x \text{ tablets} = \dfrac{1 \text{ tablet}}{250 \text{ mg}} \times \dfrac{1000 \text{ mg}}{1 \text{ g}} \times \dfrac{0.25 \text{ g}}{1}$
$= 1 \text{ tablet}$

95. $x \text{ tablets} = \dfrac{1 \text{ tablet}}{10 \text{ mg}} \times \dfrac{25 \text{ mg}}{1} = 2.5 \text{ tablets}$

96. $x \text{ tablets} = \dfrac{1 \text{ tablet}}{10 \text{ mg}} \times \dfrac{30 \text{ mg}}{1} = 3 \text{ tablets}$

97. $x \text{ tablets} = \dfrac{1 \text{ tablet}}{5 \text{ mg}} \times \dfrac{15 \text{ mg}}{1} = 3 \text{ tablets}$

98. $x \text{ capsules} = \dfrac{1 \text{ capsule}}{15 \text{ mg}} \times \dfrac{1000 \text{ mg}}{1 \text{ g}} \times \dfrac{0.015 \text{ g}}{1}$
$= 1 \text{ capsule}$

99. $x \text{ mL} = \dfrac{5 \text{ mL}}{6.7 \text{ mEq}} \times \dfrac{30 \text{ mEq}}{1} = 22.4 \text{ mL}$

2 Tbsp	30 mL
	25 mL
	20 mL
1 Tbsp	15 mL
2 tsp	10 mL
1 tsp	5 mL
½ tsp	

100. $x \text{ tablets} = \dfrac{1 \text{ tablet}}{40 \text{ mg}} \times \dfrac{20 \text{ mg}}{1} = 0.5 \text{ tablet}$

CHAPTER 11 Dimensional Analysis—Posttest 1, pp. 225–230

1. $x \text{ tablets} = \dfrac{1 \text{ tablet}}{325 \text{ mg}} \times \dfrac{975 \text{ mg}}{1} = 3 \text{ tablets}$

2. $x \text{ capsules} = \dfrac{1 \text{ capsule}}{500 \text{ mg}} \times \dfrac{1000 \text{ mg}}{1 \text{ g}} \times \dfrac{0.5 \text{g}}{1}$
$= 1 \text{ capsule}$

3. $x \text{ capsules} = \dfrac{1 \text{ capsule}}{250 \text{ mg}} \times \dfrac{1000 \text{ mg}}{1} \times \dfrac{1 \text{ g}}{1}$
$= 4 \text{ capsules}$

4. $x \text{ tablets} = \dfrac{1 \text{ tablet}}{0.03 \text{ g}} \times \dfrac{1 \text{ g}}{1000 \text{ mg}} \times \dfrac{60 \text{ mg}}{1}$
$= 2 \text{ tablets}$

5. $x \text{ tablets} = \dfrac{1 \text{ tablet}}{0.05 \text{ mg}} \times \dfrac{1 \text{ mg}}{1000 \text{ mcg}} \times \dfrac{100 \text{ mcg}}{1}$
$= 2 \text{ tablets}$

6. $x \text{ mL} = \dfrac{5 \text{ mL}}{10 \text{ mg}} \times \dfrac{25 \text{ mg}}{1} = 12.5 \text{ mL}$

2 Tbsp	30 mL
	25 mL
	20 mL
1 Tbsp	15 mL
2 tsp	10 mL
1 tsp	5 mL
½ tsp	

7. $x \text{ tablets} = \dfrac{1 \text{ tablet}}{120 \text{ mg}} \times \dfrac{60 \text{ mg}}{1} = 0.5 \text{ tablet}$

8. $x \text{ tablets} = \dfrac{1 \text{ tablet}}{30 \text{ mg}} \times \dfrac{30 \text{ mg}}{1} = 1 \text{ tablet}$

9. $x \text{ mL} = \dfrac{5 \text{ mL}}{25 \text{ mg}} \times \dfrac{50 \text{ mg}}{1} = 10 \text{ mL}$

2 Tbsp	30 mL
	25 mL
	20 mL
1 Tbsp	15 mL
2 tsp	10 mL
1 tsp	5 mL
½ tsp	

10. $x \text{ mL} = \dfrac{5 \text{ mL}}{20 \text{ mg}} \times \dfrac{30 \text{ mg}}{1} = 7.5 \text{ mL}$

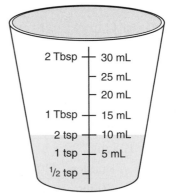

1   2   3   4   5   6   7   8   9   10 mL

ANSWERS

11. $x \text{ tablets} = \dfrac{1 \text{ tablet}}{0.2 \text{ mg}} \times \dfrac{0.1 \text{ mg}}{1} = 0.5 \text{ tablet}$

12. $x \text{ mL} = \dfrac{22.5 \text{ mL}}{30 \text{ mEq}} \times \dfrac{20 \text{ mEq}}{1} = 15 \text{ mL}$

13. $x \text{ tablets} = \dfrac{1 \text{ tablet}}{20 \text{ mg}} \times \dfrac{40 \text{ mg}}{1} = 2 \text{ tablets}$

14. $x \text{ capsules} = \dfrac{1 \text{ capsule}}{50 \text{ mg}} \times \dfrac{100 \text{ mg}}{1}$
    $= 2 \text{ capsules}$

15. $x \text{ mL} = \dfrac{1 \text{ mL}}{10 \text{ mg}} \times \dfrac{38 \text{ mg}}{1} = 3.8 \text{ mL}$

16. $x \text{ mL} = \dfrac{5 \text{ mL}}{125 \text{ mg}} \times \dfrac{100 \text{ mg}}{1} = 4 \text{ mL}$

17. $x \text{ tablets} = \dfrac{1 \text{ tablet}}{10 \text{ mg}} \times \dfrac{30 \text{ mg}}{1} = 3 \text{ tablets}$

18. $x \text{ tablets} = \dfrac{1 \text{ tablet}}{40 \text{ mg}} \times \dfrac{80 \text{ mg}}{1} = 2 \text{ tablets}$

19. $x \text{ tablets} = \dfrac{1 \text{ tablet}}{10 \text{ mg}} \times \dfrac{20 \text{ mg}}{1} = 2 \text{ tablets}$

20. $x \text{ tablets} = \dfrac{1 \text{ tablet}}{60 \text{ mg}} \times \dfrac{90 \text{ mg}}{1} = 1.5 \text{ tablets}$

$x \dfrac{\text{tablets}}{\text{day}} = \dfrac{1.5 \text{ tablets}}{1 \text{ dose}} \times \dfrac{3 \text{ doses}}{1 \text{ day}}$
    $= 4.5 \text{ tablets/day}$

21. $x \text{ tablets} = \dfrac{1 \text{ tablet}}{0.25 \text{ mg}} \times \dfrac{0.5 \text{ mg}}{1} = 2 \text{ tablets}$

22. $x \text{ tablets} = \dfrac{1 \text{ tablet}}{5 \text{ mg}} \times \dfrac{10 \text{ mg}}{1} = 2 \text{ tablets}$

23. $x \text{ tablets} = \dfrac{1 \text{ tablet}}{100 \text{ mg}} \times \dfrac{150 \text{ mg}}{1} = 1.5 \text{ tablets}$

24. $x \text{ tablets} = \dfrac{1 \text{ tablet}}{10 \text{ mg}} \times \dfrac{30 \text{ mg}}{1} = 3 \text{ tablets}$

25. $x \text{ tablets} = \dfrac{1 \text{ tablet}}{30 \text{ mg}} \times \dfrac{60 \text{ mg}}{1} = 2 \text{ tablets}$

CHAPTER 11 Dimensional Analysis—Posttest 2, pp. 231–237

1. $x \text{ capsules} = \dfrac{1 \text{ capsule}}{10 \text{ mg}} \times \dfrac{20 \text{ mg}}{1}$
   $= 2 \text{ capsules}$

2. $x \text{ mL} = \dfrac{5 \text{ mL}}{4 \text{ mg}} \times \dfrac{8 \text{ mg}}{1} = 10 \text{ mL}$

3. $x \text{ mL} = \dfrac{5 \text{ mL}}{25 \text{ mg}} \times \dfrac{60 \text{ mg}}{1} = 12 \text{ mL}$

4. $x \text{ tablets} = \dfrac{1 \text{ tablet}}{10 \text{ mg}} \times \dfrac{15 \text{ mg}}{1} = 1.5 \text{ tablets}$

5. $x \text{ mL} = \dfrac{30 \text{ mL}}{20 \text{ mEq}} \times \dfrac{5 \text{ mEq}}{1} = 7.5 \text{ mL}$

6. $x \text{ capsules} = \dfrac{1 \text{ capsule}}{250 \text{ mg}} \times \dfrac{250 \text{ mg}}{1}$
   $= 1 \text{ capsule}$

7. $x \text{ tablets} = \dfrac{1 \text{ tablet}}{2.5 \text{ mg}} \times \dfrac{7.5 \text{ mg}}{1} = 3 \text{ tablets}$

8. $x \text{ mL} = \dfrac{1 \text{ mL}}{0.05 \text{ mg}} \times \dfrac{0.05 \text{ mg}}{1} = 1 \text{ mL}$

9. $x \text{ capsules} = \dfrac{1 \text{ capsule}}{50 \text{ mg}} \times \dfrac{1000 \text{ mg}}{1 \text{ g}} \times \dfrac{0.1 \text{ g}}{1}$
   $= 2 \text{ capsules}$

10. $x \text{ tablets} = \dfrac{1 \text{ tablet}}{325 \text{ mg}} \times \dfrac{650 \text{ mg}}{1} = 2 \text{ tablets}$

11. $x \text{ tablets} = \dfrac{1 \text{ tablet}}{50 \text{ mg}} \times \dfrac{100 \text{ mg}}{1} = 2 \text{ tablets}$

12. $x \text{ mL} = \dfrac{5 \text{ mL}}{125 \text{ mg}} \times \dfrac{250 \text{ mg}}{1} = 10 \text{ mL}$

13. $x \text{ tablets} = \dfrac{1 \text{ tablet}}{5 \text{ mg}} \times \dfrac{20 \text{ mg}}{1}$
    $= 4 \text{ tablets of } 5 \text{ mg}$

14. $x \text{ tablets} = \dfrac{1 \text{ tablet}}{0.125 \text{ mg}} \times \dfrac{0.25 \text{ mg}}{1}$
    $= 2 \text{ tablets}$

15. $x \text{ mL} = \dfrac{5 \text{ mL}}{20 \text{ mg}} \times \dfrac{25 \text{ mg}}{1} = 6.25 \text{ mL}$

16. $x \text{ tablets} = \dfrac{1 \text{ tablet}}{100 \text{ mg}} \times \dfrac{1000 \text{ mg}}{1 \text{ g}} \times \dfrac{0.15 \text{ g}}{1}$
    $= 1.5 \text{ tablets}$

17. $x \text{ tablets} = \dfrac{1 \text{ tablet}}{40 \text{ mg}} \times \dfrac{80 \text{ mg}}{1} = 2 \text{ tablets}$

18. $x \text{ tablets} = \dfrac{1 \text{ tablet}}{7.5 \text{ mg}} \times \dfrac{15 \text{ mg}}{1} = 2 \text{ tablets}$

19. $x \text{ tablets} = \dfrac{1 \text{ tablet}}{15 \text{ mg}} \times \dfrac{30 \text{ mg}}{1} = 2 \text{ tablets}$

20. $x \text{ tablets} = \dfrac{1 \text{ tablet}}{250 \text{ mg}} \times \dfrac{750 \text{ mg}}{1} = 3 \text{ tablets}$

21. $x \text{ tablets} = \dfrac{1 \text{ tablet}}{5 \text{ mg}} \times \dfrac{10 \text{ mg}}{1} = 2 \text{ tablets}$

22. $x \text{ capsules} = \dfrac{1 \text{ capsule}}{75 \text{ mg}} \times \dfrac{1000 \text{ mg}}{1 \text{ g}} \times \dfrac{0.225 \text{ g}}{1}$
    $= 3 \text{ capsules}$

23. $x \text{ mL} = \dfrac{5 \text{ mL}}{50 \text{ mg}} \times \dfrac{100 \text{ mg}}{1} = 10 \text{ mL}$

24. $x \text{ tablets} = \dfrac{1 \text{ tablet}}{2.5 \text{ mg}} \times \dfrac{5 \text{ mg}}{1} = 2 \text{ tablets}$

25. $x \text{ mL} = \dfrac{5 \text{ mL}}{200 \text{ mg}} \times \dfrac{1000 \text{ mg}}{1 \text{ g}} \times \dfrac{1 \text{ g}}{1}$
    $= 25 \text{ mL}$

CHAPTER 11 Proportion/Formula Method—Worksheet, pp. 201–224

Proportion	Formula
1. $1 \text{ mg} : 1 \text{ cap} :: 2 \text{ mg} : x \text{ cap}$ $1 : 1 :: 2 : x$ $x = 2 \text{ capsules}$	$\dfrac{2 \text{ mg}}{1 \text{ mg}} \times 1 \text{ cap} = 2 \text{ capsules}$
2. $20 \text{ mg} : 5 \text{ mL} :: 30 \text{ mg} : x \text{ mL}$ $20 : 5 :: 30 : x$ $20x = 150$ $x = \dfrac{150}{20}$ $x = 7.5 \text{ mL}$	$\dfrac{30 \text{ mg}}{20 \text{ mg}} \times 5 \text{ mL} =$ $\dfrac{30}{\cancel{20}_{4}} \times \dfrac{\cancel{5}^{1}}{1} = \dfrac{30}{4}$ $\dfrac{30}{4} = 7.5 \text{ mL}$

Proportion

Formula

3. 0.05 mg : 1 tab :: 0.2 mg : x tab
0.05 : 1 :: 0.2 : x
0.05x = 0.2
$x = \dfrac{0.2}{0.05}$
x = 4 tablets
0.05 mg : 1 tab :: 0.15 mg : x tab
0.05 : 1 :: 0.15 : x
0.05x = 0.15
$x = \dfrac{0.15}{0.05}$
x = 3 tablets

$\dfrac{0.2 \text{ mg}}{0.05 \text{ mg}} \times 1 \text{ tab} =$
$\dfrac{0.2}{0.05} = 4 \text{ tablets}$
$\dfrac{0.15 \text{ mg}}{0.05 \text{ mg}} \times 1 \text{ tab} =$
$\dfrac{0.15}{0.05} = 3 \text{ tablets}$

4. 250 mg : 1 tab :: 500 mg : x tab
250 : 1 :: 500 : x
250x = 500
$x = \dfrac{500}{250}$
x = 2 tablets

$\dfrac{500}{250} \times 1 \text{ tab} =$
$\dfrac{\overset{2}{\cancel{500}}}{\underset{1}{\cancel{250}}} =$
$\dfrac{2}{1} = 2 \text{ tablets}$

5. 5 mg : 5 mL :: 2.5 mg : x mL
5 : 5 :: 2.5 : x
5x = 12.5
$x = \dfrac{12.5}{5}$
x = 2.5 mL

$\dfrac{2.5 \text{ mg}}{5 \text{ mg}} \times 5 \text{ mL} =$
$\dfrac{2.5}{\cancel{5}} \times \dfrac{\overset{1}{\cancel{5}}}{1} = \dfrac{2.5}{1} = 2.5 \text{ mL}$

6. 1 mg : 1 tab :: 2 mg : x tab
1 : 1 :: 2 : x
x = 2 tablets

$\dfrac{2 \text{ mg}}{1 \text{ mg}} \times 1 \text{ tab} =$
$\dfrac{2}{1} = 2 \text{ tablets}$

7. 10 mg : 1 tab :: 20 mg : x tab
10 : 1 :: 20 : x
10x = 20
$x = \dfrac{20}{10}$
x = 2 tablets

$\dfrac{20}{10} \times 1 \text{ tab} =$
$\dfrac{\overset{2}{\cancel{20}}}{\underset{1}{\cancel{10}}} = 2 \text{ tablets}$

8. 0.5 g : 1 tab :: 1 g : x tab
0.5 : 1 :: 1 : x
0.5x = 1
$x = \dfrac{1}{0.5}$
x = 2 tablets

$\dfrac{1 \text{ g}}{0.5 \text{ g}} \times 1 \text{ tab} =$
$\dfrac{1}{0.5} = 2 \text{ tablets}$

ANSWERS

Proportion	Formula

9. $20 \text{ mg} : 5 \text{ mL} :: 40 \text{ mg} : x \text{ mL}$
   $20 : 5 :: 40 : x$
   $20x = 200$
   $x = \dfrac{200}{20}$
   $x = 10 \text{ mL}$

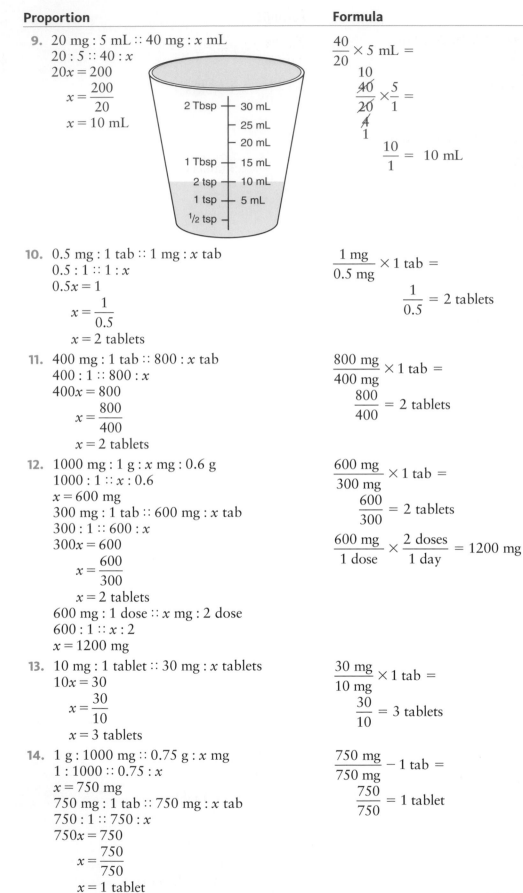

$\dfrac{40}{20} \times 5 \text{ mL} =$

$\dfrac{\overset{10}{\cancel{40}}}{\cancel{20}} \times \dfrac{5}{1} =$
$\phantom{\dfrac{40}{20}}\overset{4}{\underset{1}{}}$

$\dfrac{10}{1} = 10 \text{ mL}$

10. $0.5 \text{ mg} : 1 \text{ tab} :: 1 \text{ mg} : x \text{ tab}$
    $0.5 : 1 :: 1 : x$
    $0.5x = 1$
    $x = \dfrac{1}{0.5}$
    $x = 2 \text{ tablets}$

$\dfrac{1 \text{ mg}}{0.5 \text{ mg}} \times 1 \text{ tab} =$

$\dfrac{1}{0.5} = 2 \text{ tablets}$

11. $400 \text{ mg} : 1 \text{ tab} :: 800 : x \text{ tab}$
    $400 : 1 :: 800 : x$
    $400x = 800$
    $x = \dfrac{800}{400}$
    $x = 2 \text{ tablets}$

$\dfrac{800 \text{ mg}}{400 \text{ mg}} \times 1 \text{ tab} =$

$\dfrac{800}{400} = 2 \text{ tablets}$

12. $1000 \text{ mg} : 1 \text{ g} : x \text{ mg} : 0.6 \text{ g}$
    $1000 : 1 :: x : 0.6$
    $x = 600 \text{ mg}$
    $300 \text{ mg} : 1 \text{ tab} :: 600 \text{ mg} : x \text{ tab}$
    $300 : 1 :: 600 : x$
    $300x = 600$
    $x = \dfrac{600}{300}$
    $x = 2 \text{ tablets}$
    $600 \text{ mg} : 1 \text{ dose} :: x \text{ mg} : 2 \text{ dose}$
    $600 : 1 :: x : 2$
    $x = 1200 \text{ mg}$

$\dfrac{600 \text{ mg}}{300 \text{ mg}} \times 1 \text{ tab} =$

$\dfrac{600}{300} = 2 \text{ tablets}$

$\dfrac{600 \text{ mg}}{1 \text{ dose}} \times \dfrac{2 \text{ doses}}{1 \text{ day}} = 1200 \text{ mg}$

13. $10 \text{ mg} : 1 \text{ tablet} :: 30 \text{ mg} : x \text{ tablets}$
    $10x = 30$
    $x = \dfrac{30}{10}$
    $x = 3 \text{ tablets}$

$\dfrac{30 \text{ mg}}{10 \text{ mg}} \times 1 \text{ tab} =$

$\dfrac{30}{10} = 3 \text{ tablets}$

14. $1 \text{ g} : 1000 \text{ mg} :: 0.75 \text{ g} : x \text{ mg}$
    $1 : 1000 :: 0.75 : x$
    $x = 750 \text{ mg}$
    $750 \text{ mg} : 1 \text{ tab} :: 750 \text{ mg} : x \text{ tab}$
    $750 : 1 :: 750 : x$
    $750x = 750$
    $x = \dfrac{750}{750}$
    $x = 1 \text{ tablet}$

$\dfrac{750 \text{ mg}}{750 \text{ mg}} - 1 \text{ tab} =$

$\dfrac{750}{750} = 1 \text{ tablet}$

Proportion	Formula

15. 40 mg : 1 cap :: 80 mg : x cap
40 : 1 :: 80 : x
40x = 80
x = 2 capsules

$\dfrac{80 \text{ mg}}{40 \text{ mg}} \times 1 \text{ cap} =$

$\dfrac{80}{40} = 2$ capsules

16. 0.5 g : 1 tab :: 4 g : x tab
0.5 : 1 :: 4 : x
0.5x = 4
$x = \dfrac{4}{0.5}$
x = 8 tablets
0.5 g : 1 tab :: 2 g : x tab
0.5 : 1 :: 2 : x
0.5x = 2
$x = \dfrac{2}{0.5}$
x = 4 tablets

$\dfrac{4 \text{ g}}{0.5 \text{ g}} \times 1 \text{ tab} =$

$\dfrac{4}{0.5} = 8$ tablets

$\dfrac{2 \text{ g}}{0.5 \text{ g}} \times 1 \text{ tab} =$

$\dfrac{2}{0.5} = 4$ tablets

17. 400 mg : 1 tab :: 800 mg : x tab
400 : 1 :: 800 : x
400x = 800
$x = \dfrac{800}{400}$
x = 2 tablets

$\dfrac{800 \text{ mg}}{400 \text{ mg}} \times 1 \text{ tab} =$

$\dfrac{\overset{2}{\cancel{800}}}{\underset{1}{\cancel{400}}} = 2$ tablets

18. 30 mL : 1 dose :: x mL : 4 doses
120 mL = x
120 mL given each day

19. 12.5 mg : 5 mL :: 30 mg : x mL
12.5 : 5 :: 30 : x
12.5x = 150
$x = \dfrac{150}{12.5}$
x = 12 mL

$\dfrac{30 \text{ mg}}{12.5 \text{ mg}} \times \dfrac{5 \text{ mL}}{1} =$

$\dfrac{30}{12.5} \times \dfrac{5}{1} =$

$\dfrac{150}{12.5} = 12$ mL

20. 30 mg : 1 tab :: 60 mg : x tab
30 : 1 :: 60 : x
30x = 60
$x = \dfrac{60}{30}$
x = 2 tablets

$\dfrac{60 \text{ mg}}{30 \text{ mg}} \times 1 \text{ tab} =$

$\dfrac{60}{30} = 2$ tablets

21. 125 mg : 5 mL :: x mg : 5.5 mL
125 : 5 :: x : 5.5
5x = 687.5
$x = \dfrac{687.5}{5}$
x = 137.5 mg

$\dfrac{x \text{ mg}}{125 \text{ mg}} \times 5 \text{ mL} = 5.5 \text{ mL}$

$\dfrac{x}{\underset{25}{\cancel{125}}} \times \dfrac{\overset{1}{\cancel{5}}}{1} = 5.5$

$\dfrac{x}{25} = 5.5$

$\dfrac{\overset{1}{\cancel{25}}}{1} \times \dfrac{x}{\underset{1}{\cancel{25}}} = 5.5 \times 25$

$x = 137.5$ mg

Proportion	**Formula**

22. 40 mg : 1 tab :: 80 mg : x tab

40 : 1 :: 80 : x

$40x = 80$

$x = \dfrac{80}{40}$

$x = 2$ tablets

$\dfrac{80 \text{ mg}}{40 \text{ mg}} \times 1 \text{ tab} =$

$\dfrac{80}{40} = 2$ tablets

23. 0.4 mg : 1 tab :: x mg : 2 tab

0.4 : 1 :: x : 2

$x = 0.8$ mg

$\dfrac{x \text{ mg}}{0.4 \text{ mg}} \times 1 \text{ tab} = 2$ tablets

$\dfrac{x}{0.4} = 2$

$x = 2 \times 0.4$

$x = 0.8$ mg

24. 0.5 mg : 5 mL :: 1.5 mg : x mL

0.5 : 5 :: 1.5 : x

$0.5x = 7.5$

$x = \dfrac{7.5}{0.5}$

$x = 15$ mL

30 mL : 1 fl oz :: 15 mL : x fl oz

30 : 1 :: 15 : x

$30x = 15$

$x = \dfrac{15}{30}$

$x = \frac{1}{2}$ fl oz

$\dfrac{1.5 \text{ mg}}{0.5 \text{ mg}} \times \dfrac{5 \text{ mL}}{1} =$

$\dfrac{1.5}{0.5} \times \dfrac{5}{1} = \dfrac{7.5}{0.5}$

$\dfrac{7.5}{0.5} = 15$ mL

$15 \text{ mL} \times \dfrac{1 \text{ oz}}{30 \text{ mL}} = \dfrac{1}{2}$ fl oz

2 Tbsp — 30 mL
— 25 mL
— 20 mL
1 Tbsp — 15 mL
2 tsp — 10 mL
1 tsp — 5 mL
½ tsp —

25. 375 mg : 5 mL :: 500 mg : x mL

375 : 5 :: 500 : x

$375x = 2500$

$x = \dfrac{2500}{375}$

$x = 6.6666$ mL or 6.7 mL

$\dfrac{500 \text{ mg}}{375 \text{ mg}} \times 5 \text{ mL} =$

$\dfrac{500}{\underset{75}{375}} \times \dfrac{\overset{1}{5}}{1} =$

$\dfrac{500}{75} = 6.7$ mL

26. 50 mg : 1 tab :: 25 mg : x tab

50 : 1 :: 25 : x

$50x = 25$

$x = \dfrac{25}{50}$

$x = \frac{1}{2}$ tablet

$\dfrac{25 \text{ mg}}{50 \text{ mg}} \times 1 \text{ tab} =$

$\dfrac{25}{50} = \frac{1}{2}$ tablet

27. Supplied in 12-oz bottle

1 fl oz : 1 dose :: 12 fl oz : x dose

1 : 1 :: 12 : x

$x = 12$ doses

$\dfrac{1 \text{ dose}}{1 \text{ oz}} \times 12 \text{ oz} = 12$ doses

30 mL = 1 fl oz

Order is for 1 fl oz

ANSWERS

Proportion

Formula

28. $0.125 \text{ mg} : 1 \text{ tab} :: 0.25 \text{ mg} : x \text{ tab}$
$0.125 : 1 :: 0.25 : x$
$0.125x = 0.25$
$$x = \frac{0.25}{0.125}$$
$x = 2 \text{ tablets}$

$$\frac{0.25 \text{ mg}}{0.125 \text{ mg}} \times 1 \text{ tab} =$$
$$\frac{0.25}{0.125} = 2 \text{ tablets}$$

29. $30 \text{ mg} : 1 \text{ tab} :: 15 \text{ mg} : x \text{ tab}$
$30 : 1 :: 15 : x$
$30x = 15$
$$x = \frac{15}{30}$$
$x = \frac{1}{2} \text{ tablet}$

$$\frac{15 \text{ mg}}{30 \text{ mg}} \times 1 \text{ tab} =$$
$$\frac{15}{30} = \frac{1}{2} \text{ tablet}$$

30. $250 \text{ mg} : 5 \text{ mL} :: 125 \text{ mg} : x \text{ mL}$
$250 : 5 :: 125 : x$
$250x = 625$
$$x = \frac{625}{250}$$
$x = 2.5 \text{ mL}$

$$\frac{125 \text{ mg}}{250 \text{ mg}} \times 5 \text{ mL} =$$
$$\frac{\overset{1}{\cancel{125}}}{\underset{2}{\cancel{250}}} \times \frac{5}{1} = \frac{5}{2}$$
$$\frac{5}{2} = 2.5 \text{ mL}$$

31. $50 \text{ mg} : 1 \text{ tab} :: 25 \text{ mg} : x \text{ tab}$
$50 : 1 :: 25 : x$
$50x = 25$
$$x = \frac{25}{50}$$
$x = \frac{1}{2} \text{ tablet}$

$$\frac{25 \text{ mg}}{50 \text{ mg}} \times 1 \text{ tab} =$$
$$\frac{25}{50} = \frac{1}{2} \text{ tablet}$$

32. $1000 \text{ mg} : 1 \text{ g} :: x \text{ mg} : 0.6 \text{ g}$
$1000 : 1 :: x : 0.6$
$x = 600 \text{ mg}$
$200 \text{ mg} : 1 \text{ tab} :: 600 \text{ mg} : x \text{ tab}$
$200 : 1 :: 600 : x$
$200x = 600$
$$x = \frac{600}{200}$$
$x = 3 \text{ tablets}$
$3 \text{ tablets} : 1 \text{ dose} :: x \text{ tab} : 6 \text{ doses}$
$3 : 1 :: x : 6$
$x = 18 \text{ tablets}$

$$\frac{600 \text{ mg}}{200 \text{ mg}} = 1 \text{ tab} =$$
$$\frac{600}{200} = 3 \text{ tablets}$$
$$6 \text{ doses} \times \frac{3 \text{ tab}}{1 \text{ dose}} = 18 \text{ tablets}$$

33. $6.25 \text{ mg} : 5 \text{ mL} :: 12.5 \text{ mg} : x \text{ mL}$
$6.25 : 5 :: 12.5 : x$
$6.25x = 62.5$
$$x = \frac{62.5}{6.25}$$
$x = 10 \text{ mL}$

$$\frac{12.5 \text{ mg}}{6.25 \text{ mg}} \times 5 \text{ mL} =$$
$$\frac{\overset{2}{\cancel{12.5}}}{\underset{1}{\cancel{6.25}}} \times \frac{5}{1} =$$
$$\frac{2 \times 5}{1} = 10 \text{ mL}$$

2 Tbsp	30 mL
	25 mL
	20 mL
1 Tbsp	15 mL
2 tsp	10 mL
1 tsp	5 mL
½ tsp	

ANSWERS

Proportion

Formula

34. 500 mg : 5 mL :: 750 mg : x mL
500 : 5 :: 750 : x
500x = 3750
$x = \dfrac{3750}{500}$
x = 7.5 mL

$\dfrac{750 \text{ mg}}{500 \text{ mg}} \times 5 \text{ mL} =$

$\dfrac{\overset{15}{\cancel{750}}}{\underset{\underset{2}{100}}{\cancel{500}}} \times \dfrac{\overset{1}{\cancel{5}}}{1} =$

$\dfrac{15}{2} = 7.5 \text{ mL}$

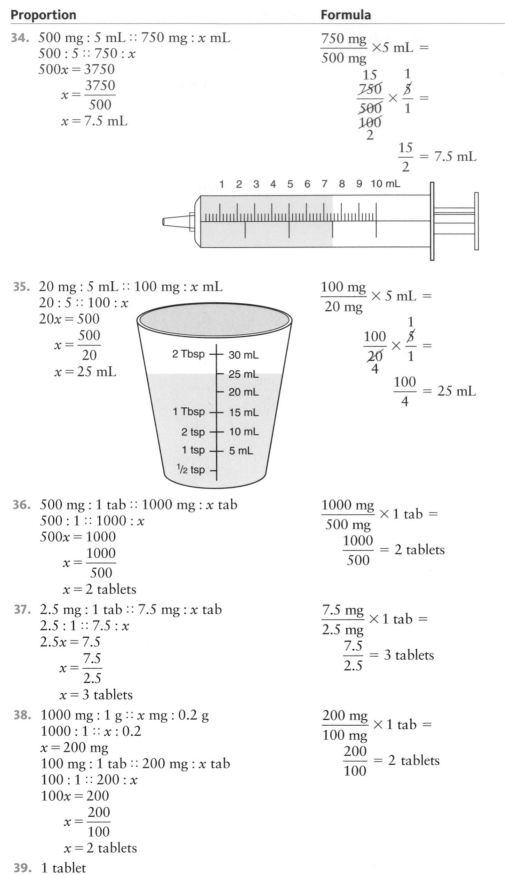

35. 20 mg : 5 mL :: 100 mg : x mL
20 : 5 :: 100 : x
20x = 500
$x = \dfrac{500}{20}$
x = 25 mL

$\dfrac{100 \text{ mg}}{20 \text{ mg}} \times 5 \text{ mL} =$

$\dfrac{100}{\underset{4}{\cancel{20}}} \times \dfrac{\overset{1}{\cancel{5}}}{1} =$

$\dfrac{100}{4} = 25 \text{ mL}$

36. 500 mg : 1 tab :: 1000 mg : x tab
500 : 1 :: 1000 : x
500x = 1000
$x = \dfrac{1000}{500}$
x = 2 tablets

$\dfrac{1000 \text{ mg}}{500 \text{ mg}} \times 1 \text{ tab} =$

$\dfrac{1000}{500} = 2 \text{ tablets}$

37. 2.5 mg : 1 tab :: 7.5 mg : x tab
2.5 : 1 :: 7.5 : x
2.5x = 7.5
$x = \dfrac{7.5}{2.5}$
x = 3 tablets

$\dfrac{7.5 \text{ mg}}{2.5 \text{ mg}} \times 1 \text{ tab} =$

$\dfrac{7.5}{2.5} = 3 \text{ tablets}$

38. 1000 mg : 1 g :: x mg : 0.2 g
1000 : 1 :: x : 0.2
x = 200 mg
100 mg : 1 tab :: 200 mg : x tab
100 : 1 :: 200 : x
100x = 200
$x = \dfrac{200}{100}$
x = 2 tablets

$\dfrac{200 \text{ mg}}{100 \text{ mg}} \times 1 \text{ tab} =$

$\dfrac{200}{100} = 2 \text{ tablets}$

39. 1 tablet
500 mg acetaminophen in each tablet

ANSWERS

Proportion	Formula
40. 0.25 mg : 1 tab :: 0.5 mg : x tab $0.25 : 1 :: 0.5 : x$ $0.25x = 0.5$ $x = \dfrac{0.5}{0.25}$ $x = 2$ tablets	$\dfrac{0.5 \text{ mg}}{0.25 \text{ mg}} \times 1 \text{ tab} =$ $\dfrac{0.5}{0.25} = 2$ tablets
41. 5 mg : 1 tab :: 10 mg : x tab $5 : 1 :: 10 : x$ $5x = 10$ $x = \dfrac{10}{5}$ $x = 2$ tablets	$\dfrac{10 \text{ mg}}{5 \text{ mg}} \times 1 \text{ tab} =$ $\dfrac{10}{5} = 2$ tablets
42. 50 mg : 1 tab :: 100 mg : x tab $50 : 1 :: 100 : x$ $50x = 100$ $x = \dfrac{100}{50}$ $x = 2$ tablets	$\dfrac{100 \text{ mg}}{50 \text{ mg}} \times 1 \text{ tab} =$ $\dfrac{100}{50} = 2$ tablets
43. 300 mg : 1 cap :: 600 mg : x cap $300 : 1 :: 600 : x$ $300x = 600$ $x = \dfrac{600}{300}$ $x = 2$ capsules	$\dfrac{600 \text{ mg}}{300 \text{ mg}} \times 1 \text{ cap} =$ $\dfrac{600}{300} = 2$ capsules
44. 0.125 mg : 1 tab :: 0.25 mg : x tab $0.125 : 1 :: 0.25 : x$ $0.125x = 0.25$ $x = \dfrac{0.25}{0.125}$ $x = 2$ tablets	$\dfrac{0.25 \text{ mg}}{0.125 \text{ mg}} \times 1 \text{ tab} =$ $\dfrac{0.25}{0.125} = 2$ tablets
45. 250 mg : 1 cap :: 500 mg : x cap $250 : 1 :: 500 : x$ $250x = 500$ $x = \dfrac{500}{250}$ $x = 2$ capsules 2 cap : 1 dose :: x cap : 4 doses $2 : 1 :: x : 4$ $x = 8$ capsules	$\dfrac{500 \text{ mg}}{250 \text{ mg}} \times 1 \text{ cap} =$ $\dfrac{500}{250} = 2$ capsules $\dfrac{2 \text{ cap}}{1 \text{ dose}} \times 4 \text{ doses} = 8$ capsules
46. 20 mg : 1 cap :: 40 mg : x cap $20 : 1 :: 40 : x$ $20x = 40$ $x = \dfrac{40}{20}$ $x = 2$ capsules	$\dfrac{40 \text{ mg}}{20 \text{ mg}} \times 1 \text{ cap} =$ $\dfrac{40}{20} = 2$ capsules

ANSWERS

Proportion   **Formula**

47. 30 mg : 1 tab :: 90 mg : x tab $\dfrac{90 \text{ mg}}{30 \text{ mg}} \times 1 \text{ tab} =$
     30 : 1 :: 90 : x
     $30x = 90$ $\dfrac{90}{30} = 3 \text{ tablets}$
     $x = \dfrac{90}{30}$
     $x = 3$ tablets

48. 75 mg : 1 tab :: 150 mg : x tab $\dfrac{150 \text{ mg}}{75 \text{ mg}} \times 1 \text{ tab} =$
     75 : 1 :: 150 : x
     $75x = 150$ $\dfrac{150}{75} = 2 \text{ tablets}$
     $x = \dfrac{150}{75}$
     $x = 2$ tablets

49. 325 mg : 1 tab :: 650 mg : x tab $\dfrac{650 \text{ mg}}{325 \text{ mg}} \times 1 \text{ tab} =$
     325 : 1 :: 650 : x
     $325x = 650$ $\dfrac{650}{325} = 2 \text{ tablets}$
     $x = \dfrac{650}{325}$
     $x = 2$ tablets

50. 15 mg : 1 mL :: 150 mg : x mL $\dfrac{150 \text{ mg}}{15 \text{ mg}} \times 1 \text{ mL} =$
     15 : 1 :: 150 : x
     $15x = 150$ $\dfrac{\overset{10}{\cancel{150}}}{\underset{1}{\cancel{15}}} = 10 \text{ mL}$
     $x = \dfrac{150}{15}$
     $x = 10$ mL

51. 250 mg : 1 tab :: 500 mg : x tab $\dfrac{500 \text{ mg}}{250 \text{ mg}} \times 1 \text{ tab} =$
     250 : 1 :: 500 : x
     $250x = 500$ $\dfrac{500}{250} = 2 \text{ tablets}$
     $x = \dfrac{500}{250}$
     $x = 2$ tablets

52. 1000 mcg : 1 mg :: x mcg : 0.2 mg $\dfrac{200 \text{ mcg}}{100 \text{ mcg}} \times 1 \text{ tab} =$
     1000 : 1 :: x : 0.2
     $x = 200$ mcg $\dfrac{200}{100} = 2 \text{ tablets}$
     100 mcg : 1 tablet :: 200 mcg : x tab
     100 : 1 :: 200 : x
     $100x = 200$
     $x = \dfrac{200}{100}$
     $x = 2$ tablets

53. 10 mg : 1 cap :: 20 mg : x cap $\dfrac{20 \text{ mg}}{10 \text{ mg}} \times 1 \text{ cap} =$
     10 : 1 :: 20 : x
     $10x = 20$ $\dfrac{20}{10} = 2 \text{ capsules}$
     $x = \dfrac{20}{10}$
     $x = 2$ capsules

ANSWERS

Proportion   **Formula**

54. $10 \text{ mg} : 5 \text{ mL} :: 30 \text{ mg} : x \text{ mL}$

$10 : 5 :: 30 : x$

$10x = 150$

$x = \dfrac{150}{10}$

$x = 15 \text{ mL}$

$\dfrac{30 \text{ mg}}{10 \text{ mg}} \times 5 \text{ mL} =$

$\dfrac{\overset{15}{\cancel{30}}}{\underset{\underset{1}{2}}{\cancel{10}}} \times \dfrac{\overset{1}{\cancel{5}}}{1} =$

$\dfrac{15}{1} = 15 \text{ mL}$

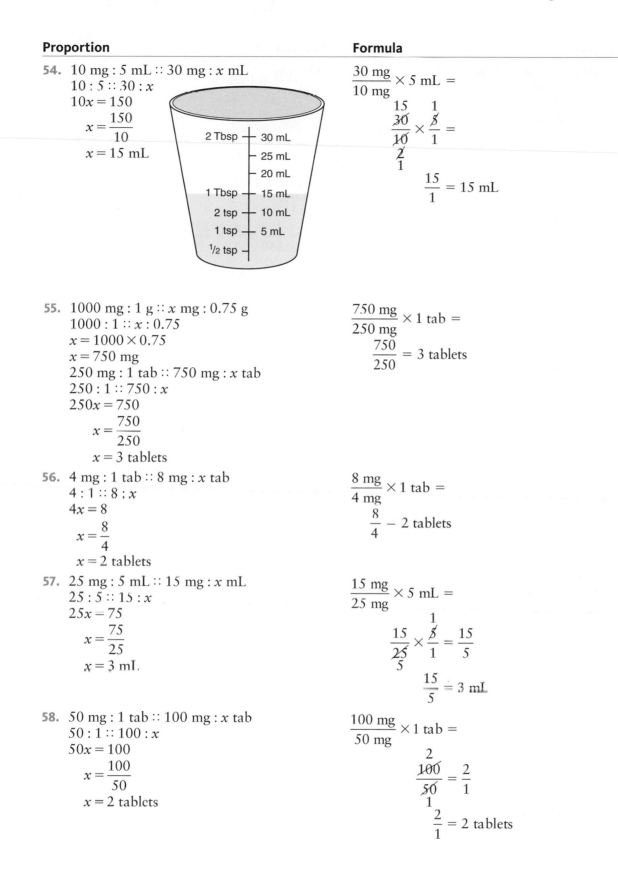

55. $1000 \text{ mg} : 1 \text{ g} :: x \text{ mg} : 0.75 \text{ g}$

$1000 : 1 :: x : 0.75$

$x = 1000 \times 0.75$

$x = 750 \text{ mg}$

$250 \text{ mg} : 1 \text{ tab} :: 750 \text{ mg} : x \text{ tab}$

$250 : 1 :: 750 : x$

$250x = 750$

$x = \dfrac{750}{250}$

$x = 3 \text{ tablets}$

$\dfrac{750 \text{ mg}}{250 \text{ mg}} \times 1 \text{ tab} =$

$\dfrac{750}{250} = 3 \text{ tablets}$

56. $4 \text{ mg} : 1 \text{ tab} :: 8 \text{ mg} : x \text{ tab}$

$4 : 1 :: 8 : x$

$4x = 8$

$x = \dfrac{8}{4}$

$x = 2 \text{ tablets}$

$\dfrac{8 \text{ mg}}{4 \text{ mg}} \times 1 \text{ tab} =$

$\dfrac{8}{4} - 2 \text{ tablets}$

57. $25 \text{ mg} : 5 \text{ mL} :: 15 \text{ mg} : x \text{ mL}$

$25 : 5 :: 15 : x$

$25x = 75$

$x = \dfrac{75}{25}$

$x = 3 \text{ mL}$

$\dfrac{15 \text{ mg}}{25 \text{ mg}} \times 5 \text{ mL} =$

$\dfrac{15}{\underset{5}{\cancel{25}}} \times \dfrac{\overset{1}{\cancel{5}}}{1} = \dfrac{15}{5}$

$\dfrac{15}{5} = 3 \text{ mL}$

58. $50 \text{ mg} : 1 \text{ tab} :: 100 \text{ mg} : x \text{ tab}$

$50 : 1 :: 100 : x$

$50x = 100$

$x = \dfrac{100}{50}$

$x = 2 \text{ tablets}$

$\dfrac{100 \text{ mg}}{50 \text{ mg}} \times 1 \text{ tab} =$

$\dfrac{\overset{2}{\cancel{100}}}{\underset{1}{\cancel{50}}} = \dfrac{2}{1}$

$\dfrac{2}{1} = 2 \text{ tablets}$

ANSWERS

Proportion	**Formula**

59. $500 \text{ mg} : 1 \text{ tab} :: 1000 \text{ mg} : x \text{ tab}$
$500 : 1 :: 1000 : x$
$500x = 1000$
$x = \dfrac{1000}{500}$
$x = 2 \text{ tablets}$

$\dfrac{1000 \text{ mg}}{500 \text{ mg}} \times 1 \text{ tab} =$
$\dfrac{1000}{500} = 2 \text{ tablets}$

60. $150 \text{ mg} : 5 \text{ mL} :: 250 \text{ mg} : x \text{ mL}$
$150 : 5 :: 250 : x$
$150x = 1250$
$x = \dfrac{1250}{150}$
$x = 8.33 \text{ mL or } 8.3 \text{ mL}$

$\dfrac{250 \text{ mg}}{150 \text{ mg}} \times 5 \text{ mL} =$
$\dfrac{250}{\underset{30}{\cancel{150}}} \times \dfrac{\overset{1}{\cancel{5}}}{1} = \dfrac{250}{30}$
$\dfrac{250}{30} = 8.33 \text{ mL or } 8.3 \text{ mL}$

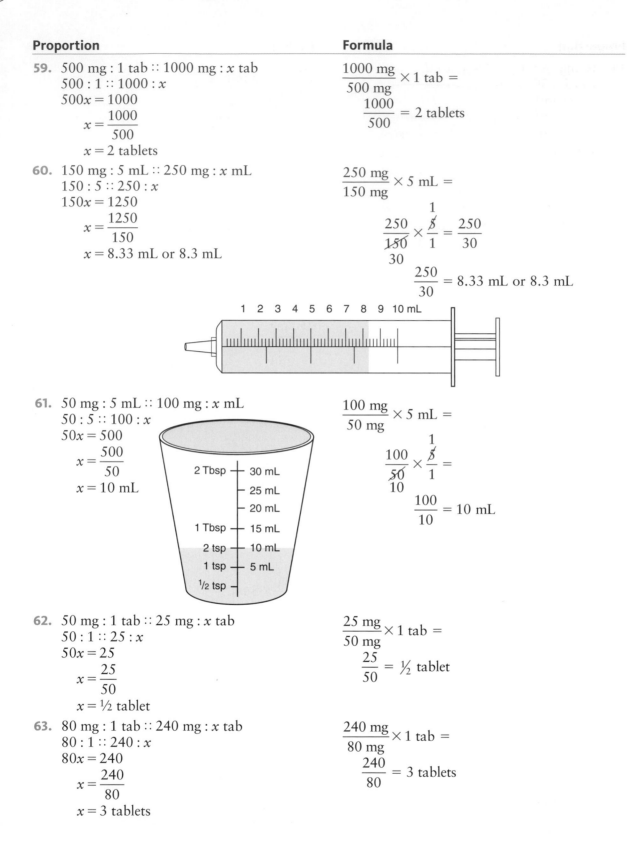

61. $50 \text{ mg} : 5 \text{ mL} :: 100 \text{ mg} : x \text{ mL}$
$50 : 5 :: 100 : x$
$50x = 500$
$x = \dfrac{500}{50}$
$x = 10 \text{ mL}$

$\dfrac{100 \text{ mg}}{50 \text{ mg}} \times 5 \text{ mL} =$
$\dfrac{100}{\underset{10}{\cancel{50}}} \times \dfrac{\overset{1}{\cancel{5}}}{1} =$
$\dfrac{100}{10} = 10 \text{ mL}$

62. $50 \text{ mg} : 1 \text{ tab} :: 25 \text{ mg} : x \text{ tab}$
$50 : 1 :: 25 : x$
$50x = 25$
$x = \dfrac{25}{50}$
$x = \frac{1}{2} \text{ tablet}$

$\dfrac{25 \text{ mg}}{50 \text{ mg}} \times 1 \text{ tab} =$
$\dfrac{25}{50} = \frac{1}{2} \text{ tablet}$

63. $80 \text{ mg} : 1 \text{ tab} :: 240 \text{ mg} : x \text{ tab}$
$80 : 1 :: 240 : x$
$80x = 240$
$x = \dfrac{240}{80}$
$x = 3 \text{ tablets}$

$\dfrac{240 \text{ mg}}{80 \text{ mg}} \times 1 \text{ tab} =$
$\dfrac{240}{80} = 3 \text{ tablets}$

ANSWERS

Proportion	Formula

64. $1000 \text{ mcg} : 1 \text{ mg} :: x \text{ mcg} : 0.05 \text{ mg}$
$1000 : 1 :: x : 0.05$
$x = 50 \text{ mcg}$
$50 \text{ mcg} : 1 \text{ mL} :: 90 \text{ mcg} : x \text{ mL}$
$50 : 1 :: 90 : x$
$50x = 90$
$x = \dfrac{90}{50}$
$x = 1.8 \text{ mL}$

$\dfrac{90 \text{ mcg}}{50 \text{ mcg}} \times 1 \text{ mL} =$
$\dfrac{90}{50} = 1.8 \text{ mL}$

65. $12.5 \text{ mg} : 5 \text{ mL} :: x \text{ mg} : 10 \text{ mL}$
$12.5 : 5 :: x : 10$
$5x = 125$
$x = \dfrac{125}{5}$
$x = 25 \text{ mg}$

$\dfrac{x \text{ mg}}{12.5 \text{ mg}} \times 5 \text{ mL} = 10 \text{ mL}$
$\dfrac{x}{12.5} \times \dfrac{5}{1} = 10$
$\dfrac{\overset{1}{\cancel{12.5}}}{1} \times \dfrac{x}{\underset{1}{\cancel{12.5}}} \times \dfrac{5}{1} = \dfrac{10}{1} \times 12.5$
$5x = 125$
$x = \dfrac{125}{5}$
$x = 25 \text{ mg}$

66. $25 \text{ mg} : 1 \text{ cap} :: 50 \text{ mg} : x \text{ cap}$
$25 : 1 :: 50 : x$
$25x = 50$
$x = \dfrac{50}{25}$
$x = 2 \text{ capsules}$

$\dfrac{50 \text{ mg}}{25 \text{ mg}} \times 1 \text{ cap} =$
$\dfrac{50}{25} = 2 \text{ capsules}$

67. $30 \text{ mg} : 1 \text{ cap} :: 90 \text{ mg} : x \text{ cap}$
$30 : 1 :: 90 : x$
$30x = 90$
$x = \dfrac{90}{30}$
$x = 3 \text{ capsules}$

$\dfrac{90 \text{ mg}}{30 \text{ mg}} \times 1 \text{ cap} =$
$\dfrac{90}{30} = 3 \text{ capsules}$

68. 40-mg tablet
$40 \text{ mg} : 1 \text{ tab} :: 40 \text{ mg} : x \text{ tab}$
$40 : 1 :: 40 : x$
$40x = 40$
$x = \dfrac{40}{40}$
$x = 1 \text{ tablet}$

40-mg tablets. The other strengths of the medication would require swallowing more pills.
$40 \text{ mg} \times \dfrac{1 \text{ tab}}{40 \text{ mg}} = 1 \text{ tablet}$

69. $20 \text{ mEq} : 15 \text{ mL} :: 10 \text{ mEq} : x \text{ mL}$
$20 : 15 :: 10 : x$
$20x = 150$
$x = \dfrac{150}{20}$
$x = 7.5 \text{ mL}$

$\dfrac{10 \text{ mEq}}{20 \text{ mEq}} \times \dfrac{15 \text{ mL}}{1} =$
$\dfrac{10}{\underset{4}{\cancel{20}}} \times \dfrac{\overset{3}{\cancel{15}}}{1} = \dfrac{30}{4}$
$\dfrac{30}{4} = 7.5 \text{ mL}$

1 2 3 4 5 6 7 8 9 10 mL

ANSWERS

Proportion   **Formula**

70. 0.5 mg : 1 tab :: 1.5 mg : x tab

0.5 : 1 :: 1.5 : x

0.5x = 1.5

$x = \dfrac{1.5}{0.5}$

x = 3 tablets

$\dfrac{1.5 \text{ mg}}{0.5 \text{ mg}} \times 1 \text{ tab} =$

$\dfrac{1.5}{0.5}$ = 3 tablets

71. 0.25 mg : 1 tab :: 0.5 mg : x tab

0.25 : 1 :: 0.5 : x

0.25x = 0.5

$x = \dfrac{0.5}{0.25}$

x = 2 tablets

$\dfrac{0.5 \text{ mg}}{0.25 \text{ mg}} \times 1 \text{ tab} =$

$\dfrac{0.5}{0.25}$ = 2 tablets

72. 325 mg : 1 tab :: 650 mg : x tab

325 : 1 :: 650 : x

325x = 650

$x = \dfrac{650}{325}$

x = 2 tablets

$\dfrac{\overset{2}{\cancel{650}} \text{ mg}}{\underset{1}{\cancel{325}} \text{ mg}} \times 1 \text{ tab} =$

$\dfrac{2}{1}$ = 2 tablets

73. 0.25 mg : 1 tab :: 0.5 mg : x tab

0.25 : 1 :: 0.5 : x

0.25x = 0.5

$x = \dfrac{0.5}{0.25}$

x = 2 tablets

$\dfrac{0.5 \text{ mg}}{0.25 \text{ mg}} \times 1 \text{ tab} =$

$\dfrac{0.5}{0.25}$ = 2 tablets

74. 375 mg : x mL :: 125 mg : 5 mL

375 : x :: 125 : 5

125x = 1875

x = 15 mL

$\dfrac{375 \text{ mg}}{125 \text{ mg}} \times 5 \text{ mL} = 15 \text{ mL}$

75. 30 mg : 1 tab :: 30 mg : x tab

30 : 1 :: 30 : x

30x = 30

$x = \dfrac{30}{30}$

x = 1 tab

$\dfrac{30 \text{ mg}}{30 \text{ mg}} \times 1 \text{ tab} =$

$\dfrac{30}{30}$ = 1 tablet

76. 0.15 mg : 1 tab :: 0.3 mg : x tab

0.15 : 1 :: 0.3 : x

0.15x = 0.3

$x = \dfrac{0.3}{0.15}$

x = 2 tablets of 0.15 mg

$\dfrac{0.3 \text{ mg}}{0.15 \text{ mg}} \times 1 \text{ tab} =$

$\dfrac{0.3}{0.15}$ = 2 tablets of 0.15 mg

77. 5 mg : 1 tab :: 7.5 mg : x tab

5 : 1 :: 7.5 : x

5x = 7.5

$x = \dfrac{7.5}{5}$

x = 1.5 tablets

$\dfrac{7.5 \text{ mg}}{5 \text{ mg}} \times 1 \text{ tab} =$

$\dfrac{7.5}{5}$ = 1.5 tablets

ANSWERS

Proportion   **Formula**

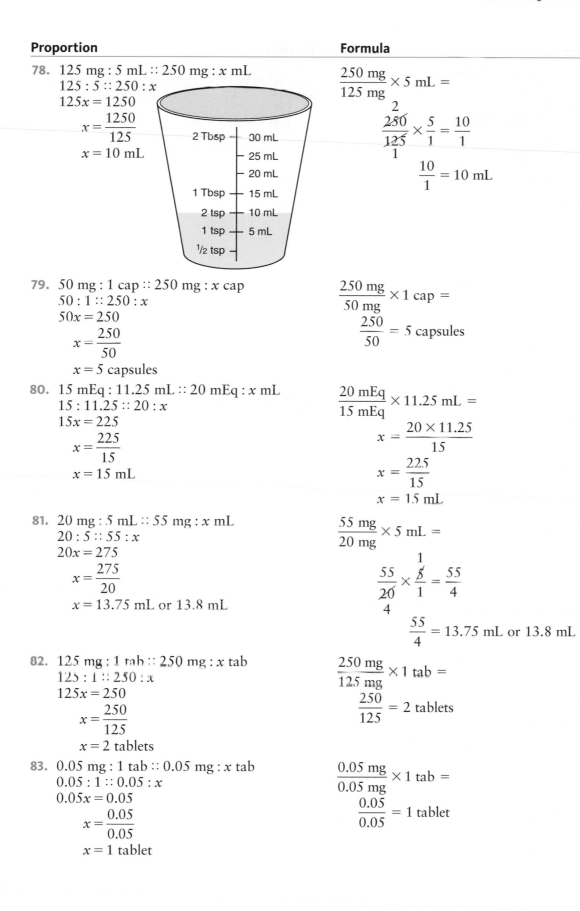

78. 125 mg : 5 mL :: 250 mg : x mL
125 : 5 :: 250 : x
$125x = 1250$
$x = \dfrac{1250}{125}$
$x = 10$ mL

$\dfrac{250\text{ mg}}{125\text{ mg}} \times 5\text{ mL} =$

$\dfrac{\overset{2}{\cancel{250}}}{\underset{1}{\cancel{125}}} \times \dfrac{5}{1} = \dfrac{10}{1}$

$\dfrac{10}{1} = 10$ mL

79. 50 mg : 1 cap :: 250 mg : x cap
50 : 1 :: 250 : x
$50x = 250$
$x = \dfrac{250}{50}$
$x = 5$ capsules

$\dfrac{250\text{ mg}}{50\text{ mg}} \times 1\text{ cap} =$

$\dfrac{250}{50} = 5$ capsules

80. 15 mEq : 11.25 mL :: 20 mEq : x mL
15 : 11.25 :: 20 : x
$15x = 225$
$x = \dfrac{225}{15}$
$x = 15$ mL

$\dfrac{20\text{ mEq}}{15\text{ mEq}} \times 11.25\text{ mL} =$

$x = \dfrac{20 \times 11.25}{15}$

$x = \dfrac{225}{15}$

$x = 15$ mL

81. 20 mg : 5 mL :: 55 mg : x mL
20 : 5 :: 55 : x
$20x = 275$
$x = \dfrac{275}{20}$
$x = 13.75$ mL or 13.8 mL

$\dfrac{55\text{ mg}}{20\text{ mg}} \times 5\text{ mL} =$

$\dfrac{55}{\underset{4}{\cancel{20}}} \times \dfrac{\overset{1}{\cancel{5}}}{1} = \dfrac{55}{4}$

$\dfrac{55}{4} = 13.75$ mL or 13.8 mL

82. 125 mg : 1 tab :: 250 mg : x tab
125 : 1 :: 250 : x
$125x = 250$
$x = \dfrac{250}{125}$
$x = 2$ tablets

$\dfrac{250\text{ mg}}{125\text{ mg}} \times 1\text{ tab} =$

$\dfrac{250}{125} = 2$ tablets

83. 0.05 mg : 1 tab :: 0.05 mg : x tab
0.05 : 1 :: 0.05 : x
$0.05x = 0.05$
$x = \dfrac{0.05}{0.05}$
$x = 1$ tablet

$\dfrac{0.05\text{ mg}}{0.05\text{ mg}} \times 1\text{ tab} =$

$\dfrac{0.05}{0.05} = 1$ tablet

ANSWERS

Proportion	Formula
84. $1000 \text{ mg} : 1 \text{ g} :: x \text{ mg} : 0.2 \text{ g}$ $1000 : 1 :: x : 0.2$ $x = 200 \text{ mg}$ Give 1 tablet of 200 mg $200 \text{ mg} : 1 \text{ dose} :: x \text{ mg} : 3 \text{ doses}$ $x = 600 \text{ mg}$ will be given per day	$\dfrac{200 \text{ mg}}{200 \text{ mg}} \times 1 \text{ tab} =$ $\dfrac{200}{200} = 1 \text{ tablet}$ $\dfrac{200 \text{ mg}}{1 \text{ dose}} \times 3 \text{ doses} = 600 \text{ mg}$
85. $5 \text{ mg} : 1 \text{ tab} :: 15 \text{ mg} : x \text{ tab}$ $5 : 1 :: 15 : x$ $5x = 15$ $x = \dfrac{15}{5}$ $x = 3 \text{ tablets}$	$\dfrac{15 \text{ mg}}{5 \text{ mg}} \times 1 \text{ tab} =$ $\dfrac{15}{5} = 3 \text{ tablets}$
86. $400 \text{ mg} : 1 \text{ tab} :: 800 \text{ mg} : x \text{ tab}$ $400 : 1 :: 800 : x$ $400x = 800$ $x = \dfrac{800}{400}$ $x = 2 \text{ tablets}$	$\dfrac{800 \text{ mg}}{400 \text{ mg}} \times 1 \text{ tab} =$ $\dfrac{800}{400} = 2 \text{ tablets}$
87. $250 \text{ mg} : 1 \text{ cap} :: 500 \text{ mg} : x \text{ cap}$ $250 : 1 :: 500 : x$ $250x = 500$ $x = \dfrac{500}{250}$ $x = 2 \text{ capsules}$	$\dfrac{500 \text{ mg}}{250 \text{ mg}} \times 1 \text{ cap} =$ $\dfrac{500}{250} = 2 \text{ capsules}$
88. $25 \text{ mg} : 1 \text{ tab} :: 50 \text{ mg} : x \text{ tab}$ $25 : 1 :: 50 : x$ $25x = 50$ $x = \dfrac{50}{25}$ $x = 2 \text{ tablets}$	$\dfrac{50 \text{ mg}}{25 \text{ mg}} \times 1 \text{ tab} =$ $\dfrac{50}{25} = 2 \text{ tablets}$
89. $10 \text{ mg} : 1 \text{ pill} :: 30 \text{ mg} : x \text{ pills}$ $10 : 1 :: 30 : x$ $10x = 30$ $x = \dfrac{30}{10}$ $x = 3 \text{ pills}$	$\dfrac{30 \text{ mg}}{10 \text{ mg}} \times 1 \text{ pill} =$ $\dfrac{30}{10} = 3 \text{ pills}$
90. $10 \text{ mg} : 1 \text{ mL} : 6 \text{ mg} : x \text{ mL}$ $10 : 1 :: 6 : x$ $10x = 6$ $x = \dfrac{6}{10}$ $x = 0.6 \text{ mL}$	$\dfrac{6 \text{ mg}}{10 \text{ mg}} \times 1 \text{ mL} = 0.6 \text{ mL}$
91. $75 \text{ mg} : 1 \text{ cap} :: 150 \text{ mg} : x \text{ cap}$ $75 : 1 :: 150 : x$ $75x = 150$ $x = \dfrac{150}{75}$ $x = 2 \text{ capsules}$	$\dfrac{150 \text{ mg}}{75 \text{ mg}} \times 1 \text{ cap} =$ $\dfrac{150}{75} = 2 \text{ capsules}$

ANSWERS

Proportion	**Formula**

92. 100 mg : 1 cap :: 200 mg : x cap
  100 : 1 :: 200 : x
  $100x = 200$
  $x = \dfrac{200}{100}$
  $x = 2$ capsules

$\dfrac{200 \text{ mg}}{100 \text{ mg}} \times 1 \text{ cap} =$
$\dfrac{200}{100} = 2$ capsules

93. 2.5 mg : 1 tab :: 10 mg : x tab
  2.5 : 1 :: 10 : x
  $2.5x = 10$
  $x = \dfrac{10}{2.5}$
  $x = 4$ tablets

$\dfrac{10 \text{ mg}}{2.5 \text{ mg}} \times 1 \text{ tab} =$
$\dfrac{10}{2.5} = 4$ tablets

94. 1000 mg : 1 g :: x mg : 0.25 g
  1000 : 1 :: x : 0.25
  $x = 250$ mg
  250 mg : 1 tab :: 250 mg : x tab
  250 : 1 :: 250 : x
  $250x = 250$
  $x = 1$ tablet

$\dfrac{250 \text{ mg}}{250 \text{ mg}} \times 1 \text{ tab} =$
$\dfrac{250}{250} = 1$ tablet

95. 10 mg : 1 tab :: 25 mg : x tab
  10 : 1 :: 25 : x
  $10x = 25$
  $x = \dfrac{25}{10}$
  $x = 2.5$ tablets

$\dfrac{25 \text{ mg}}{10 \text{ mg}} \times 1 \text{ tab} =$
$\dfrac{25}{10} = 2.5$ tablets

96. 10 mg : 1 tab :: 30 mg : x tab
  10 : 1 :: 30 : x
  $10x = 30$
  $x = \dfrac{30}{10}$
  $x = 3$ tablets

$\dfrac{30 \text{ mg}}{10 \text{ mg}} \times 1 \text{ tab} =$
$\dfrac{\overset{3}{\cancel{30}}}{\underset{1}{\cancel{10}}} = 3$ tablets

97. 5 mg : 1 tab :: 15 mg : x tab
  5 : 1 :: 15 : x
  $5x = 15$
  $x = \dfrac{15}{5}$
  $x = 3$ tablets

$\dfrac{15 \text{ mg}}{5 \text{ mg}} \times 1 \text{ tab} =$
$\dfrac{15}{5} = 3$ tablets

98. 1000 mg : 1 g :: x mg : 0.015 g
  1000 : 1 :: x : 0.015
  $x = 15$ mg
  15 mg : 1 cap :: 15 mg : x cap
  15 : 1 :: 15 : x
  $15x = 15$
  $x = \dfrac{15}{15}$
  $x = 1$ capsule

$\dfrac{15 \text{ mg}}{15 \text{ mg}} \times 1 \text{ cap} =$
$\dfrac{15}{15} = 1$ capsule

ANSWERS

Proportion	Formula

99. 6.7 mEq : 5 mL :: 30 mEq : x mL
6.7 : 5 :: 30 : x
6.7x = 150
$x = \dfrac{150}{6.7}$
x = 22.4 mL

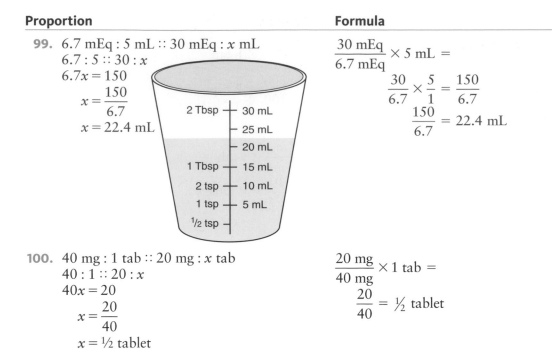

2 Tbsp — 30 mL
— 25 mL
— 20 mL
1 Tbsp — 15 mL
2 tsp — 10 mL
1 tsp — 5 mL
½ tsp —

$\dfrac{30 \text{ mEq}}{6.7 \text{ mEq}} \times 5 \text{ mL} =$
$\dfrac{30}{6.7} \times \dfrac{5}{1} = \dfrac{150}{6.7}$
$\dfrac{150}{6.7} = 22.4$ mL

100. 40 mg : 1 tab :: 20 mg : x tab
40 : 1 :: 20 : x
40x = 20
$x = \dfrac{20}{40}$
x = ½ tablet

$\dfrac{20 \text{ mg}}{40 \text{ mg}} \times 1 \text{ tab} =$
$\dfrac{20}{40} = $ ½ tablet

CHAPTER 11 Proportion/Formula Method—Posttest 1, pp. 225–230

Proportion	Formula

1. 325 : 1 tab :: 975 : x tab
325 : 1 :: 975 : x
325x = 975
$x = \dfrac{975}{325}$
x = 3 tablets

$\dfrac{975 \text{ mg}}{325 \text{ mg}} \times 1 \text{ tab} =$
$\dfrac{975}{325} = 3$ tablets

2. 1000 mg : 1 g :: x mg : 0.5 g
1000 : 1 :: x : 0.5
x = 500 mg
500 mg : 1 cap :: 500 mg : x cap
500 : 1 :: 500 : x
500x = 500
$x = \dfrac{500}{500}$
x = 1 capsule

$\dfrac{500 \text{ mg}}{500 \text{ mg}} \times 1 \text{ cap} =$
$\dfrac{500}{500} = 1$ capsule

3. 250 mg : 1 cap :: 1000 mg : x cap
250 : 1 :: 1000 : x
250x = 1000
$x = \dfrac{1000}{250}$
x = 4 capsules

$\dfrac{1000 \text{ mg}}{250 \text{ mg}} \times 1 \text{ cap} =$
$\dfrac{1000}{250} = 4$ capsules

ANSWERS

Proportion | **Formula**

4. 30 mg : 1 tab :: 60 mg : x tab
30 : 1 :: 60 : x
$30x = 60$
$x = \dfrac{\overset{2}{\cancel{60}}}{\underset{1}{\cancel{30}}}$
$x = 2$ tablets

$\dfrac{60 \text{ mg}}{30 \text{ mg}} \times 1 \text{ tab} =$
$\dfrac{\overset{2}{\cancel{60}}}{\underset{1}{\cancel{30}}} = 2$ tablets

5. 100 mcg = 0.1 mg
0.05 mg : 1 tab :: 0.1 : x tab
0.05 : 1 :: 0.1 : x
$0.05x = 0.1$
$x = \dfrac{0.1}{0.05}$
$x = 2$ tablets

$\dfrac{0.1 \text{ mg}}{0.05 \text{ mg}} \times 1 \text{ tab} =$
$\dfrac{0.1}{0.05} = 2$ tablets

6. 10 mg : 5 mL :: 25 mg : x mL
10 : 5 :: 25 : x
$10x = 125$
$x = \dfrac{125}{10}$
$x = 12.5$ mL

$\dfrac{25 \text{ mg}}{10 \text{ mg}} \times 5 \text{ mL} =$
$\dfrac{25}{\underset{2}{\cancel{10}}} \times \dfrac{\overset{1}{\cancel{5}}}{1} = \dfrac{25}{2}$
$\dfrac{25}{2} = 12.5$ mL

7. 120 mg : 1 tab :: 60 mg : x tab
120 : 1 :: 60 : x
$120x = 60$
$x = \dfrac{60}{120}$
$x = \frac{1}{2}$ tablet

$\dfrac{60 \text{ mg}}{120 \text{ mg}} \times 1 \text{ tab} =$
$\dfrac{\overset{1}{\cancel{60}}}{\underset{2}{\cancel{120}}} = \frac{1}{2}$ tablet

8. 30 mg : 1 tab :: 30 mg : x tab
30 : 1 :: 30 : x
$30x = 30$
$x = \dfrac{30}{30}$
$x = 1$ tablet

$\dfrac{30 \text{ mg}}{30 \text{ mg}} \times 1 \text{ tab} =$
$\dfrac{30}{30} = 1$ tablet

ANSWERS

Proportion	Formula

9. $25 \text{ mg} : 5 \text{ mL} :: 50 \text{ mg} : x \text{ mL}$
$25 : 5 :: 50 : x$
$25x = 250$
$x = \dfrac{250}{25}$
$x = 10 \text{ mL}$

$\dfrac{50 \text{ mg}}{25 \text{ mg}} \times 5 \text{ mL} =$

$\dfrac{\overset{5}{\cancel{50}}}{\underset{5}{\cancel{25}}} \times \dfrac{\overset{1}{\cancel{5}}}{1} =$

$\dfrac{10}{1} = 10 \text{ mL}$

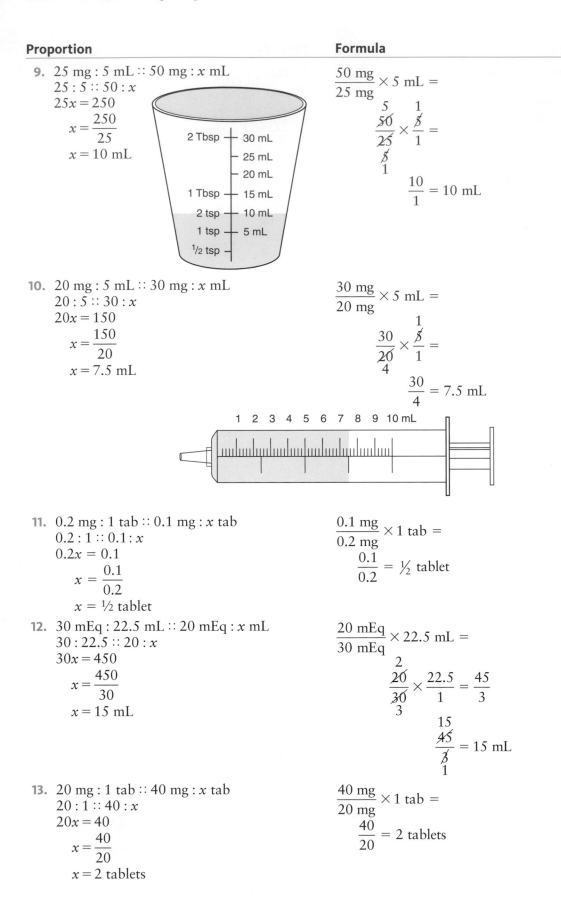

10. $20 \text{ mg} : 5 \text{ mL} :: 30 \text{ mg} : x \text{ mL}$
$20 : 5 :: 30 : x$
$20x = 150$
$x = \dfrac{150}{20}$
$x = 7.5 \text{ mL}$

$\dfrac{30 \text{ mg}}{20 \text{ mg}} \times 5 \text{ mL} =$

$\dfrac{30}{\underset{4}{\cancel{20}}} \times \dfrac{\overset{1}{\cancel{5}}}{1} =$

$\dfrac{30}{4} = 7.5 \text{ mL}$

11. $0.2 \text{ mg} : 1 \text{ tab} :: 0.1 \text{ mg} : x \text{ tab}$
$0.2 : 1 :: 0.1 : x$
$0.2x = 0.1$
$x = \dfrac{0.1}{0.2}$
$x = \frac{1}{2} \text{ tablet}$

$\dfrac{0.1 \text{ mg}}{0.2 \text{ mg}} \times 1 \text{ tab} =$

$\dfrac{0.1}{0.2} = \frac{1}{2} \text{ tablet}$

12. $30 \text{ mEq} : 22.5 \text{ mL} :: 20 \text{ mEq} : x \text{ mL}$
$30 : 22.5 :: 20 : x$
$30x = 450$
$x = \dfrac{450}{30}$
$x = 15 \text{ mL}$

$\dfrac{20 \text{ mEq}}{30 \text{ mEq}} \times 22.5 \text{ mL} =$

$\dfrac{\overset{2}{\cancel{20}}}{\underset{3}{\cancel{30}}} \times \dfrac{22.5}{1} = \dfrac{45}{3}$

$\dfrac{\overset{15}{\cancel{45}}}{\underset{1}{\cancel{3}}} = 15 \text{ mL}$

13. $20 \text{ mg} : 1 \text{ tab} :: 40 \text{ mg} : x \text{ tab}$
$20 : 1 :: 40 : x$
$20x = 40$
$x = \dfrac{40}{20}$
$x = 2 \text{ tablets}$

$\dfrac{40 \text{ mg}}{20 \text{ mg}} \times 1 \text{ tab} =$

$\dfrac{40}{20} = 2 \text{ tablets}$

ANSWERS

Proportion	**Formula**

14. 50 mg : 1 cap :: 100 mg : x cap
50 : 1 :: 100 : x
50x = 100
$x = \dfrac{100}{50}$
x = 2 capsules

$\dfrac{100 \text{ mg}}{50 \text{ mg}} \times 1 \text{ cap} =$
$\dfrac{100}{50} = 2 \text{ capsules}$

15. 10 mg : 1 mL :: 38 mg : x mL
10 : 1 :: 38 : x
10x = 38
$x = \dfrac{38}{10}$
x = 3.8 mL

$\dfrac{38 \text{ mg}}{10 \text{ mg}} \times 1 \text{ mL} =$
$\dfrac{38}{10} = 3.8 \text{ mL}$

16. 125 mg : 5 mL :: 100 mg : x mL
125 : 5 :: 100 : x
125x = 500
$x = \dfrac{500}{125}$
x = 4 mL

$\dfrac{100 \text{ mg}}{125 \text{ mg}} \times 5 \text{ mL} =$
$\dfrac{100}{\underset{25}{\cancel{125}}} \times \dfrac{\overset{1}{\cancel{5}}}{1} = \dfrac{100}{25}$
$\dfrac{100}{25} = 4 \text{ mL}$

17. 10 mg : 1 tab :: 30 mg : x tab
10 : 1 :: 30 : x
10x = 30
$x = \dfrac{30}{10}$
x = 3 tablets

$\dfrac{30 \text{ mg}}{10 \text{ mg}} \times 1 \text{ tab} =$
$\dfrac{30}{10} = 3 \text{ tablets}$

18. 40 mg : 1 tab :: 80 mg : x tab
40 : 1 :: 80 : x
40x = 80
$x = \dfrac{80}{40}$
x = 2 tablets

$\dfrac{80 \text{ mg}}{40 \text{ mg}} \times 1 \text{ tab} =$
$\dfrac{80}{40} = 2 \text{ tablets}$

19. 10 mg : 1 tab :: 20 mg : x tab
10 : 1 :: 20 : x
10x = 20
$x = \dfrac{20}{10}$
x = 2 tablets

$\dfrac{20 \text{ mg}}{10 \text{ mg}} \times 1 \text{ tab} =$
$\dfrac{20}{10} = 2 \text{ tablets}$

ANSWERS

Proportion	Formula

20. 60 mg : 1 tab :: 90 mg : x tab
60 : 1 :: 90 : x
$60x = 90$
$x = \dfrac{90}{60}$
$x = 1\frac{1}{2}$ tablets per dose
$1\frac{1}{2}$ tab : 1 dose :: x tab : 3 doses
$\frac{3}{2} : 1 :: x : 3$
$x = \dfrac{3}{2} \times \dfrac{3}{1}$
$x = \dfrac{9}{2}$
$x = 4\frac{1}{2}$ tablets/day

$\dfrac{90 \text{ mg}}{60 \text{ mg}} \times 1 \text{ tab} =$
$\dfrac{90}{60} = 1\frac{1}{2}$ tablets per dose

21. 0.25 mg : 1 tab :: 0.5 mg : x tab
0.25 : 1 :: 0.5 : x
$0.25x = 0.5$
$x = \dfrac{0.5}{0.25}$
$x = 2$ tablets

$\dfrac{0.5 \text{ mg}}{0.25 \text{ mg}} \times 1 \text{ tab} =$
$\dfrac{0.5}{0.25} = 2$ tablets

22. 5 mg : 1 tab :: 10 mg : x tab
5 : 1 :: 10 : x
$5x = 10$
$x = \dfrac{10}{5}$
$x = 2$ tablets

$\dfrac{10 \text{ mg}}{5 \text{ mg}} \times 1 \text{ tab} =$
$\dfrac{10}{5} = 2$ tablets

23. 100 mg : 1 tab :: 150 mg : x tab
100 : 1 :: 150 : x
$100x = 150$
$x = \dfrac{150}{100}$
$x = 1\frac{1}{2}$ tablets

$\dfrac{150 \text{ mg}}{100 \text{ mg}} \times 1 \text{ tab} =$
$\dfrac{150}{100} = 1\frac{1}{2}$ tablets

24. 10 mg : 1 tab :: 30 mg : x tab
10 : 1 :: 30 : x
$10x = 30$
$x = \dfrac{30}{10}$
$x = 3$ tablets

$\dfrac{30 \text{ mg}}{10 \text{ mg}} \times 1 \text{ tab} =$
$\dfrac{30}{10} = 3$ tablets

25. 30 mg : 1 tab :: 60 mg : x tab
30 : 1 :: 60 : x
$30x = 60$
$x = \dfrac{60}{30}$
$x = 2$ tablets

$\dfrac{60 \text{ mg}}{30 \text{ mg}} \times 1 \text{ tab} =$
$\dfrac{60}{30} = 2$ tablets

CHAPTER 11 Proportion/Formula Method—Posttest 2, pp. 231–237

Proportion	Formula

1. 10 mg : 1 cap :: 20 mg : x cap
10 : 1 :: 20 : x
$10x = 20$
$x = \dfrac{20}{10}$
$x = 2$ capsules

$\dfrac{20 \text{ mg}}{10 \text{ mg}} \times 1 \text{ cap} =$
$\dfrac{20}{10} = 2$ capsules

2. 4 mg : 5 mL :: 8 mg : x mL
4 : 5 :: 8 : x
$4x = 40$
$x = \dfrac{40}{4}$
$x = 10$ mL

$\dfrac{8 \text{ mg}}{4 \text{ mg}} \times 5 \text{ mL} =$
$\dfrac{\overset{2}{\cancel{8}}}{\underset{1}{\cancel{4}}} \times \dfrac{5}{1} = \dfrac{10}{1} = 10$ mL

3. 25 mg : 5 mL :: 60 mg : x mL
25 : 5 :: 60 : x
$25x = 300$
$x = \dfrac{300}{25}$
$x = 12$ mL

$\dfrac{60 \text{ mg}}{25 \text{ mg}} \times 5 \text{ mL} =$
$\dfrac{60}{\underset{5}{\cancel{25}}} \times \dfrac{\overset{1}{\cancel{5}}}{1} = \dfrac{60}{5}$
$\dfrac{60}{5} = 12$ mL

4. 10 mg : 1 tab :: 15 mg : x tab
10 : 1 :: 15 : x
$10x = 15$
$x = \dfrac{15}{10}$
$x = 1\frac{1}{2}$ tablets

$\dfrac{15 \text{ mg}}{10 \text{ mg}} \times 1 \text{ tab} =$
$\dfrac{15}{10} = 1\frac{1}{2}$ tablets

5. 20 mEq : 30 mL :: 5 mEq : x mL
20 : 30 :: 5 : x
$20x = 150$
$x = \dfrac{150}{20}$
$x = 7.5$ mL

$\dfrac{5 \text{ mEq}}{20 \text{ mEq}} \times 30 \text{ mL} =$
$\dfrac{5}{\underset{2}{\cancel{20}}} \times \dfrac{\overset{3}{\cancel{30}}}{1} = \dfrac{15}{2}$
$\dfrac{15}{2} = 7.5$ mL

2 Tbsp — 30 mL
— 25 mL
— 20 mL
1 Tbsp — 15 mL
2 tsp — 10 mL
1 tsp — 5 mL
½ tsp —

6. 1000 mg : 1 g :: x mg : 0.25 g
1000 : 1 :: x : 0.25
$x = 250$ mg
250 mg : 1 cap :: 250 mg : x cap
250 : 1 :: 250 : x
$250x = 250$
$x = \dfrac{250}{250}$
$x = 1$ capsule

$\dfrac{250 \text{ mg}}{250 \text{ mg}} \times 1 \text{ cap} =$
$\dfrac{250}{250} = 1$ capsule

ANSWERS

Proportion   **Formula**

7. 2.5 mg : 1 tab :: 7.5 mg : x tab $\dfrac{7.5 \text{ mg}}{2.5 \text{ mg}} \times 1 \text{ cap} =$
    2.5 : 1 :: 7.5 : x
    $2.5x = 7.5$ $\dfrac{7.5}{2.5} = 3 \text{ tablets}$
    $x = \dfrac{7.5}{2.5}$
    $x = 3$ tablets

8. 0.05 mg : 1 mL :: 0.05 mg : x mL $\dfrac{0.05 \text{ mg}}{0.05 \text{ mg}} \times 1 \text{ mL} =$
    0.05 : 1 :: 0.05 : x
    $0.05x = 0.05$ $\dfrac{0.05}{0.05} = 1 \text{ mL}$
    $x = \dfrac{0.05}{0.05}$
    $x = 1$ mL

9. 1000 mg : 1 g :: x mg : 0.1 g $\dfrac{100 \text{ mg}}{50 \text{ mg}} \times 1 \text{ cap} =$
    1000 : 1 :: x : 0.1
    $x = 100$ mg $\dfrac{100}{50} = 2 \text{ capsules}$
    50 mg : 1 cap :: 100 mg : x cap
    50 : 1 :: 100 : x
    $50x = 100$
    $x = \dfrac{100}{50}$
    $x = 2$ capsules

10. 325 mg : 1 tab :: 650 mg : x tab $\dfrac{650 \text{ mg}}{325 \text{ mg}} \times 1 \text{ tab} =$
    325 : 1 :: 650 : x
    $325x = 650$ $\dfrac{650}{325} = 2 \text{ tablets}$
    $x = \dfrac{650}{325}$
    $x = 2$ tablets

11. 50 mg : 1 tab :: 100 mg : x tab $\dfrac{100 \text{ mg}}{50 \text{ mg}} \times 1 \text{ tab} =$
    50 : 1 :: 100 : x
    $50x = 100$ $\dfrac{100}{50} = 2 \text{ tablets}$
    $x = \dfrac{100}{50}$
    $x = 2$ tablets

12. 125 mg : 5 mL :: 250 mg : x mL $\dfrac{250 \text{ mg}}{125 \text{ mg}} \times 5 \text{ mL} =$
    125 : 5 :: 250 : x
    $125x = 1250$ $\dfrac{250}{\overset{25}{\cancel{125}}} \times \dfrac{\overset{1}{\cancel{5}}}{1} = \dfrac{250}{25}$
    $x = \dfrac{1250}{125}$
    $x = 10$ mL $\dfrac{250}{25} = 10 \text{ mL}$

2 Tbsp — 30 mL
        — 25 mL
        — 20 mL
1 Tbsp — 15 mL
2 tsp — 10 mL
1 tsp — 5 mL
½ tsp —

ANSWERS

Proportion	Formula

13. 5 mg : 1 tab :: 20 mg : x tab
5 : 1 :: 20 : x
$5x = 20$
$x = \dfrac{20}{5}$
$x = 4$ tablets of 5 mg/tab

$\dfrac{20 \text{ mg}}{5 \text{ mg}} \times 1 \text{ tab} =$
$\dfrac{20}{5} = 4$ tablets of 5 mg/tab

14. 0.125 mg : 1 tab :: 0.25 mg : x tab
0.125 : 1 :: 0.25 : x
$0.125x = 0.25$
$x = \dfrac{0.25}{0.125}$
$x = 2$ tablets

$\dfrac{0.25 \text{ mg}}{0.125 \text{ mg}} \times 1 \text{ tab} =$
$\dfrac{0.25}{0.125} = 2$ tablets

15. 20 mg : 5 mL :: 25 mg : x mL
20 : 5 :: 25 : x
$20x = 125$
$x = \dfrac{125}{20}$
$x = 6.25$ mL or 6.3 mL

$\dfrac{25 \text{ mg}}{20 \text{ mg}} \times 5 \text{ mL} =$
$\dfrac{25}{\overset{4}{\cancel{20}}} \times \dfrac{\overset{1}{\cancel{5}}}{1} = \dfrac{25}{4}$
$\dfrac{25}{4} = 6.25$ mL or 6.3 mL

16. 1000 mg : 1 g :: x mg : 0.15 g
$x = 150$ mg
100 mg : 1 tab :: 150 mg : x tab
100 : 1 :: 150 : x
$100x = 150$
$x = \dfrac{150}{100}$
$x = 1.5$ tablets

$\dfrac{150 \text{ mg}}{100 \text{ mg}} \times 1 \text{ tab}$
$\dfrac{150}{100} = 1.5$ tablets

17. 40 mg : 1 tab :: 80 mg : x tab
40 : 1 :: 80 : x
$40x = 80$
$x = \dfrac{80}{40}$
$x = 2$ tablets

$\dfrac{80 \text{ mg}}{40 \text{ mg}} \times 1 \text{ tab} =$
$\dfrac{\overset{2}{\cancel{80}}}{\underset{1}{\cancel{40}}} = 2$ tablets

18. 7.5 mg : 1 tab :: 15 mg : x tab
7.5 : 1 :: 15 : x
$7.5x = 15$
$x = \dfrac{15}{7.5}$
$x = 2$ tablets

$\dfrac{15 \text{ mg}}{7.5 \text{ mg}} \times 1 \text{ tab} =$
$\dfrac{15}{7.5} = 2$ tablets

19. 15 mg : 1 tab :: 30 mg : x tab
15 : 1 :: 30 : x
$15x = 30$
$x = \dfrac{30}{15}$
$x = 2$ tablets

$\dfrac{30 \text{ mg}}{15 \text{ mg}} \times 1 \text{ tab} =$
$\dfrac{30}{15} = 2$ tablets

ANSWERS

Proportion	**Formula**

20. $250 \text{ mg} : 1 \text{ tab} :: 750 \text{ mg} : x \text{ tab}$
$250 : 1 :: 750 : x$
$250x = 750$
$x = \dfrac{750}{250}$
$x = 3 \text{ tablets}$

$\dfrac{750 \text{ mg}}{250 \text{ mg}} \times 1 \text{ tab} =$
$\dfrac{750}{250} = 3 \text{ tablets}$

21. $5 \text{ mg} : 1 \text{ tab} :: 10 \text{ mg} : x \text{ tab}$
$5 : 1 :: 10 : x$
$5x = 10$
$x = \dfrac{10}{5}$
$x = 2 \text{ tablets}$

$\dfrac{10 \text{ mg}}{5 \text{ mg}} \times 1 \text{ tab} =$
$\dfrac{10}{5} = 2 \text{ tablets}$

22. $75 \text{ mg} : 1 \text{ capsule} :: 225 \text{ mg} : x \text{ tab}$
$75 : 1 :: 225 : x$
$75x = 225$
$x = \dfrac{225}{75}$
$x = 3 \text{ capsules}$

$\dfrac{225 \text{ mg}}{75 \text{ mg}} \times 1 \text{ capsule} =$
$\dfrac{225}{75} = 3 \text{ capsules}$

23. $50 \text{ mg} : 5 \text{ mL} :: 100 \text{ mg} : x \text{ mL}$
$50 : 5 :: 100 : x$
$50x = 500$
$x = \dfrac{500}{50}$
$x = 10 \text{ mL}$

$\dfrac{100 \text{ mg}}{50 \text{ mg}} \times 5 \text{ mL} =$
$\dfrac{\overset{}{100}}{\underset{10}{\cancel{50}}} \times \dfrac{\overset{1}{\cancel{5}}}{1} =$
$\dfrac{100}{10} = 10 \text{ mL}$

2 Tbsp — 30 mL
— 25 mL
— 20 mL
1 Tbsp — 15 mL
2 tsp — 10 mL
1 tsp — 5 mL
½ tsp —

24. $2.5 \text{ mg} : 1 \text{ tab} :: 5 \text{ mg} : x \text{ tab}$
$2.5 : 1 :: 5 : x$
$2.5x = 5$
$x = \dfrac{5}{2.5}$
$x = 2 \text{ tablets}$

$\dfrac{5 \text{ mg}}{2.5 \text{ mg}} \times 1 \text{ tab} =$
$\dfrac{5}{2.5} = 2 \text{ tablets}$

25. $200 \text{ mg} : 5 \text{ mL} :: 1000 \text{ mg} : x \text{ mL}$
$200 : 5 :: 1000 : x$
$200x = 5000$
$x = \dfrac{5000}{200}$
$x = 25 \text{ mL}$

$\dfrac{1000 \text{ mg}}{200 \text{ mg}} \times 5 \text{ mL} =$
$\dfrac{\overset{}{1000}}{\underset{40}{\cancel{200}}} \times \dfrac{\overset{1}{\cancel{5}}}{1} =$
$\dfrac{1000}{40} = 25 \text{ mL}$

ANSWERS

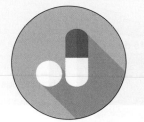

Parenteral Dosages

LEARNING OBJECTIVES

Upon completion of the materials provided in this chapter, you will be able to perform computations accurately by mastering the following mathematical concepts:

1 Using the dimensional analysis method to solve parenteral dosage problems

2 Converting all measures within the problem to equivalent measures in one system of measurement if required

3 Using a proportion to solve parenteral dosage problems

4 Using the stated formula as an alternative method of solving parenteral dosage problems

Parenteral refers to outside the alimentary canal or gastrointestinal tract. Medications may be given parenterally when they cannot be taken by mouth or when rapid action is desired. Some medications are not available by any other method of administration. Parenteral medications are absorbed directly into the bloodstream; therefore the amount of drug needed can be determined more accurately. This type of administration of medications is necessary for the uncooperative or unconscious patient, or for a patient who has been designated *NPO*. An advantage of intravenous (IV) parenteral medications is that the patient does not have to endure the discomfort of multiple injections, especially when the medications are used for pain control.

Parenteral medications are administered by (1) subcutaneous injection—beneath the skin, in fat; (2) intramuscular (IM) injection—within the muscle; or (3) intradermal injection—within the skin (Figure 12-1). Parenteral medications may also be given intravenously (IV)—within the vein. IV drugs may be diluted and administered by themselves, in conjunction with existing IV fluids, or in addition to IV fluids. Any time that the integrity of the skin—the body's prime defense against microorganisms—is threatened, infection may occur. Thus the nurse must use sterile technique when preparing and administering parenteral medications.

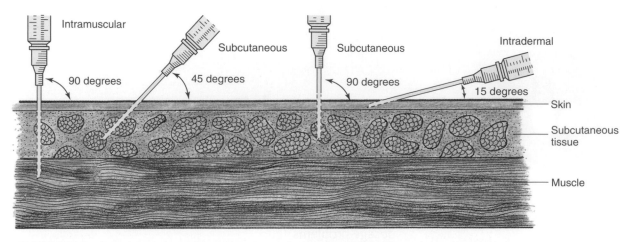

FIGURE 12-1 Intramuscular, subcutaneous, and intradermal injections, with comparison of the angles of insertion. (From Potter PA, Perry AG, Stockert PA, Hall AM: *Fundamentals of nursing,* ed 8, St Louis, 2013, Mosby.)

Drugs for parenteral use are supplied as liquids or powders. The medications are packaged in a variety of forms. A liquid may be contained in an ampule, which is a single-dose container that must be broken at the neck to withdraw the drug (Figures 12-2 and 12-3).

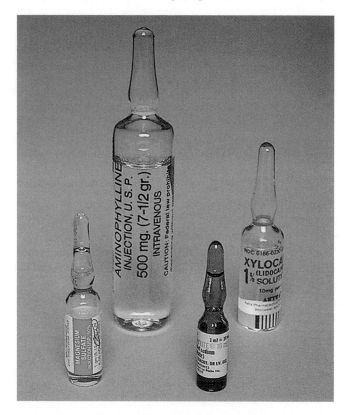

FIGURE 12-2 Examples of ampules. (From Potter PA, Perry AG, Stockert PA, Hall AM: *Fundamentals of nursing,* ed 8, St Louis, 2013, Mosby.)

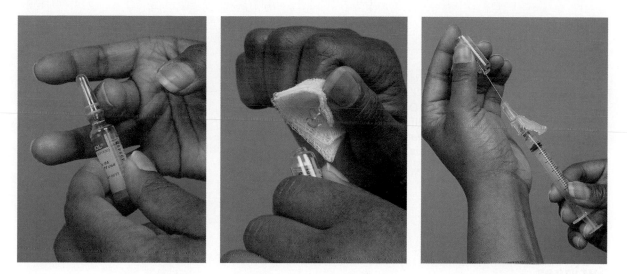

FIGURE 12-3 Breaking the ampule to withdraw the medication. (From Potter PA, Perry AG, Stockert PA, Hall AM: *Fundamentals of nursing,* ed 8, St Louis, 2013, Mosby.)

Vials are also used to package parenteral medications in liquid or powder form. A vial is a glass or plastic container that is sealed with a rubber stopper (Figure 12-4). Because vials usually contain more than one dose of a medication, the amount desired is withdrawn by inserting a needle through the rubber stopper and removing the required amount (Figure 12-5).

Some of the more unstable drugs may be supplied in vials that have a compartment containing the liquid diluent. Pressure applied to the top of the vial releases the stopper between the compartments and allows the drug to be dissolved. These are called *Mix-O-Vials* (Figure 12-6).

Medications may also be supplied in either prefilled disposable syringes or a plastic reusable syringe with a disposable cartridge and a needle unit. Such units contain a specific amount of medication. If the medication order is less than the amount supplied, discard the unneeded portion before administering the medication to the patient. If the discard is a narcotic, follow your institution's rules for documentation.

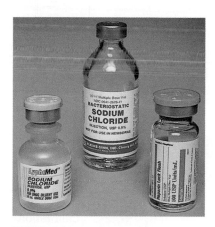

FIGURE 12-4 Examples of vials. (From Potter PA, Perry AG, Stockert PA, Hall AM: *Fundamentals of nursing,* ed 8, St Louis, 2013, Mosby.)

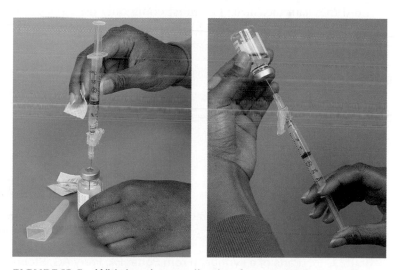

FIGURE 12-5 Withdrawing medication from a vial through the rubber stopper. (From Potter PA, Perry AG, Stockert PA, Hall AM: *Fundamentals of nursing,* ed 8, St Louis, 2013, Mosby.)

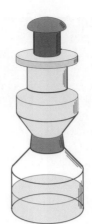

FIGURE 12-6 A Mix-O-Vial or Act-O-Vial. (From Clayton BD, Willihnganz MJ: *Basic pharmacology for nurses,* ed 16, St Louis, 2013, Mosby.)

Syringes

For accurate measurement of medications that are to be administered by the parenteral route, a syringe must be used. Each syringe is supplied in a sterile package. Although syringes may be made of glass or plastic, plastic syringes are more commonly used. All are designed to be used only once and then discarded. Figure 12-7 shows the parts of a syringe.

1. TIP. The tip is located at the end of the syringe. This is the part that holds the needle.
2. BARREL. This is the outer part of the syringe and the part that holds the medication. The various calibrations are printed on the outside of the barrel.
3. PLUNGER. This is the interior part of the syringe, which slides within the barrel. The plunger is moved backward to withdraw and measure the medication. Then it is pushed forward to inject the medication into the patient.

Syringes come in a variety of sizes. The size used depends on the amount and type of medication to be administered. There are three types of syringes: hypodermic, tuberculin, and insulin syringes.

Hypodermic Syringes. Hypodermic syringes vary in size as to the amount of fluid they can measure. The most commonly used sizes are 2-, 2½-, 3-, and 5-mL syringes (Figure 12-8). Hypodermic syringes are also available in 10-, 20-, 30-, and 50-mL sizes.

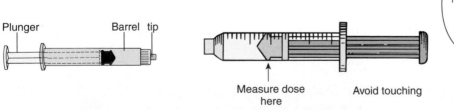

Plunger   Barrel   tip

Measure dose here   Avoid touching

FIGURE 12-7 Parts of a syringe. (From Potter PA, Perry AG, Stockert PA, Hall AM: *Fundamentals of nursing,* ed 8, St Louis, 2013, Mosby.)

FIGURE 12-8 Calibrations on a 3-mL syringe. (From Clayton BD, Willihnganz MJ: *Basic pharmacology for nurses,* ed 16, St Louis, 2013, Mosby.)

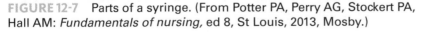

Syringes that are smaller in capacity can easily be used to measure decimal fractions of a milliliter. Longer lines mark the half- and whole-number milliliters, and shorter lines mark the decimal fractions. Each line indicates one tenth of a milliliter. With larger-capacity syringes, each mark may represent a 0.2-mL increment or whole milliliter increments. The larger-capacity syringes are not appropriate for measuring smaller quantities of medication for administration. The nurse must select the proper size of syringe for the calculated volume of medication.

Tuberculin Syringes. A tuberculin syringe is a thin, 1-mL syringe (Figure 12-9). The mL side of the syringe includes markings for hundredths of a milliliter. These syringes are commonly used in pediatrics and also to measure medications given in very small amounts, such as heparin. Tuberculin syringes should not be confused with insulin syringes.

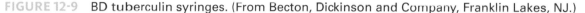

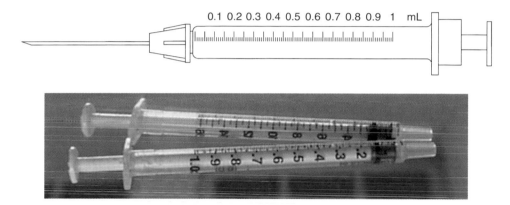

FIGURE 12-9   BD tuberculin syringes. (From Becton, Dickinson and Company, Franklin Lakes, NJ.)

Needleless System. The Occupational Safety and Health Administration has recommended administration of parenteral medications with the use of a needleless system. This recommendation is for the protection of both patients and nurses from needlesticks. Needleless systems provide a shield that protects the needle device and are only for IV use (Figure 12-10).

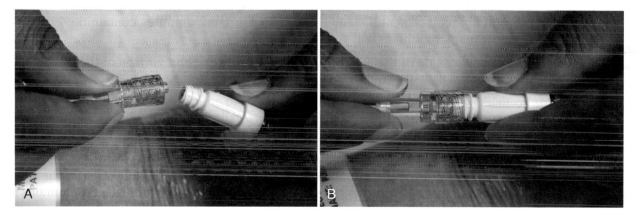

FIGURE 12-10   **A,** Needleless infusion system. **B,** Connection into an injection port. (From Perry AG, Potter PA, Ostendorf WR: *Clinical nursing skills and techniques,* ed 8, St Louis, 2014, Mosby.)

Calculation of Parenteral Drug Dosages: Dimensional Analysis Method

EXAMPLE 1: The physician orders Apresoline 30 mg IM. Apresoline 20 mg/mL is available. How many milliliters will the nurse administer?

a. On the left side of the equation, place the name or abbreviation of the drug form of *x*, or what you are solving for.

$$x \text{ mL} =$$

73. The physician orders Monocid 800 mg IM daily. How many milliliters will the nurse administer? _____

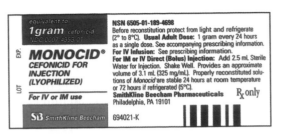

74. Mr. Paley receives promethazine 30 mg IM at 0930 for relief of nausea after a colonoscopy. How many milliliters will the nurse administer? _____

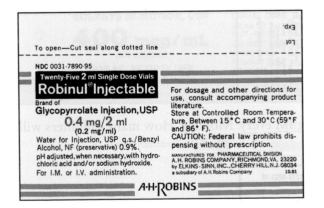

75. Your patient receives Robinul 0.28 mg IM at 0600. How many milliliters will you administer? _____

76. Mrs. Lopez has Ativan 3 mg IM ordered at bedtime for insomnia. Ativan is supplied in a 4 mg/mL prefilled syringe. How many milliliters will the nurse administer? _____

77. The physician orders D₅W 1000 mL plus NaCl 15 mEq at 30 mL IV per hour. NaCl is supplied in a 40-mL vial containing 100 mEq. How many milliliters of NaCl will be added to the 1000 mL of D₅W? _____

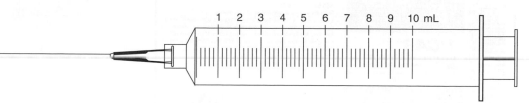

78. Mr. Neal receives Kefzol 250 mg IV q 6 h for 12 doses after an ethmoidectomy. How many milliliters will the nurse prepare? _____

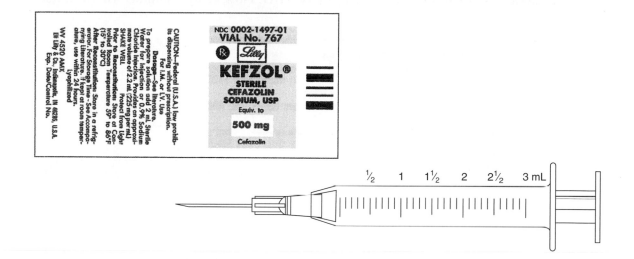

79. Your patient receives the antibiotic Cleocin phosphate 300 mg IV q 6 h for treatment of diphtheria. How many milliliters will you prepare? _____

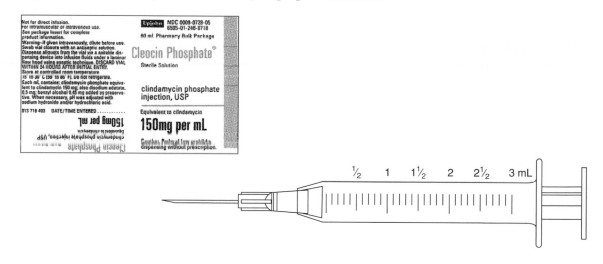

80. The physician orders lidocaine 75 mg IV STAT. Lidocaine is available in a 5-mL vial containing 100 mg/5 mL. How many milliliters will the nurse prepare? _____

81. The physician orders Ticar 0.8 g IM q 6 h. How many milliliters will the nurse prepare? _____

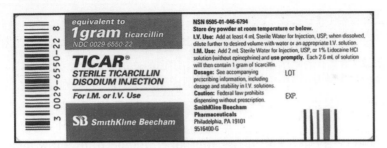

82. The physician orders Solu-Medrol 100 mg IV STAT. How many milliliters will the nurse prepare? _____

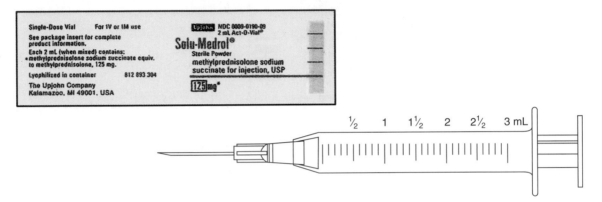

83. Mr. Scott takes Cerebyx 300 mg IV STAT for grand mal seizures. Cerebyx 75 mg/mL in a 10-mL vial is available. How many milliliters will the patient receive? _____

84. The physician orders scopolamine 0.4 mg subcutaneous at 0700. How many milliliters will the nurse administer? _____

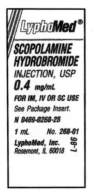

85. The physician orders for your patient promethazine 10 mg IM STAT for relief of nausea and vomiting. How many milliliters will the patient receive? _____

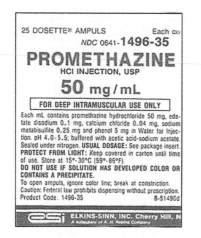

86. The physician orders Dilaudid 1 mg IV q 4 h prn. How many milliliters will the nurse administer? _____

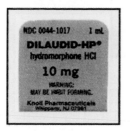

87. Your patient requires Vistaril 50 mg IM q 4 h prn for severe agitation. How many milliliters will you administer? _____

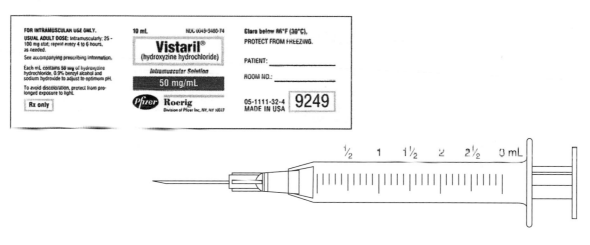

88. Ms. Jones has fentanyl citrate 60 mcg IM ordered q 2 h prn for pain. How many milliliters will the nurse administer? _____

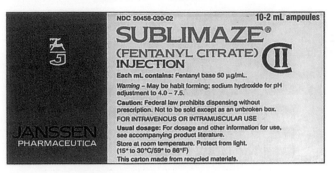

89. Atropine 0.5 mg IM STAT is ordered. How many milliliters will the nurse administer? _____

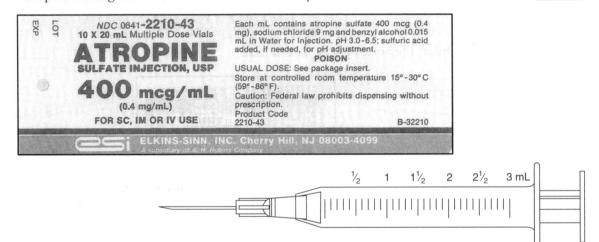

90. Your patient has Thorazine 15 mg IM q 6 h ordered for severe agitation. How many milliliters will you administer? _____

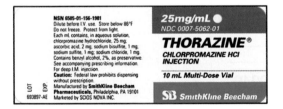

91. The physician orders Tigan 150 mg IM for treatment of nausea. How many milliliters will the nurse prepare? _____

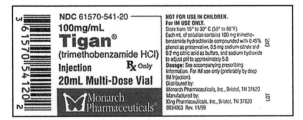

92. Mr. Garcia has Robinul 75 mcg IM ordered 30 minutes before surgery. Robinul 0.2 mg/mL is available. How many milliliters will the nurse administer? _____

93. Your patient with delirium tremens receives diazepam 2 mg IM q 6 h. How many milliliters will you administer? _____

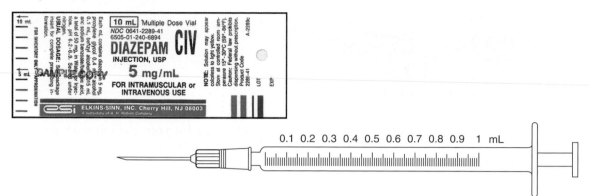

94. The physician orders Flagyl 500 mg IV q 6 h to treat Ms. King's yeast infection. After reconstitution you have Flagyl 100 mg/mL. How many milliliters will you prepare? _____

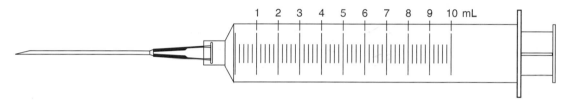

95. The physician orders streptomycin 0.64 g IM daily. After reconstitution you have streptomycin 400 mg/mL. How many milliliters will you administer? _____

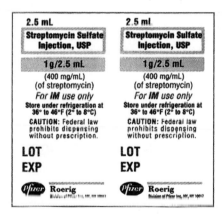

96. Your patient receives nafcillin 500 mg IM q 6 h for treatment of a *Staphylococcus aureus* infection. You have nafcillin 250 mg/mL. How many milliliters will you administer? _____

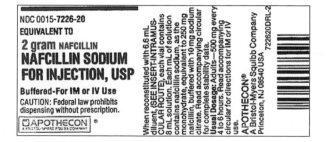

97. The physician orders Stadol 0.5 mg IV q 4 h for pain. How many milliliters will the nurse administer? _____

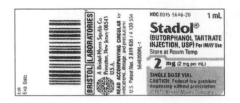

98. The physician orders Imferon 100 mg IM every other day for your patient with pernicious anemia. The drug is supplied in ampules containing 25 mg/0.5 mL. How many milliliters will you administer? _____

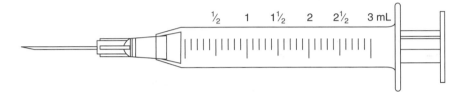

99. Your patient with arthritis receives Solganal 10 mg IM. Solganal is supplied as 50 mg/mL. How many milliliters will you administer? _____

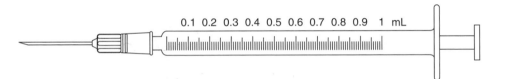

100. Mrs. Sutter has Versed 3.5 mg IM ordered 1 hour before her surgery. You have Versed 5 mg/mL supplied in a 2-mL vial. How many milliliters will you administer? _____

ANSWERS ON PP. 319–328 AND 332–349.

NAME _____

DATE _____

ACCEPTABLE SCORE ___19___

YOUR SCORE _____

HW ✓ 6/13

POSTTEST 1 ✚

DIRECTIONS: The medication order is listed at the beginning of each problem. Calculate the parenteral doses. Show your work. Shade the syringe when provided to indicate the correct dose.

1. The physician orders Vistaril 25 mg IM three times a day q 6 h prn to enhance the effects of pain medication for your patient with a thyroidectomy. How many milliliters will you administer? _0.5mL_

$$\frac{25mg}{1} = \frac{1mL}{50mg} = \frac{25}{50}$$

0.5

FOR INTRAMUSCULAR USE ONLY.
USUAL ADULT DOSE: Intramuscularly: 25 -
100 mg stat; repeat every 4 to 6 hours,
as needed.
See accompanying prescribing information.

Each mL contains 50 mg of hydroxyzine
hydrochloride, 0.9% benzyl alcohol and
sodium hydroxide to adjust to optimum pH.

To avoid discoloration, protect from prolonged exposure to light.

Rx only

10 mL   NDC 0049-5460-74

Vistaril®
(hydroxyzine hydrochloride)
Intramuscular Solution
50 mg/mL

Pfizer **Roerig**
Division of Pfizer Inc, NY, NY 10017

Store below 86°F (30°C).
PROTECT FROM FREEZING.

PATIENT: _____

ROOM NO.: _____

05-1111-32-4 **9249**
MADE IN USA

2. Your patient with a septoplasty complains of nausea and has promethazine 25 mg IM four times a day ordered. How many milliliters will you administer? _0.5mL_

$$\frac{25mg}{1} = \frac{1mL}{50mg} = \frac{25}{50} = 0.5$$

25 DOSETTE® AMPULS   Each co
NDC 0641-**1496-35**

PROMETHAZINE
HCl INJECTION, USP

50 mg/mL

FOR DEEP INTRAMUSCULAR USE ONLY

Each mL contains promethazine hydrochloride 50 mg, ede-
tate disodium 0.1 mg, calcium chloride 0.04 mg, sodium
metabisulfite 0.25 mg and phenol 5 mg in Water for Injec-
tion. pH 4.0-5.5; buffered with acetic acid-sodium acetate.
Sealed under nitrogen. USUAL DOSAGE: See package insert.
PROTECT FROM LIGHT: Keep covered in carton until time
of use. Store at 15°-30°C (59°-86°F).
DO NOT USE IF SOLUTION HAS DEVELOPED COLOR OR
CONTAINS A PRECIPITATE.
To open ampuls, ignore color line; break at constriction.
Caution: Federal law prohibits dispensing without prescription.
Product Code: 1496-35   B-51496d

ELKINS-SINN INC. Cherry Hill, NJ
A Subsidiary of A. H. Robins Company

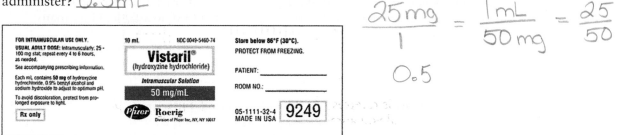

3. Your patient who has undergone tympanomastoidectomy complains of pain and has codeine 30 mg IM q 2 h prn ordered. Codeine is supplied in a 1-mL ampule containing 15 mg. How many milliliters will you administer? _2 ml_

$$\frac{30mg}{1} = \frac{1mL}{15mg} = \frac{30}{15} =$$

2

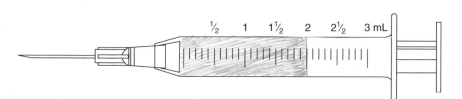

4. The physician orders Keflin 500 mg IM q 6 h for your patient with a *Klebsiella* infection. Keflin 1 g/10 mL is available. How many milliliters will you administer? 5mL

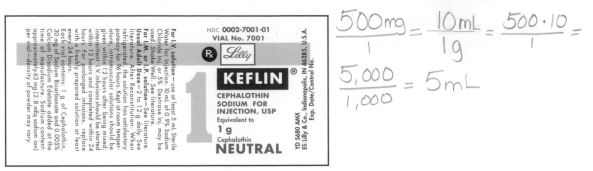

$$\frac{500mg}{1} = \frac{10mL}{1g} = \frac{500 \cdot 10}{1} =$$

$$\frac{5,000}{1,000} = 5mL$$

5. Your patient, who has undergone medullary carcinoma excision, has hydrocortisone 50 mg IM twice a day ordered. You have hydrocortisone 100 mg/2 mL available. How many milliliters will you administer? 1 mL

$$\frac{50mg}{1} = \frac{2mL}{100mg} = \frac{100}{100} = 1$$

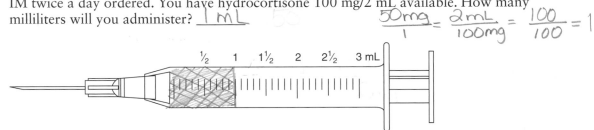

6. The physician orders Dilaudid 0.5 mg IM q 4 h prn for pain. How many milliliters will the nurse administer? 0.25 mL

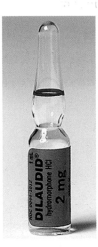

$$\frac{0.5mg}{1} = \frac{1}{2mg} = \frac{0.5}{2} =$$

$$0.25$$

7. Mr. Harrison has Toradol 15 mg IM ordered q 6 h for pain after a hip replacement. A prefilled syringe with Toradol 30 mg/mL is available. How many milliliters will the nurse administer? 0.5 mL

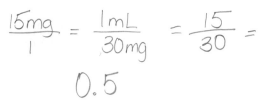

$$\frac{15mg}{1} = \frac{1mL}{30mg} = \frac{15}{30} =$$

$$0.5$$

8. The physician orders scopolamine 0.2 mg IM at 0600 before surgery. How many milliliters will the nurse administer? __0.5 mL__

$$\frac{0.2mg}{1} = \frac{1mL}{0.4} = \frac{0.2}{0.4} = 0.5$$

SCOPOLAMINE HYDROBROMIDE
INJECTION, USP
0.4 mg/mL
FOR IM, IV OR SC USE
See Package Insert.
N 0469-0268-25
1 mL   No. 268-01
LyphoMed, Inc.
Rosemont, IL 60018
LyphoMed®

0.1 0.2 0.3 0.4 0.5 0.6 0.7 0.8 0.9 1 mL

9. The physician orders Thorazine 100 mg IM STAT. Thorazine is supplied in a 10-mL vial containing 25 mg/mL. How many milliliters will the nurse administer? __4 mL__

$$\frac{100\ mg}{1} = \frac{1mL}{25mg} = \frac{100}{25} = 4$$

NSN 6505-01-156-1981
Dilute before I.V. use. Store below 86°F
Do not freeze. Protect from light.
Each mL contains, in aqueous solution,
chlorpromazine hydrochloride, 25 mg;
ascorbic acid, 2 mg; sodium bisulfite, 1 mg;
sodium sulfite, 1 mg; sodium chloride, 1 mg.
Contains benzyl alcohol, 2%, as preservative.
See accompanying prescribing information.
For deep I.M. injection.
Caution: Federal law prohibits dispensing
without prescription.
Manufactured by **SmithKline Beecham**
Pharmaceuticals, Philadelphia, PA 19101
Marketed by SCIOS NOVA INC.

25mg/mL ●
NDC 0007-5062-01
THORAZINE®
CHLORPROMAZINE HCl
INJECTION
10 mL Multi-Dose Vial
SB SmithKline Beecham

10. Your severely agitated patient has diazepam 2 mg IM q 6 h prn ordered. How many milliliters will you administer? __0.4 mL__

$$\frac{2mg}{1} = \frac{1mL}{5mg} = \frac{2}{5} = 0.4$$

10 mL Multiple Dose Vial
NDC 0641-2289-41
6505-01-240-6894
DIAZEPAM CIV
INJECTION, USP
5 mg/mL
FOR INTRAMUSCULAR or
INTRAVENOUS USE
ELKINS-SINN, INC. Cherry Hill, NJ 08003

0.1 0.2 0.3 0.4 0.5 0.6 0.7 0.8 0.9 1 mL

11. Atropine 0.7 mg IM STAT is ordered for your patient before surgery. You have atropine 0.5 mg/mL. How many milliliters will you administer? __1.4 mL__

$$\frac{0.7\ mg}{1} = \frac{1mL}{0.5mg} = \frac{0.7}{0.5} = 1.4$$

12. Your patient with a medication reaction complains of pruritus and has Benadryl 25 mg IM prn ordered. You have Benadryl 50 mg/mL available. How many milliliters will you administer? 0.5 mL

$$\frac{25\,mg}{1} = \frac{1\,mL}{50\,mg} = \frac{25}{50} = 0.5$$

N 0071-4402-10

Benadryl®
(Diphenhydramine Hydro-
chloride Injection, USP)
50 mg per mL
HIGH POTENCY
10 mL

Ⓟ **PARKE-DAVIS**

13. The physician orders Depo-Medrol 50 mg IM twice a day. How many milliliters will the nurse administer? 0.625 mL

$$\frac{50\,mg}{1} = \frac{1\,mL}{80\,mg} = \frac{50}{80} = 0.625$$

NDC 0009-0306-01
1 ml
Depo-Medrol®
Sterile Aqueous Suspension
sterile methylprednisolone
acetate suspension, USP
80 mg per ml

For IM, intrasynovial and soft
tissue injection only.
Not for IV use.
See package insert for
complete product
information.
Shake well immediately
before using.
812-312-201
The Upjohn Company
Kalamazoo, MI 49001, USA

14. The physician orders Tagamet 600 mg IV q 6 h. How many milliliters will the nurse administer? 4 mL

$$\frac{600\,mg}{1} = \frac{2\,mL}{300\,mg} = \frac{1,200}{300} = 4$$

Store at controlled room temperature
(59° to 86°F). Do not refrigerate.
Each 2 mL contains, in aqueous solution,
cimetidine hydrochloride equivalent to
cimetidine, 300 mg; phenol, 10 mg.
For I.M. injection; dilute for slow I.V. use.
Dosage: See accompanying prescribing
information.
Caution: Federal law prohibits dispensing
without prescription.
U.S. Patents 3,950,333 and 4,024,271
SmithKline Beecham Pharmaceuticals
Philadelphia, PA 19101

2mL=300mg
NDC 0108-5022-01
TAGAMET®
**CIMETIDINE HCl
INJECTION**
8 mL Multi-Dose Vial
SⒷ SmithKline Beecham

LOT
EXP.
693957-P

15. The physician orders Ancef 300 mg IV q 8 h. You have Ancef 1 g/50 mL available. How many milliliters will you administer? 15 mL

$$\frac{300\,mg}{1} = \frac{50\,mL}{1\,g} = \frac{15,000}{1,000} = 15$$

16. The physician orders morphine 6 mg IM q 3 h prn. How many milliliters will the nurse administer? _0.6 mL_

$$\frac{6mg}{1} = \frac{1mL}{10mg} = \frac{6}{10} = 0.6$$

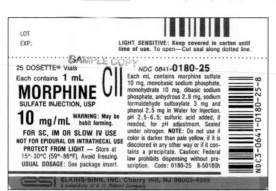

17. The physician orders dexamethasone 6 mg IM STAT. You have dexamethasone 10 mg/mL. How many milliliters will you administer? _0.6 mL_

$$\frac{6mg}{1} = \frac{1mL}{10mg} = \frac{6}{10} = 0.6$$

18. Your patient with congestive heart failure has furosemide 20 mg IV daily ordered. How many milliliters will you administer? _2 mL_

$$\frac{20mg}{1} = \frac{4mL}{40mg} = \frac{80}{40} = 2$$

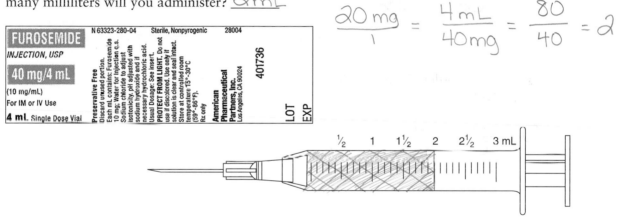

19. The physician orders digoxin 0.3 mg IM now. How many milliliters will the nurse administer? _1.2 mL_

$$\frac{0.3mg}{1} = \frac{2mL}{500mcg} = \frac{0.6}{500} = 1.2$$

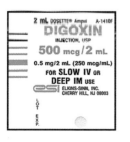

20. Mrs. Joyce has verapamil 5-mg IV bolus ordered to be given over 2 minutes now for dysrhythmia. Verapamil 2.5 mg/mL is supplied. How many milliliters will Mrs. Joyce receive? _2 mL_

$$\frac{5mg}{1} = \frac{1mL}{2.5mg} = \frac{5}{2.5} = 2$$

ANSWERS ON PP. 328–330 AND 349–352.

NAME _____

DATE _____

ACCEPTABLE SCORE __19__

YOUR SCORE _____

POSTTEST 2 +

DIRECTIONS: The medication order is listed at the beginning of each problem. Calculate the parenteral doses. Show your work. Shade the syringe when provided to indicate the correct dose.

1. Your patient, who was involved in a motor vehicle accident, complains of pain and has Dilaudid 2 mg IM q 3 h prn ordered. How many milliliters will you administer? _____

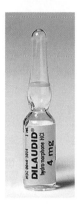

2. Your preoperative patient complains of anxiety and has Ativan 2 mg IM q 6 h ordered. Ativan is supplied 4 mg/mL. How many milliliters will you administer? _____

3. The physician orders erythromycin 0.4 g IV today. The drug is supplied in vials containing 500 mg/10 mL. How many milliliters will the nurse prepare? _____

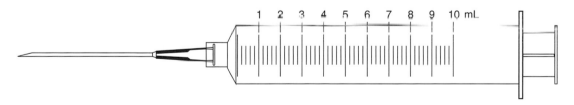

4. Mrs. Jesse has Cardizem 20 mg IV ordered STAT for hypertension. How many milliliters will the nurse administer? _____

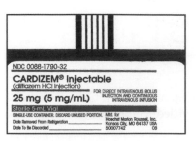

5. Your patient who has had a lumpectomy has codeine 60 mg IM q 3 h ordered. How many milliliters will you administer? _____

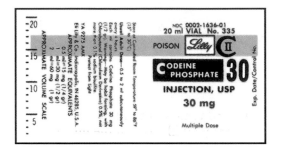

6. Mr. Ryan has Tigan 200 mg IM ordered three times a day for nausea and vomiting. How many milliliters will you administer? _____

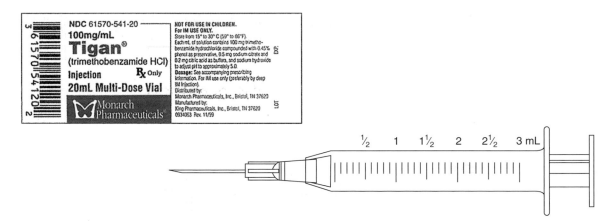

7. The physician orders atropine 0.2 mg IM at 0600. How many milliliters will the nurse administer? _____

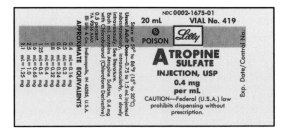

8. The physician orders Benadryl 25 mg IV STAT for your patient with a mild medication reaction. How many milliliters will you prepare? _____

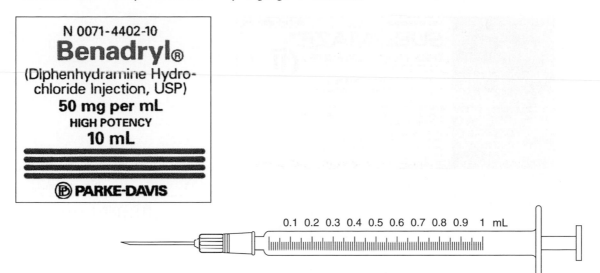

9. Ms. Straw has Anzemet 100 mg IV ordered to be given 30 minutes before her chemotherapy. Anzemet 20 mg/mL is available. How many milliliters will the nurse administer? _____

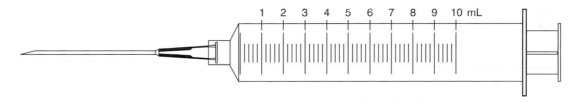

10. Mr. Trent has hydroxyzine 75 mg IM STAT ordered for severe motion sickness. You have hydroxyzine 50 mg/mL. How many milliliters will you administer? _____

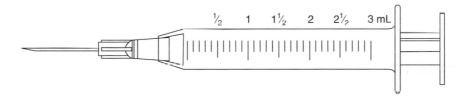

11. Your postsurgical patient has Sublimaze 70 mcg IM ordered q 2 h prn for pain. How many milliliters will you prepare? _____

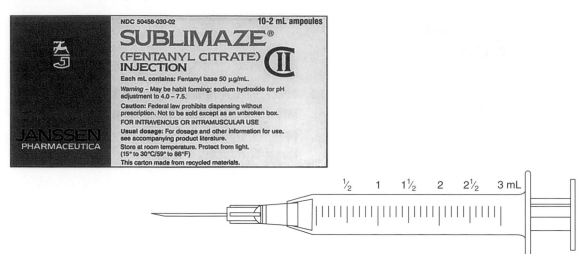

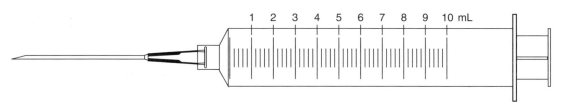

12. The physician orders scopolamine 0.4 mg IM at 0700. Scopolamine 0.3 mg/mL is available. How many milliliters will the nurse administer? _____

13. The physician orders piperacillin 2 g IV q 8 h for your patient with sepsis. Piperacillin 1 g/2.5 mL is available. How many milliliters will you prepare? _____

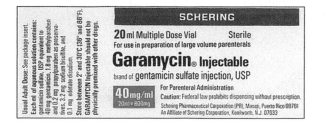

14. The physician orders gentamicin 26 mg IV q 8 h. How many milliliters will the nurse prepare? _____

15. The physician orders Lovenox 85 mg subcutaneous q 12 h. The drug is available as 40 mg/0.4 mL. How many milliliters will the nurse administer? _____

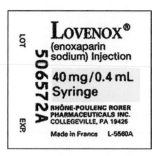

16. Your patient, who has undergone tricuspid valve repair, has Lanoxin 80 mcg IM twice a day ordered. How many milliliters will you administer? _____

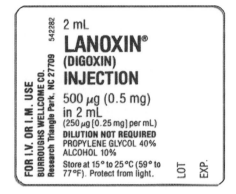

17. The physician orders morphine 4 mg subcutaneous q 4 h prn. Morphine is supplied in a 1-mL ampule containing 8 mg. How many milliliters will the nurse administer? _____

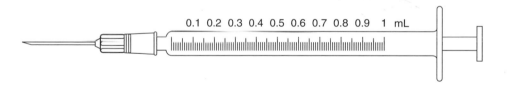

18. Your patient with a history of seizures has Dilantin 100 mg IV q 8 h ordered. Dilantin 50 mg/2 mL is available. How many milliliters will you prepare? _____

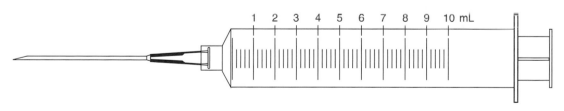

19. Mr. Richards has Floxin 300 mg IV q 12 h ordered to treat his prostatitis. Floxin 400 mg/100 mL is available. How many milliliters will the nurse administer? _____

20. The physician orders D$_5$W 500 mL plus calcium chloride (CaCl$_2$) 10 mEq at 10 mL per hour IV. CaCl$_2$ is supplied in a 10-mL ampule containing 13.6 mEq. How many milliliters of CaCl$_2$ will be added to the 500 mL of D$_5$W? _____

ANSWERS ON PP. 330–332 AND 352–355.

evolve   For additional practice problems, refer to the Basic Calculations section of *Drug Calculations Companion,* Version 5, on Evolve.

ANSWERS

CHAPTER 12 Dimensional Analysis—Worksheet, pp. 283–306

1. $x \text{ mL} = \dfrac{1 \text{ mL}}{400 \text{ mg}} \times \dfrac{500 \text{ mg}}{1} = 1.25 \text{ mL}$

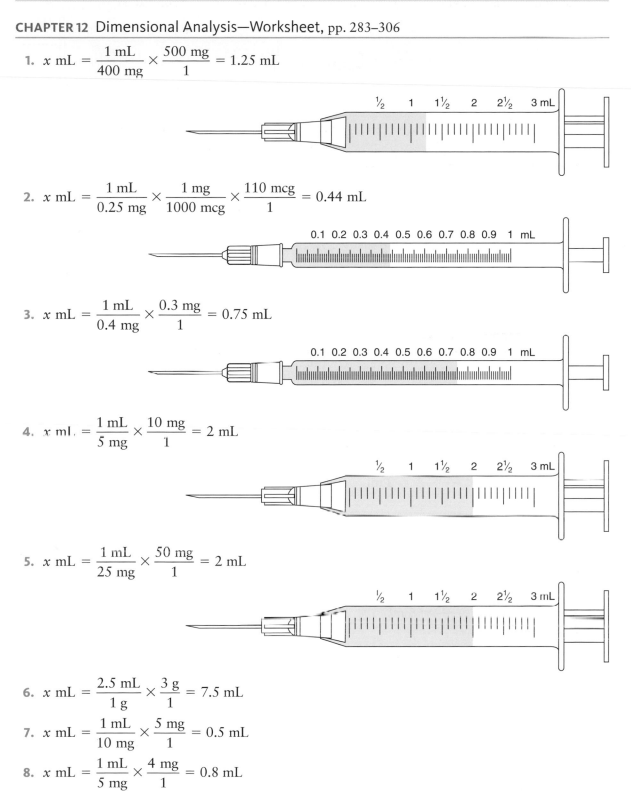

2. $x \text{ mL} = \dfrac{1 \text{ mL}}{0.25 \text{ mg}} \times \dfrac{1 \text{ mg}}{1000 \text{ mcg}} \times \dfrac{110 \text{ mcg}}{1} = 0.44 \text{ mL}$

3. $x \text{ mL} = \dfrac{1 \text{ mL}}{0.4 \text{ mg}} \times \dfrac{0.3 \text{ mg}}{1} = 0.75 \text{ mL}$

4. $x \text{ mL} = \dfrac{1 \text{ mL}}{5 \text{ mg}} \times \dfrac{10 \text{ mg}}{1} = 2 \text{ mL}$

5. $x \text{ mL} = \dfrac{1 \text{ mL}}{25 \text{ mg}} \times \dfrac{50 \text{ mg}}{1} = 2 \text{ mL}$

6. $x \text{ mL} = \dfrac{2.5 \text{ mL}}{1 \text{ g}} \times \dfrac{3 \text{ g}}{1} = 7.5 \text{ mL}$

7. $x \text{ mL} = \dfrac{1 \text{ mL}}{10 \text{ mg}} \times \dfrac{5 \text{ mg}}{1} = 0.5 \text{ mL}$

8. $x \text{ mL} = \dfrac{1 \text{ mL}}{5 \text{ mg}} \times \dfrac{4 \text{ mg}}{1} = 0.8 \text{ mL}$

9. $x \text{ mL} = \dfrac{1 \text{ mL}}{10 \text{ mg}} \times \dfrac{30 \text{ mg}}{1} = 3 \text{ mL}$

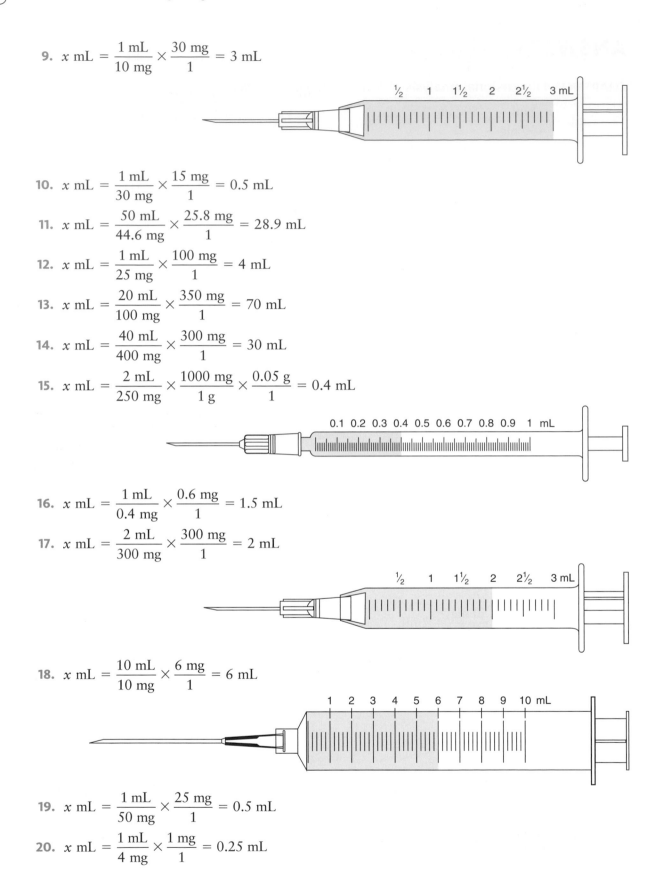

10. $x \text{ mL} = \dfrac{1 \text{ mL}}{30 \text{ mg}} \times \dfrac{15 \text{ mg}}{1} = 0.5 \text{ mL}$

11. $x \text{ mL} = \dfrac{50 \text{ mL}}{44.6 \text{ mg}} \times \dfrac{25.8 \text{ mg}}{1} = 28.9 \text{ mL}$

12. $x \text{ mL} = \dfrac{1 \text{ mL}}{25 \text{ mg}} \times \dfrac{100 \text{ mg}}{1} = 4 \text{ mL}$

13. $x \text{ mL} = \dfrac{20 \text{ mL}}{100 \text{ mg}} \times \dfrac{350 \text{ mg}}{1} = 70 \text{ mL}$

14. $x \text{ mL} = \dfrac{40 \text{ mL}}{400 \text{ mg}} \times \dfrac{300 \text{ mg}}{1} = 30 \text{ mL}$

15. $x \text{ mL} = \dfrac{2 \text{ mL}}{250 \text{ mg}} \times \dfrac{1000 \text{ mg}}{1 \text{ g}} \times \dfrac{0.05 \text{ g}}{1} = 0.4 \text{ mL}$

16. $x \text{ mL} = \dfrac{1 \text{ mL}}{0.4 \text{ mg}} \times \dfrac{0.6 \text{ mg}}{1} = 1.5 \text{ mL}$

17. $x \text{ mL} = \dfrac{2 \text{ mL}}{300 \text{ mg}} \times \dfrac{300 \text{ mg}}{1} = 2 \text{ mL}$

18. $x \text{ mL} = \dfrac{10 \text{ mL}}{10 \text{ mg}} \times \dfrac{6 \text{ mg}}{1} = 6 \text{ mL}$

19. $x \text{ mL} = \dfrac{1 \text{ mL}}{50 \text{ mg}} \times \dfrac{25 \text{ mg}}{1} = 0.5 \text{ mL}$

20. $x \text{ mL} = \dfrac{1 \text{ mL}}{4 \text{ mg}} \times \dfrac{1 \text{ mg}}{1} = 0.25 \text{ mL}$

ANSWERS

21. $x \text{ mL} = \dfrac{1 \text{ mL}}{20 \text{ mg}} \times \dfrac{10 \text{ mg}}{1} = 0.5 \text{ mL}$

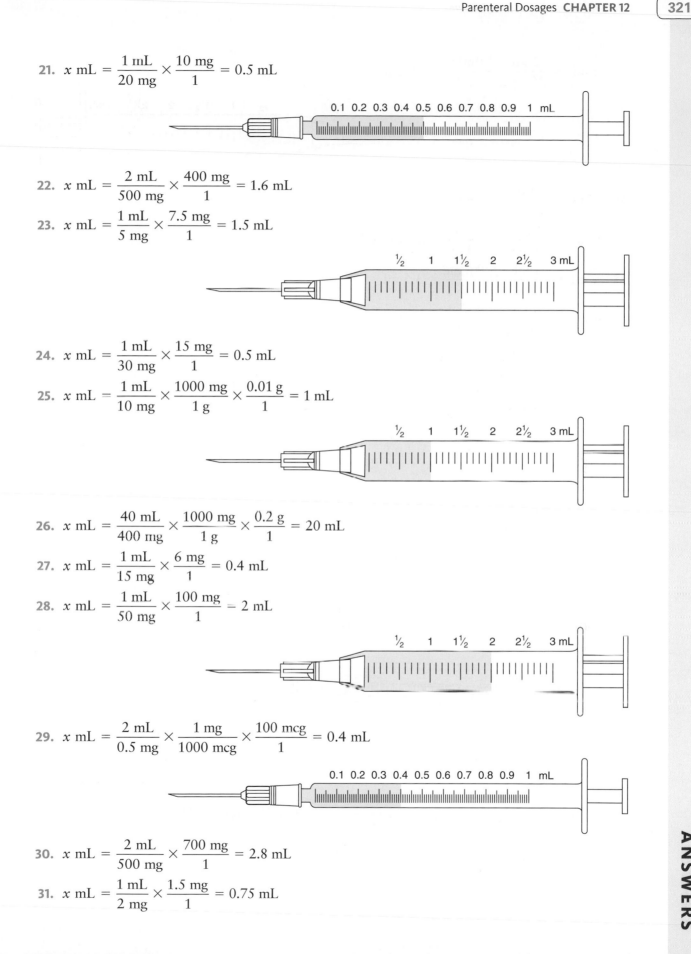

22. $x \text{ mL} = \dfrac{2 \text{ mL}}{500 \text{ mg}} \times \dfrac{400 \text{ mg}}{1} = 1.6 \text{ mL}$

23. $x \text{ mL} = \dfrac{1 \text{ mL}}{5 \text{ mg}} \times \dfrac{7.5 \text{ mg}}{1} = 1.5 \text{ mL}$

24. $x \text{ mL} = \dfrac{1 \text{ mL}}{30 \text{ mg}} \times \dfrac{15 \text{ mg}}{1} = 0.5 \text{ mL}$

25. $x \text{ mL} = \dfrac{1 \text{ mL}}{10 \text{ mg}} \times \dfrac{1000 \text{ mg}}{1 \text{ g}} \times \dfrac{0.01 \text{ g}}{1} = 1 \text{ mL}$

26. $x \text{ mL} = \dfrac{40 \text{ mL}}{400 \text{ mg}} \times \dfrac{1000 \text{ mg}}{1 \text{ g}} \times \dfrac{0.2 \text{ g}}{1} = 20 \text{ mL}$

27. $x \text{ mL} = \dfrac{1 \text{ mL}}{15 \text{ mg}} \times \dfrac{6 \text{ mg}}{1} = 0.4 \text{ mL}$

28. $x \text{ mL} = \dfrac{1 \text{ mL}}{50 \text{ mg}} \times \dfrac{100 \text{ mg}}{1} = 2 \text{ mL}$

29. $x \text{ mL} = \dfrac{2 \text{ mL}}{0.5 \text{ mg}} \times \dfrac{1 \text{ mg}}{1000 \text{ mcg}} \times \dfrac{100 \text{ mcg}}{1} = 0.4 \text{ mL}$

30. $x \text{ mL} = \dfrac{2 \text{ mL}}{500 \text{ mg}} \times \dfrac{700 \text{ mg}}{1} = 2.8 \text{ mL}$

31. $x \text{ mL} = \dfrac{1 \text{ mL}}{2 \text{ mg}} \times \dfrac{1.5 \text{ mg}}{1} = 0.75 \text{ mL}$

Copyright © 2016 by Mosby, an imprint of Elsevier Inc.

ANSWERS

32. x mL $= \dfrac{2 \text{ mL}}{250 \text{ mg}} \times \dfrac{100 \text{ mg}}{1} = 0.8$ mL

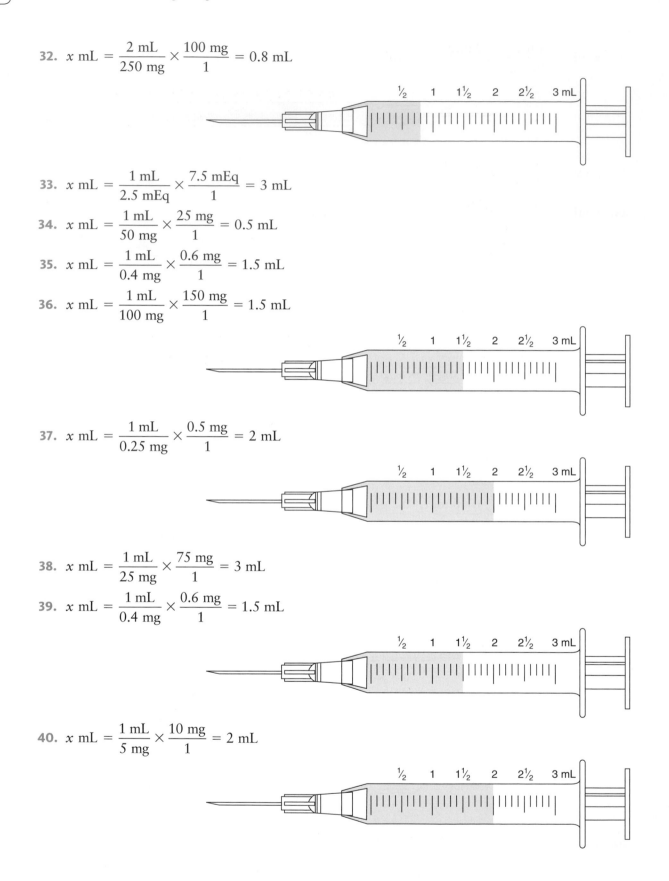

33. x mL $= \dfrac{1 \text{ mL}}{2.5 \text{ mEq}} \times \dfrac{7.5 \text{ mEq}}{1} = 3$ mL

34. x mL $= \dfrac{1 \text{ mL}}{50 \text{ mg}} \times \dfrac{25 \text{ mg}}{1} = 0.5$ mL

35. x mL $= \dfrac{1 \text{ mL}}{0.4 \text{ mg}} \times \dfrac{0.6 \text{ mg}}{1} = 1.5$ mL

36. x mL $= \dfrac{1 \text{ mL}}{100 \text{ mg}} \times \dfrac{150 \text{ mg}}{1} = 1.5$ mL

37. x mL $= \dfrac{1 \text{ mL}}{0.25 \text{ mg}} \times \dfrac{0.5 \text{ mg}}{1} = 2$ mL

38. x mL $= \dfrac{1 \text{ mL}}{25 \text{ mg}} \times \dfrac{75 \text{ mg}}{1} = 3$ mL

39. x mL $= \dfrac{1 \text{ mL}}{0.4 \text{ mg}} \times \dfrac{0.6 \text{ mg}}{1} = 1.5$ mL

40. x mL $= \dfrac{1 \text{ mL}}{5 \text{ mg}} \times \dfrac{10 \text{ mg}}{1} = 2$ mL

ANSWERS

41. $x \text{ mL} = \dfrac{2 \text{ mL}}{100 \text{ mg}} \times \dfrac{25 \text{ mg}}{1} = 0.5 \text{ mL}$

0.1 0.2 0.3 0.4 0.5 0.6 0.7 0.8 0.9 1 mL

42. $x \text{ mL} = \dfrac{40 \text{ mL}}{400 \text{ mg}} \times \dfrac{200 \text{ mg}}{1} = 20 \text{ mL}$

43. $x \text{ mL} = \dfrac{1 \text{ mL}}{500 \text{ mg}} \times \dfrac{1000 \text{ mg}}{1 \text{ g}} \times \dfrac{0.25 \text{ g}}{1} = 0.5 \text{ mL}$

44. $x \text{ mL} = \dfrac{10 \text{ mL}}{13.6 \text{ mEq}} \times \dfrac{5 \text{ mEq}}{1} = 3.68 \text{ mL}$

45. $x \text{ mL} = \dfrac{1 \text{ mL}}{130 \text{ mg}} \times \dfrac{70 \text{ mg}}{1} = 0.54 \text{ mL}$

0.1 0.2 0.3 0.4 0.5 0.6 0.7 0.8 0.9 1 mL

46. $x \text{ mL} = \dfrac{1 \text{ mL}}{10 \text{ mg}} \times \dfrac{200 \text{ mg}}{1} = 20 \text{ mL}$

47. $x \text{ mL} = \dfrac{1 \text{ mL}}{4 \text{ mg}} \times \dfrac{2 \text{ mg}}{1} = 0.5 \text{ mL}$

48. $x \text{ mL} = \dfrac{2 \text{ mL}}{0.5 \text{ mg}} \times \dfrac{0.2 \text{ mg}}{1} = 0.8 \text{ mL}$

0.1 0.2 0.3 0.4 0.5 0.6 0.7 0.8 0.9 1 mL

49. $x \text{ mL} = \dfrac{1 \text{ mL}}{15 \text{ mg}} \times \dfrac{10 \text{ mg}}{1} = 0.67 \text{ mL}$

50. $x \text{ mL} = \dfrac{1 \text{ mL}}{50 \text{ mg}} \times \dfrac{25 \text{ mg}}{1} = 0.5 \text{ mL}$

0.1 0.2 0.3 0.4 0.5 0.6 0.7 0.8 0.9 1 mL

ANSWERS

51. $x \text{ mL} = \dfrac{1.2 \text{ mL}}{500 \text{ mg}} \times \dfrac{600 \text{ mg}}{1} = 1.44 \text{ mL}$

52. $x \text{ mL} = \dfrac{1 \text{ mL}}{0.4 \text{ mg}} \times \dfrac{0.9 \text{ mg}}{1} = 2.25 \text{ mL}$

53. $x \text{ mL} = \dfrac{1 \text{ mL}}{30 \text{ mg}} \times \dfrac{30 \text{ mg}}{1} = 1 \text{ mL}$

54. $x \text{ mL} = \dfrac{1 \text{ mL}}{4 \text{ mg}} \times \dfrac{3 \text{ mg}}{1} = 0.75 \text{ mL}$

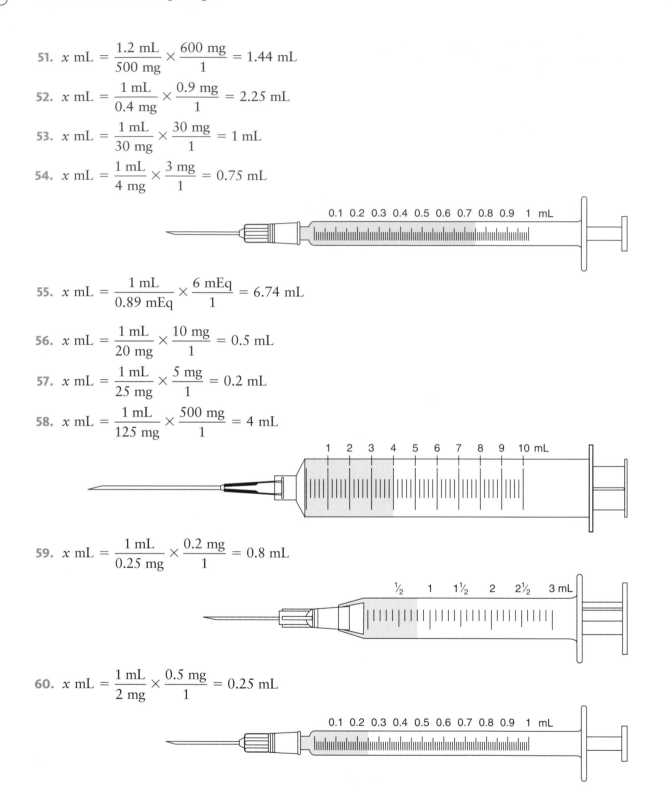

55. $x \text{ mL} = \dfrac{1 \text{ mL}}{0.89 \text{ mEq}} \times \dfrac{6 \text{ mEq}}{1} = 6.74 \text{ mL}$

56. $x \text{ mL} = \dfrac{1 \text{ mL}}{20 \text{ mg}} \times \dfrac{10 \text{ mg}}{1} = 0.5 \text{ mL}$

57. $x \text{ mL} = \dfrac{1 \text{ mL}}{25 \text{ mg}} \times \dfrac{5 \text{ mg}}{1} = 0.2 \text{ mL}$

58. $x \text{ mL} = \dfrac{1 \text{ mL}}{125 \text{ mg}} \times \dfrac{500 \text{ mg}}{1} = 4 \text{ mL}$

59. $x \text{ mL} = \dfrac{1 \text{ mL}}{0.25 \text{ mg}} \times \dfrac{0.2 \text{ mg}}{1} = 0.8 \text{ mL}$

60. $x \text{ mL} = \dfrac{1 \text{ mL}}{2 \text{ mg}} \times \dfrac{0.5 \text{ mg}}{1} = 0.25 \text{ mL}$

61. $x \text{ mL} = \dfrac{20 \text{ mL}}{500 \text{ mg}} \times \dfrac{1000 \text{ mg}}{1 \text{ g}} \times \dfrac{0.2 \text{ g}}{1} = 8 \text{ mL}$

62. $x \text{ mL} = \dfrac{1 \text{ mL}}{30 \text{ mg}} \times \dfrac{15 \text{ mg}}{1} = 0.5 \text{ mL}$

63. $x \text{ mL} = \dfrac{1 \text{ mL}}{50 \text{ mg}} \times \dfrac{100 \text{ mg}}{1} = 2 \text{ mL}$

64. $x \text{ mL} = \dfrac{2 \text{ mL}}{0.5 \text{ mg}} \times \dfrac{0.25 \text{ mg}}{1} = 1 \text{ mL}$

65. $x \text{ mL} = \dfrac{1 \text{ mL}}{1 \text{ mg}} \times \dfrac{1 \text{ mg}}{1000 \text{ mcg}} \times \dfrac{500 \text{ mcg}}{1} = 0.5 \text{ mL}$

66. $x \text{ mL} = \dfrac{10 \text{ mL}}{4.8 \text{ mEq}} \times \dfrac{5 \text{ mEq}}{1} = 10.42 \text{ mL}$

67. $x \text{ mL} = \dfrac{1 \text{ mL}}{150 \text{ mg}} \times \dfrac{50 \text{ mg}}{1} = 0.333 \text{ mL}$

68. $x \text{ mL} = \dfrac{1 \text{ mL}}{0.4 \text{ mg}} \times \dfrac{0.2 \text{ mg}}{1} = 0.5 \text{ mL}$

69. $x \text{ mL} = \dfrac{2 \text{ mL}}{80 \text{ mg}} \times \dfrac{55 \text{ mg}}{1} = 1.38 \text{ mL}$

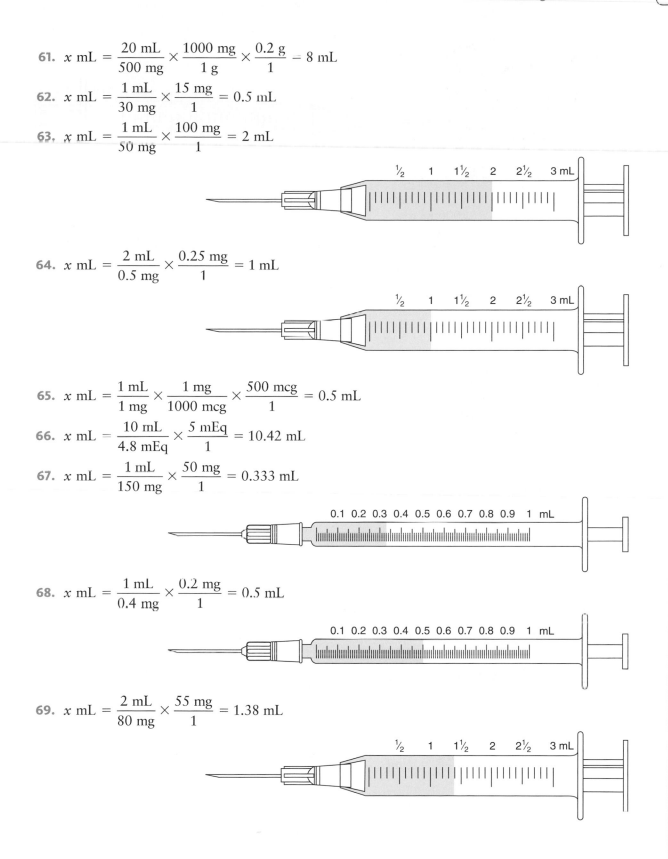

Copyright © 2016 by Mosby, an imprint of Elsevier Inc.

ANSWERS

70. $x \text{ mL} = \dfrac{2 \text{ mL}}{500 \text{ mg}} \times \dfrac{600 \text{ mg}}{1} = 2.4 \text{ mL}$

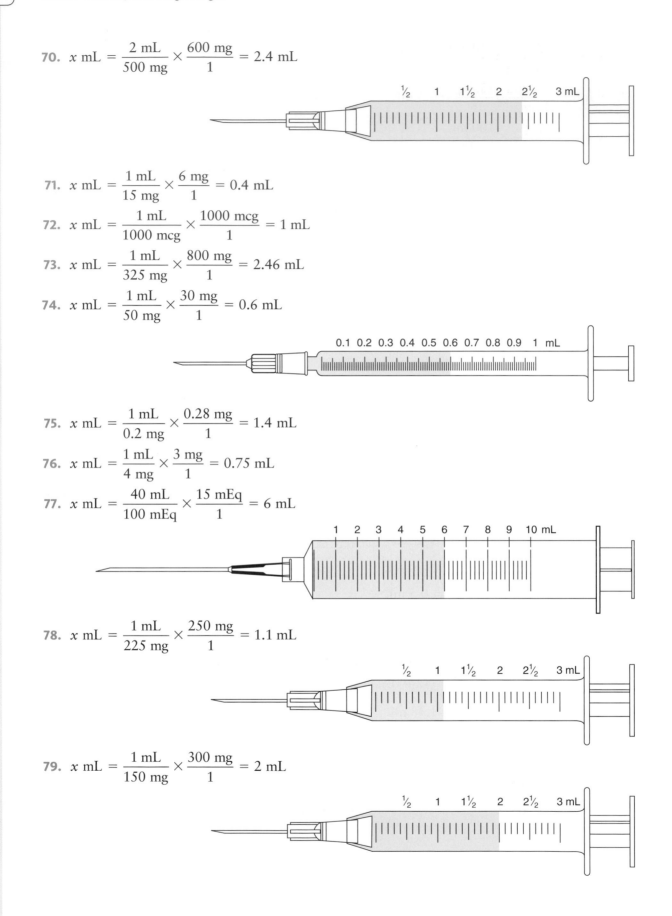

71. $x \text{ mL} = \dfrac{1 \text{ mL}}{15 \text{ mg}} \times \dfrac{6 \text{ mg}}{1} = 0.4 \text{ mL}$

72. $x \text{ mL} = \dfrac{1 \text{ mL}}{1000 \text{ mcg}} \times \dfrac{1000 \text{ mcg}}{1} = 1 \text{ mL}$

73. $x \text{ mL} = \dfrac{1 \text{ mL}}{325 \text{ mg}} \times \dfrac{800 \text{ mg}}{1} = 2.46 \text{ mL}$

74. $x \text{ mL} = \dfrac{1 \text{ mL}}{50 \text{ mg}} \times \dfrac{30 \text{ mg}}{1} = 0.6 \text{ mL}$

75. $x \text{ mL} = \dfrac{1 \text{ mL}}{0.2 \text{ mg}} \times \dfrac{0.28 \text{ mg}}{1} = 1.4 \text{ mL}$

76. $x \text{ mL} = \dfrac{1 \text{ mL}}{4 \text{ mg}} \times \dfrac{3 \text{ mg}}{1} = 0.75 \text{ mL}$

77. $x \text{ mL} = \dfrac{40 \text{ mL}}{100 \text{ mEq}} \times \dfrac{15 \text{ mEq}}{1} = 6 \text{ mL}$

78. $x \text{ mL} = \dfrac{1 \text{ mL}}{225 \text{ mg}} \times \dfrac{250 \text{ mg}}{1} = 1.1 \text{ mL}$

79. $x \text{ mL} = \dfrac{1 \text{ mL}}{150 \text{ mg}} \times \dfrac{300 \text{ mg}}{1} = 2 \text{ mL}$

ANSWERS

80. $x \text{ mL} = \dfrac{5 \text{ mL}}{100 \text{ mg}} \times \dfrac{75 \text{ mg}}{1} = 3.75 \text{ mL}$

81. $x \text{ mL} = \dfrac{2.6 \text{ mL}}{1 \text{ g}} \times \dfrac{0.8 \text{ g}}{1} = 2.08 \text{ mL}$

82. $x \text{ mL} = \dfrac{2 \text{ mL}}{125 \text{ mg}} \times \dfrac{100 \text{ mg}}{1} = 1.6 \text{ mL}$

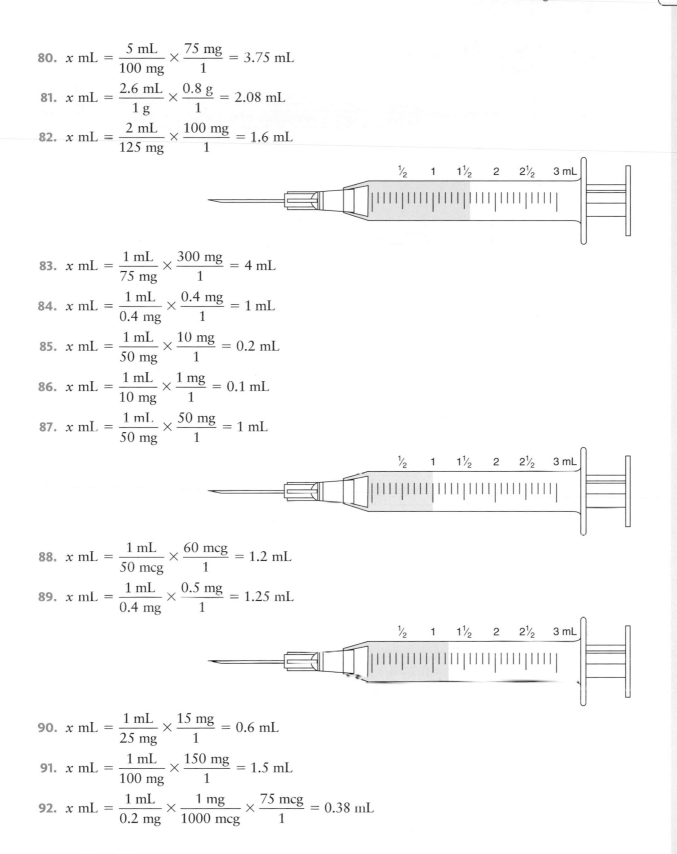

83. $x \text{ mL} = \dfrac{1 \text{ mL}}{75 \text{ mg}} \times \dfrac{300 \text{ mg}}{1} = 4 \text{ mL}$

84. $x \text{ mL} = \dfrac{1 \text{ mL}}{0.4 \text{ mg}} \times \dfrac{0.4 \text{ mg}}{1} = 1 \text{ mL}$

85. $x \text{ mL} = \dfrac{1 \text{ mL}}{50 \text{ mg}} \times \dfrac{10 \text{ mg}}{1} = 0.2 \text{ mL}$

86. $x \text{ mL} = \dfrac{1 \text{ mL}}{10 \text{ mg}} \times \dfrac{1 \text{ mg}}{1} = 0.1 \text{ mL}$

87. $x \text{ mL} = \dfrac{1 \text{ mL}}{50 \text{ mg}} \times \dfrac{50 \text{ mg}}{1} = 1 \text{ mL}$

88. $x \text{ mL} = \dfrac{1 \text{ mL}}{50 \text{ mcg}} \times \dfrac{60 \text{ mcg}}{1} = 1.2 \text{ mL}$

89. $x \text{ mL} = \dfrac{1 \text{ mL}}{0.4 \text{ mg}} \times \dfrac{0.5 \text{ mg}}{1} = 1.25 \text{ mL}$

90. $x \text{ mL} = \dfrac{1 \text{ mL}}{25 \text{ mg}} \times \dfrac{15 \text{ mg}}{1} = 0.6 \text{ mL}$

91. $x \text{ mL} = \dfrac{1 \text{ mL}}{100 \text{ mg}} \times \dfrac{150 \text{ mg}}{1} = 1.5 \text{ mL}$

92. $x \text{ mL} = \dfrac{1 \text{ mL}}{0.2 \text{ mg}} \times \dfrac{1 \text{ mg}}{1000 \text{ mcg}} \times \dfrac{75 \text{ mcg}}{1} = 0.38 \text{ mL}$

ANSWERS

93. $x \text{ mL} = \dfrac{1 \text{ mL}}{5 \text{ mg}} \times \dfrac{2 \text{ mg}}{1} = 0.4 \text{ mL}$

94. $x \text{ mL} = \dfrac{1 \text{ mL}}{100 \text{ mg}} \times \dfrac{500 \text{ mg}}{1} = 5 \text{ mL}$

95. $x \text{ mL} = \dfrac{2.5 \text{ mL}}{1000 \text{ mg}} \times \dfrac{640 \text{ mg}}{1} = 1.6 \text{ mL}$

96. $x \text{ mL} = \dfrac{1 \text{ mL}}{250 \text{ mg}} \times \dfrac{500 \text{ mg}}{1} = 2 \text{ mL}$

97. $x \text{ mL} = \dfrac{1 \text{ mL}}{2 \text{ mg}} \times \dfrac{0.5 \text{ mg}}{1} = 0.25 \text{ mL}$

98. $x \text{ mL} = \dfrac{0.5 \text{ mL}}{25 \text{ mg}} \times \dfrac{100 \text{ mg}}{1} = 2 \text{ mL}$

99. $x \text{ mL} = \dfrac{1 \text{ mL}}{50 \text{ mg}} \times \dfrac{10 \text{ mg}}{1} = 0.2 \text{ mL}$

100. $x \text{ mL} = \dfrac{1 \text{ mL}}{5 \text{ mg}} \times \dfrac{3.5 \text{ mg}}{1} = 0.7 \text{ mL}$

CHAPTER 12 Dimensional Analysis—Posttest 1, pp. 307–311

1. $x \text{ mL} = \dfrac{1 \text{ mL}}{50 \text{ mg}} \times \dfrac{25 \text{ mg}}{1} = 0.5 \text{ mL}$

2. $x \text{ mL} = \dfrac{1 \text{ mL}}{50 \text{ mg}} \times \dfrac{25 \text{ mg}}{1} = 0.5 \text{ mL}$

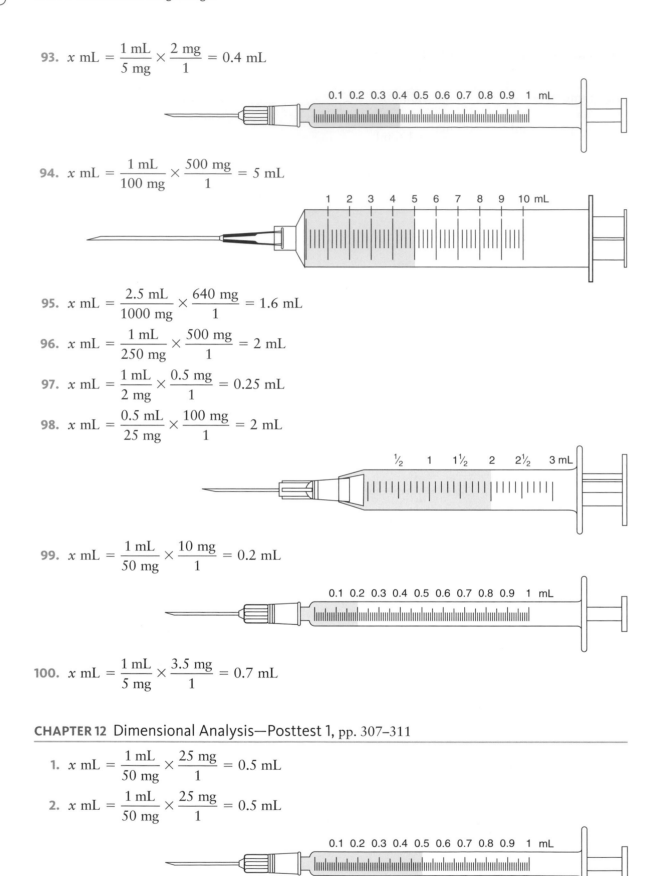

3. $x \text{ mL} = \dfrac{1 \text{ mL}}{15 \text{ mg}} \times \dfrac{30 \text{ mg}}{1} = 2 \text{ mL}$

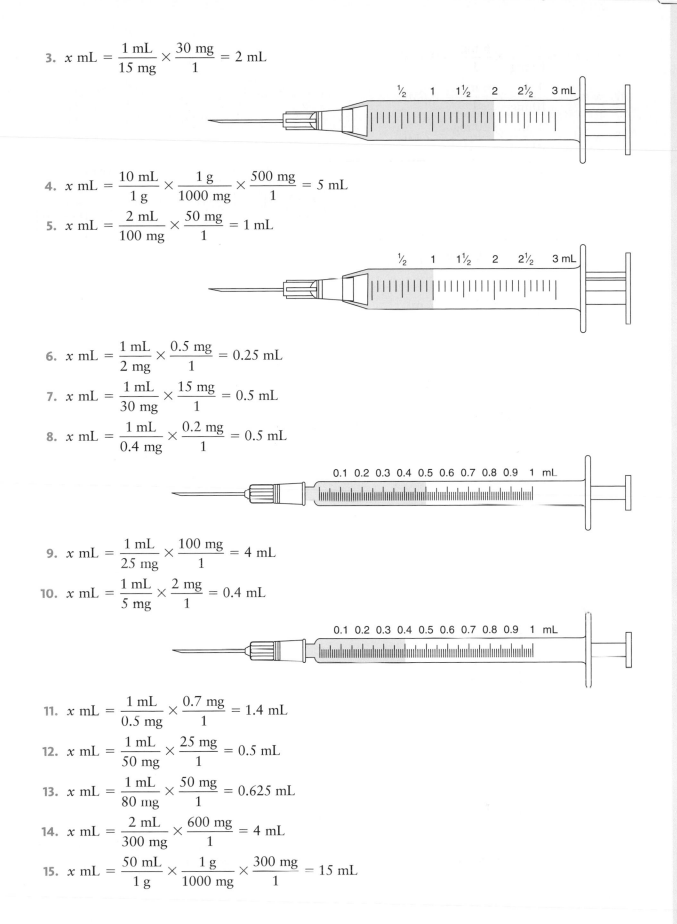

4. $x \text{ mL} = \dfrac{10 \text{ mL}}{1 \text{ g}} \times \dfrac{1 \text{ g}}{1000 \text{ mg}} \times \dfrac{500 \text{ mg}}{1} = 5 \text{ mL}$

5. $x \text{ mL} = \dfrac{2 \text{ mL}}{100 \text{ mg}} \times \dfrac{50 \text{ mg}}{1} = 1 \text{ mL}$

6. $x \text{ mL} = \dfrac{1 \text{ mL}}{2 \text{ mg}} \times \dfrac{0.5 \text{ mg}}{1} = 0.25 \text{ mL}$

7. $x \text{ mL} = \dfrac{1 \text{ mL}}{30 \text{ mg}} \times \dfrac{15 \text{ mg}}{1} = 0.5 \text{ mL}$

8. $x \text{ mL} = \dfrac{1 \text{ mL}}{0.4 \text{ mg}} \times \dfrac{0.2 \text{ mg}}{1} = 0.5 \text{ mL}$

9. $x \text{ mL} = \dfrac{1 \text{ mL}}{25 \text{ mg}} \times \dfrac{100 \text{ mg}}{1} = 4 \text{ mL}$

10. $x \text{ mL} = \dfrac{1 \text{ mL}}{5 \text{ mg}} \times \dfrac{2 \text{ mg}}{1} = 0.4 \text{ mL}$

11. $x \text{ mL} = \dfrac{1 \text{ mL}}{0.5 \text{ mg}} \times \dfrac{0.7 \text{ mg}}{1} = 1.4 \text{ mL}$

12. $x \text{ mL} = \dfrac{1 \text{ mL}}{50 \text{ mg}} \times \dfrac{25 \text{ mg}}{1} = 0.5 \text{ mL}$

13. $x \text{ mL} = \dfrac{1 \text{ mL}}{80 \text{ mg}} \times \dfrac{50 \text{ mg}}{1} = 0.625 \text{ mL}$

14. $x \text{ mL} = \dfrac{2 \text{ mL}}{300 \text{ mg}} \times \dfrac{600 \text{ mg}}{1} = 4 \text{ mL}$

15. $x \text{ mL} = \dfrac{50 \text{ mL}}{1 \text{ g}} \times \dfrac{1 \text{ g}}{1000 \text{ mg}} \times \dfrac{300 \text{ mg}}{1} = 15 \text{ mL}$

ANSWERS

16. $x \text{ mL} = \dfrac{1 \text{ mL}}{10 \text{ mg}} \times \dfrac{6 \text{ mg}}{1} = 0.6 \text{ mL}$

17. $x \text{ mL} = \dfrac{1 \text{ mL}}{10 \text{ mg}} \times \dfrac{6 \text{ mg}}{1} = 0.6 \text{ mL}$

18. $x \text{ mL} = \dfrac{1 \text{ mL}}{10 \text{ mg}} \times \dfrac{20 \text{ mg}}{1} = 2 \text{ mL}$

19. $x \text{ mL} = \dfrac{2 \text{ mL}}{0.5 \text{ mg}} \times \dfrac{0.3 \text{ mg}}{1} = 1.2 \text{ mL}$

20. $x \text{ mL} = \dfrac{1 \text{ mL}}{2.5 \text{ mg}} \times \dfrac{5 \text{ mg}}{1} = 2 \text{ mL}$

CHAPTER 12 Dimensional Analysis—Posttest 2, pp. 313–318

1. $x \text{ mL} = \dfrac{1 \text{ mL}}{4 \text{ mg}} \times \dfrac{2 \text{ mg}}{1} = 0.5 \text{ mL}$

2. $x \text{ mL} = \dfrac{1 \text{ mL}}{4 \text{ mg}} \times \dfrac{2 \text{ mg}}{1} = 0.5 \text{ mL}$

3. $x \text{ mL} = \dfrac{10 \text{ mL}}{500 \text{ mg}} \times \dfrac{1000 \text{ mg}}{1 \text{ g}} \times \dfrac{0.4 \text{ g}}{1} = 8 \text{ mL}$

4. $x \text{ mL} = \dfrac{1 \text{ mL}}{5 \text{ mg}} \times \dfrac{20 \text{ mg}}{1} = 4 \text{ mL}$

5. $x \text{ mL} = \dfrac{1 \text{ mL}}{30 \text{ mg}} \times \dfrac{60 \text{ mg}}{1} = 2 \text{ mL}$

6. $x \text{ mL} = \dfrac{1 \text{ mL}}{100 \text{ mg}} \times \dfrac{200 \text{ mg}}{1} = 2 \text{ mL}$

7. $x \text{ mL} = \dfrac{1 \text{ mL}}{0.4 \text{ mg}} \times \dfrac{0.2 \text{ mg}}{1} = 0.5 \text{ mL}$

ANSWERS

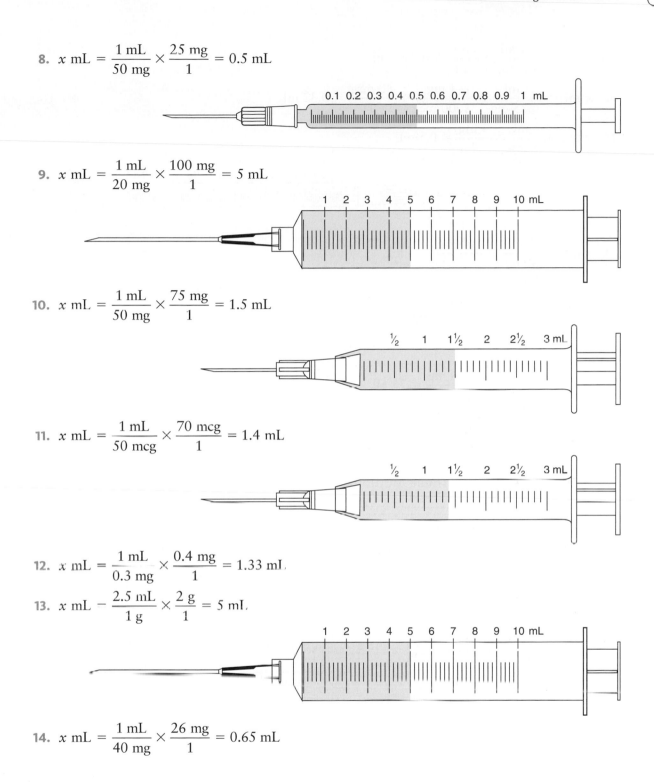

8. $x \text{ mL} = \dfrac{1 \text{ mL}}{50 \text{ mg}} \times \dfrac{25 \text{ mg}}{1} = 0.5 \text{ mL}$

9. $x \text{ mL} = \dfrac{1 \text{ mL}}{20 \text{ mg}} \times \dfrac{100 \text{ mg}}{1} = 5 \text{ mL}$

10. $x \text{ mL} = \dfrac{1 \text{ mL}}{50 \text{ mg}} \times \dfrac{75 \text{ mg}}{1} = 1.5 \text{ mL}$

11. $x \text{ mL} = \dfrac{1 \text{ mL}}{50 \text{ mcg}} \times \dfrac{70 \text{ mcg}}{1} = 1.4 \text{ mL}$

12. $x \text{ mL} = \dfrac{1 \text{ mL}}{0.3 \text{ mg}} \times \dfrac{0.4 \text{ mg}}{1} = 1.33 \text{ mL}$

13. $x \text{ mL} = \dfrac{2.5 \text{ mL}}{1 \text{ g}} \times \dfrac{2 \text{ g}}{1} = 5 \text{ mL}$

14. $x \text{ mL} = \dfrac{1 \text{ mL}}{40 \text{ mg}} \times \dfrac{26 \text{ mg}}{1} = 0.65 \text{ mL}$

15. $x \text{ mL} = \dfrac{0.4 \text{ mL}}{40 \text{ mg}} \times \dfrac{85 \text{ mg}}{1} = 0.85 \text{ mL}$

16. $x \text{ mL} = \dfrac{1 \text{ mL}}{0.25 \text{ mg}} \times \dfrac{1 \text{ mg}}{1000 \text{ mcg}} \times \dfrac{80 \text{ mcg}}{1} = 0.32 \text{ mL}$

17. $x \text{ mL} = \dfrac{1 \text{ mL}}{8 \text{ mg}} \times \dfrac{4 \text{ mg}}{1} = 0.5 \text{ mL}$

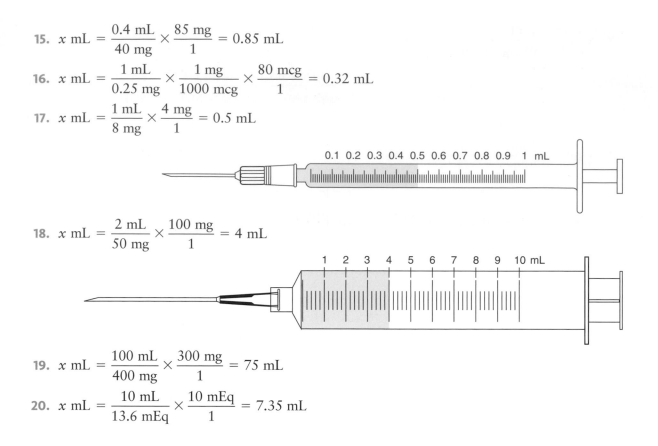

18. $x \text{ mL} = \dfrac{2 \text{ mL}}{50 \text{ mg}} \times \dfrac{100 \text{ mg}}{1} = 4 \text{ mL}$

19. $x \text{ mL} = \dfrac{100 \text{ mL}}{400 \text{ mg}} \times \dfrac{300 \text{ mg}}{1} = 75 \text{ mL}$

20. $x \text{ mL} = \dfrac{10 \text{ mL}}{13.6 \text{ mEq}} \times \dfrac{10 \text{ mEq}}{1} = 7.35 \text{ mL}$

CHAPTER 12 Proportion/Formula Method—Worksheet, pp. 283–306

Proportion	Formula
1. 400 mg : 1 mL :: 500 mg : x mL $400x = 500$ $x = \dfrac{500}{400}$ $x = 1.25$ mL or 1.3 mL	$\dfrac{500 \text{ mg}}{400 \text{ mg}} \times 1 \text{ mL} = 1.25 \text{ mL or } 1.3 \text{ mL}$

Proportion	Formula

2. 500 mcg : 2 mL :: 110 mcg : x mL
$500x = 220$
$x = \dfrac{220}{500}$
$x = 0.44$ mL

$\dfrac{110 \text{ mcg}}{500 \text{ mcg}} \times 2 \text{ mL} = \dfrac{220}{500} = 0.44 \text{ mL}$

0.1 0.2 0.3 0.4 0.5 0.6 0.7 0.8 0.9 1 mL

3. 0.4 mg : 1 mL :: 0.3 mg : x mL
$0.4x = 0.3$
$x = \dfrac{0.3}{0.4}$
$x = 0.75$ mL

$\dfrac{0.3 \text{ mg}}{0.4 \text{ mg}} \times 1 \text{ mL} = 0.75 \text{ mL}$

0.1 0.2 0.3 0.4 0.5 0.6 0.7 0.8 0.9 1 mL

4. 5 mg : 1 mL :: 10 mg : x mL
$5x = 10$
$x = \dfrac{10}{5}$
$x = 2$ mL

$\dfrac{10 \text{ mg}}{5 \text{ mg}} \times 1 \text{ mL} = 2 \text{ mL}$

½ 1 1½ 2 2½ 3 mL

5. 25 mg : 1 mL :: 50 mg : x mL
$25x = 50$
$x = \dfrac{50}{25}$
$x = 2$ mL

$\dfrac{50 \text{ mg}}{25 \text{ mg}} \times 1 \text{ mL} = \dfrac{50}{25} = 2 \text{ mL}$

½ 1 1½ 2 2½ 3 mL

6. 1 g : 2.5 mL :: 3 g : x mL
$x = 2.5 \times 3$
$x = 7.5$ mL

$\dfrac{3 \text{ g}}{1 \text{ g}} \times 2.5 \text{ mL} = 7.5 \text{ mL}$

7. 10 mg : 1 mL :: 5 mg : x mL
$10x = 5$
$x = \dfrac{5}{10}$
$x = 0.5$ mL

$\dfrac{5 \text{ mg}}{10 \text{ mg}} \times 1 \text{ mL} = 0.5 \text{ mL}$

ANSWERS

Proportion	**Formula**

8. 5 mg : 1 mL :: 4 mg : x mL

$5x = 4$

$x = \dfrac{4}{5}$

$x = 0.8$ mL

$\dfrac{4 \text{ mg}}{5 \text{ mg}} \times 1 \text{ mL} = \dfrac{4}{5} = 0.8 \text{ mL}$

9. 40 mg : 4 mL :: 30 mg : x mL

$40x = 120$

$x = \dfrac{120}{40}$

$x = 3$ mL

$\dfrac{30 \text{ mg}}{\underset{10}{\cancel{40}} \text{ mg}} \times \dfrac{\overset{1}{\cancel{4}} \text{ mL}}{1} = \dfrac{30}{10} = 3 \text{ mL}$

10. 30 mg : 1 mL :: 15 mg : x mL

$30x = 15$

$x = \dfrac{15}{30}$

$x = 0.5$ mL

$\dfrac{\overset{1}{\cancel{15}} \text{ mg}}{\underset{2}{\cancel{30}} \text{ mg}} \times 1 \text{ mL} = \tfrac{1}{2} \text{ or } 0.5 \text{ mL}$

11. 44.6 mEq : 50 mL :: 25.8 mEq : x mL

$44.6x = 1290$

$x = \dfrac{1290}{44.6}$

$x = 28.9$ mL or 29 mL

$\dfrac{25.8 \text{ mEq}}{44.6 \text{ mEq}} \times 50 \text{ mL} =$

$0.58 \times 50 = 28.9 \text{ mL or } 29 \text{ mL}$

12. 25 mg : 1 mL :: 100 mg : x mL

$25x = 100$

$x = \dfrac{100}{25}$

$x = 4$ mL

$\dfrac{100 \text{ mg}}{25 \text{ mg}} \times 1 \text{ mL} = 4 \text{ mL}$

13. 100 mg : 20 mL :: 350 mg : x mL

$100x = 7000$

$x = \dfrac{7000}{100}$

$x = 70$ mL

$\dfrac{\overset{70}{\cancel{350}} \text{ mg}}{\underset{1}{\underset{\cancel{5}}{\cancel{100}}} \text{ mg}} \times \dfrac{\overset{1}{\cancel{20}} \text{ mL}}{1} =$

$\dfrac{70}{1} = 70 \text{ mL}$

14. 400 mg : 40 mL :: 300 mg : x mL

$400x = 12{,}000$

$x = \dfrac{12{,}000}{400}$

$x = 30$ mL

$\dfrac{300 \text{ mg}}{400 \text{ mg}} \times 40 \text{ mL} =$

$\dfrac{300}{\underset{10}{\cancel{400}}} \times \dfrac{\overset{1}{\cancel{40}}}{1} =$

$\dfrac{300}{10} = 30 \text{ mL}$

Proportion	**Formula**

15. 250 mg : 2 mL :: 50 mg : x mL
250x = 100
$x = \dfrac{100}{250}$
$x = 0.4$ mL

$$\dfrac{50 \text{ mg}}{\underset{125}{\cancel{250}} \text{ mg}} \times \dfrac{\overset{1}{\cancel{2}} \text{ mL}}{1} = \dfrac{50}{125} = 0.4 \text{ mL}$$

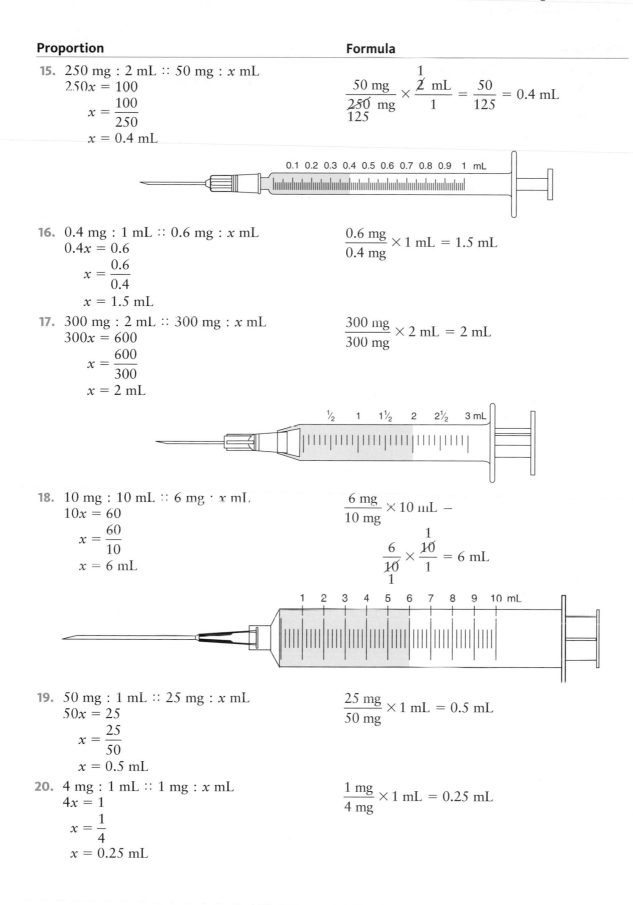

16. 0.4 mg : 1 mL :: 0.6 mg : x mL
0.4x = 0.6
$x = \dfrac{0.6}{0.4}$
$x = 1.5$ mL

$$\dfrac{0.6 \text{ mg}}{0.4 \text{ mg}} \times 1 \text{ mL} = 1.5 \text{ mL}$$

17. 300 mg : 2 mL :: 300 mg : x mL
300x = 600
$x = \dfrac{600}{300}$
$x = 2$ mL

$$\dfrac{300 \text{ mg}}{300 \text{ mg}} \times 2 \text{ mL} = 2 \text{ mL}$$

18. 10 mg : 10 mL :: 6 mg : x mL
10x = 60
$x = \dfrac{60}{10}$
$x = 6$ mL

$$\dfrac{6 \text{ mg}}{10 \text{ mg}} \times 10 \text{ mL} -$$

$$\dfrac{6}{\underset{1}{\cancel{10}}} \times \dfrac{\overset{1}{\cancel{10}}}{1} = 6 \text{ mL}$$

19. 50 mg : 1 mL :: 25 mg : x mL
50x = 25
$x = \dfrac{25}{50}$
$x = 0.5$ mL

$$\dfrac{25 \text{ mg}}{50 \text{ mg}} \times 1 \text{ mL} = 0.5 \text{ mL}$$

20. 4 mg : 1 mL :: 1 mg : x mL
4x = 1
$x = \dfrac{1}{4}$
$x = 0.25$ mL

$$\dfrac{1 \text{ mg}}{4 \text{ mg}} \times 1 \text{ mL} = 0.25 \text{ mL}$$

ANSWERS

Proportion	Formula
21. 20 mg : 1 mL :: 10 mg : x mL $20x = 10$ $x = \dfrac{10}{20}$ $x = 0.5$ mL	$\dfrac{10 \text{ mg}}{20 \text{ mg}} \times 1 \text{ mL} = 0.5 \text{ mL}$

0.1 0.2 0.3 0.4 0.5 0.6 0.7 0.8 0.9 1 mL

Proportion	Formula
22. 500 mg : 2 mL :: 400 mg : x mL $500x = 800$ $x = \dfrac{800}{500}$ $x = 1.6$ mL	$\dfrac{400 \text{ mg}}{500 \text{ mg}} \times 2 \text{ mL} =$ $\dfrac{800}{500} = 1.6 \text{ mL}$
23. 5 mg : 1 mL :: 7.5 mg : x mL $5x = 7.5$ $x = \dfrac{7.5}{5}$ $x = 1.5$ mL	$\dfrac{7.5 \text{ mg}}{5 \text{ mg}} \times 1 \text{ mL} = 1.5 \text{ mL}$

½ 1 1½ 2 2½ 3 mL

Proportion	Formula
24. 30 mg : 1 mL :: 15 mg : x mL $30x = 15$ $x = \dfrac{15}{30}$ $x = \tfrac{1}{2}$ $x = 0.5$ mL	$\dfrac{15 \text{ mg}}{30 \text{ mg}} \times 1 \text{ mL} = 0.5 \text{ mL}$
25. 10 mg : 1 mL :: 10 mg : x mL $10x = 10$ $x = \dfrac{10}{10}$ $x = 1$ mL	$\dfrac{10 \text{ mg}}{10 \text{ mg}} \times 1 \text{ mL} = 1 \text{ mL}$

½ 1 1½ 2 2½ 3 mL

Proportion	Formula
26. 400 mg : 40 mL :: 200 mg : x mL $400x = 8000$ $x = \dfrac{8000}{400}$ $x = 20$ mL	$\dfrac{200 \text{ mg}}{400 \text{ mg}} \times \dfrac{40 \text{ mL}}{1} = 20 \text{ mL}$

Proportion   **Formula**

27. 15 mg : 1 mL :: 6 mg : x mL
     15x = 6
     $$x = \frac{6}{15}$$
     x = 0.4 mL

$$\frac{6 \text{ mg}}{15 \text{ mg}} \times 1 \text{ mL} = 0.4 \text{ mL}$$

28. 50 mg : 1 mL :: 100 mg : x mL
     50x = 100
     $$x = \frac{100}{50}$$
     x = 2 mL

$$\frac{100 \text{ mg}}{50 \text{ mg}} \times 1 \text{ mL} = 2 \text{ mL}$$

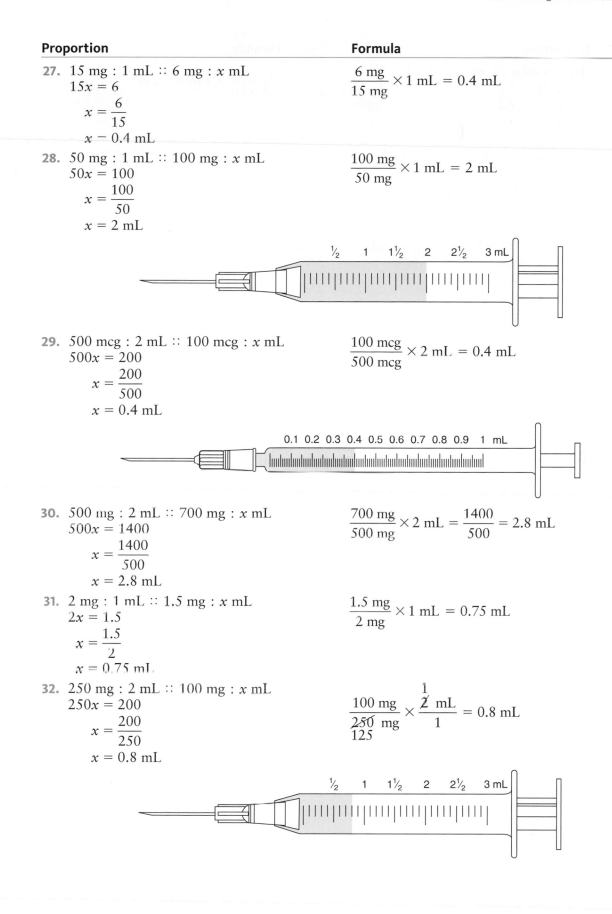

29. 500 mcg : 2 mL :: 100 mcg : x mL
     500x = 200
     $$x = \frac{200}{500}$$
     x = 0.4 mL

$$\frac{100 \text{ mcg}}{500 \text{ mcg}} \times 2 \text{ mL} = 0.4 \text{ mL}$$

30. 500 mg : 2 mL :: 700 mg : x mL
     500x = 1400
     $$x = \frac{1400}{500}$$
     x = 2.8 mL

$$\frac{700 \text{ mg}}{500 \text{ mg}} \times 2 \text{ mL} = \frac{1400}{500} = 2.8 \text{ mL}$$

31. 2 mg : 1 mL :: 1.5 mg : x mL
     2x = 1.5
     $$x = \frac{1.5}{2}$$
     x = 0.75 mL

$$\frac{1.5 \text{ mg}}{2 \text{ mg}} \times 1 \text{ mL} = 0.75 \text{ mL}$$

32. 250 mg : 2 mL :: 100 mg : x mL
     250x = 200
     $$x = \frac{200}{250}$$
     x = 0.8 mL

$$\frac{100 \text{ mg}}{\underset{125}{\cancel{250} \text{ mg}}} \times \frac{\overset{1}{\cancel{2}} \text{ mL}}{1} = 0.8 \text{ mL}$$

Proportion	Formula
33. $2.5 \text{ mEq} : 1 \text{ mL} :: 7.5 \text{ mEq} : x \text{ mL}$ $2.5x = 7.5$ $x = \dfrac{7.5}{2.5}$ $x = 3 \text{ mL}$	$\dfrac{7.5 \text{ mEq}}{2.5 \text{ mEq}} \times 1 \text{ mL} = 3 \text{ mL}$
34. $50 \text{ mg} : 1 \text{ mL} :: 25 \text{ mg} : x \text{ mL}$ $50x = 25$ $x = \dfrac{25}{50}$ $x = 0.5 \text{ mL}$	$\dfrac{25 \text{ mg}}{50 \text{ mg}} \times 1 \text{ mL} = 0.5 \text{ mL}$
35. $0.4 \text{ mg} : 1 \text{ mL} :: 0.6 \text{ mg} : x \text{ mL}$ $0.4x = 0.6$ $x = \dfrac{0.6}{0.4}$ $x = 1.5 \text{ mL}$	$\dfrac{0.6 \text{ mg}}{0.4 \text{ mg}} \times 1 \text{ mL} = 1.5 \text{ mL}$
36. $100 \text{ mg} : 1 \text{ mL} :: 150 \text{ mg} : x \text{ mL}$ $100x = 150$ $x = \dfrac{150}{100}$ $x = 1.5 \text{ mL}$	$\dfrac{150 \text{ mg}}{100 \text{ mg}} \times 1 \text{ mL} = 1.5 \text{ mL}$

Proportion	Formula
37. $0.25 \text{ mg} : 1 \text{ mL} :: 0.5 \text{ mg} : x \text{ mL}$ $0.25x = 0.5$ $x = \dfrac{0.5}{0.25}$ $x = 2 \text{ mL}$	$\dfrac{0.5 \text{ mg}}{0.25 \text{ mg}} \times 1 \text{ mL} = 2 \text{ mL}$

Proportion	Formula
38. $25 \text{ mg} : 1 \text{ mL} :: 75 \text{ mg} : x \text{ mL}$ $25x = 75$ $x = \dfrac{75}{25}$ $x = 3 \text{ mL}$	$\dfrac{75 \text{ mg}}{25 \text{ mg}} \times 1 \text{ mL} = 3 \text{ mL}$

Proportion	Formula

39. $0.4 \text{ mg} : 1 \text{ mL} :: 0.6 \text{ mg} : x \text{ mL}$
$0.4x = 0.6$
$x = \dfrac{0.6}{0.4}$
$x = 1.5 \text{ mL}$

$\dfrac{0.6 \text{ mg}}{0.4 \text{ mg}} \times \dfrac{1 \text{ mL}}{1} = 1.5 \text{ mL}$

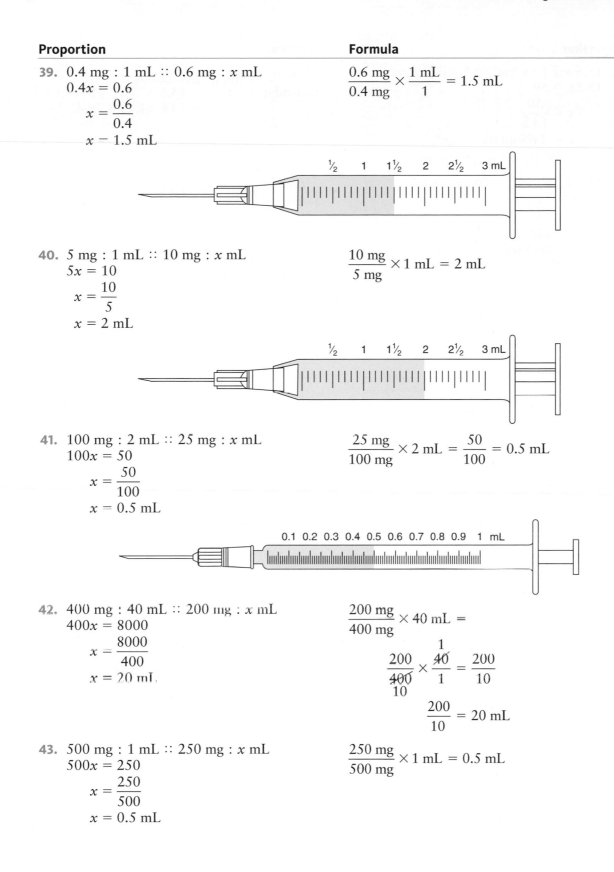

40. $5 \text{ mg} : 1 \text{ mL} :: 10 \text{ mg} : x \text{ mL}$
$5x = 10$
$x = \dfrac{10}{5}$
$x = 2 \text{ mL}$

$\dfrac{10 \text{ mg}}{5 \text{ mg}} \times 1 \text{ mL} = 2 \text{ mL}$

41. $100 \text{ mg} : 2 \text{ mL} :: 25 \text{ mg} : x \text{ mL}$
$100x = 50$
$x = \dfrac{50}{100}$
$x = 0.5 \text{ mL}$

$\dfrac{25 \text{ mg}}{100 \text{ mg}} \times 2 \text{ mL} = \dfrac{50}{100} = 0.5 \text{ mL}$

42. $400 \text{ mg} : 40 \text{ mL} :: 200 \text{ mg} : x \text{ mL}$
$400x = 8000$
$x = \dfrac{8000}{400}$
$x = 20 \text{ mL}$

$\dfrac{200 \text{ mg}}{400 \text{ mg}} \times 40 \text{ mL} =$
$\dfrac{200}{\underset{10}{400}} \times \dfrac{\overset{1}{40}}{1} = \dfrac{200}{10}$
$\dfrac{200}{10} = 20 \text{ mL}$

43. $500 \text{ mg} : 1 \text{ mL} :: 250 \text{ mg} : x \text{ mL}$
$500x = 250$
$x = \dfrac{250}{500}$
$x = 0.5 \text{ mL}$

$\dfrac{250 \text{ mg}}{500 \text{ mg}} \times 1 \text{ mL} = 0.5 \text{ mL}$

ANSWERS

Proportion   **Formula**

44. 13.6 mEq : 10 mL :: 5 mEq : x mL
$13.6x = 50$
$x = \dfrac{50}{13.6}$
$x = 3.68$ mL or 3.7 mL

$\dfrac{5 \text{ mEq}}{13.6 \text{ mEq}} \times 10 \text{ mL} = \dfrac{50}{13.6}$
$= 3.68$ mL or 3.7 mL

45. 130 mg : 1 mL :: 70 mg : x mL
$130x = 70$
$x = \dfrac{70}{130}$
$x = 0.54$ mL

$\dfrac{70 \text{ mg}}{130 \text{ mg}} \times 1 \text{ mL} = 0.54$ mL

46. 10 mg : 1 mL :: 200 mg : x mL
$10x = 200$
$x = \dfrac{200}{10}$
$x = 20$ mL

$\dfrac{200 \text{ mg}}{10 \text{ mg}} \times 1 \text{ mL} = 20$ mL

47. 4 mg : 1 mL :: 2 mg : x mL
$4x = 2$
$x = \dfrac{2}{4} = 0.5$ mL

$\dfrac{2 \text{ mg}}{4 \text{ mg}} \times 1 \text{ mL} = \dfrac{2}{4} = 0.5$ mL

48. 0.5 mg : 2 mL :: 0.2 mg : x mL
$0.5x = 0.4$
$x = \dfrac{0.4}{0.5}$
$x = 0.8$ mL

$\dfrac{0.2 \text{ mg}}{0.5 \text{ mg}} \times 2 \text{ mL} = \dfrac{0.4}{0.5} = 0.8$ mL

49. 15 mg : 1 mL :: 10 mg : x mL
$15x = 10$
$x = \dfrac{10}{15}$
$x = 0.67$ mL

$\dfrac{10 \text{ mg}}{15 \text{ mg}} \times 1 \text{ mL} = 0.67$ mL

ANSWERS

Proportion	Formula

50. 50 mg : 1 mL :: 25 mg : x mL
$50x = 25$
$x = \dfrac{25}{50}$
$x = 0.5$ mL

$\dfrac{25 \text{ mg}}{50 \text{ mg}} \times 1 \text{ mL} = 0.5 \text{ mL}$

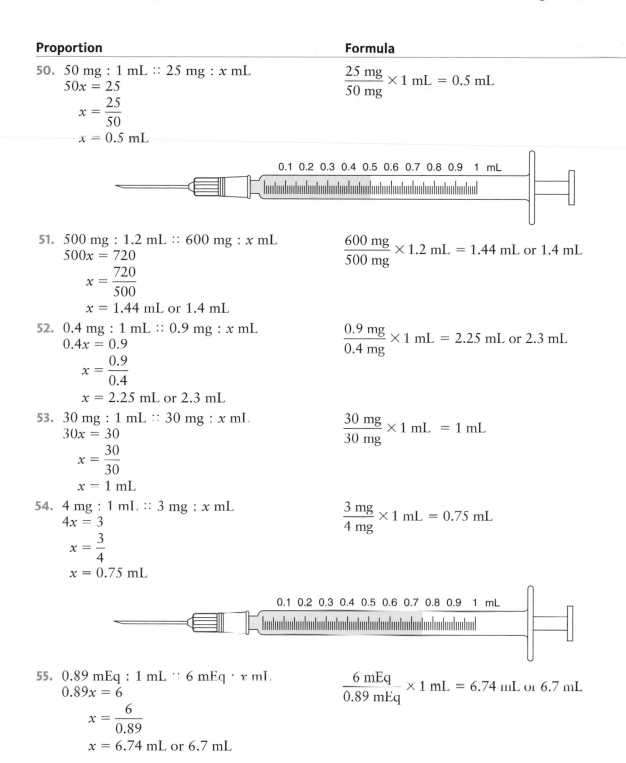

51. 500 mg : 1.2 mL :: 600 mg : x mL
$500x = 720$
$x = \dfrac{720}{500}$
$x = 1.44$ mL or 1.4 mL

$\dfrac{600 \text{ mg}}{500 \text{ mg}} \times 1.2 \text{ mL} = 1.44 \text{ mL or } 1.4 \text{ mL}$

52. 0.4 mg : 1 mL :: 0.9 mg : x mL
$0.4x = 0.9$
$x = \dfrac{0.9}{0.4}$
$x = 2.25$ mL or 2.3 mL

$\dfrac{0.9 \text{ mg}}{0.4 \text{ mg}} \times 1 \text{ mL} = 2.25 \text{ mL or } 2.3 \text{ mL}$

53. 30 mg : 1 mL :: 30 mg : x mL
$30x = 30$
$x = \dfrac{30}{30}$
$x = 1$ mL

$\dfrac{30 \text{ mg}}{30 \text{ mg}} \times 1 \text{ mL} = 1 \text{ mL}$

54. 4 mg : 1 mL :: 3 mg : x mL
$4x = 3$
$x = \dfrac{3}{4}$
$x = 0.75$ mL

$\dfrac{3 \text{ mg}}{4 \text{ mg}} \times 1 \text{ mL} = 0.75 \text{ mL}$

55. 0.89 mEq : 1 mL :: 6 mEq : x mL
$0.89x = 6$
$x = \dfrac{6}{0.89}$
$x = 6.74$ mL or 6.7 mL

$\dfrac{6 \text{ mEq}}{0.89 \text{ mEq}} \times 1 \text{ mL} = 6.74 \text{ mL or } 6.7 \text{ mL}$

ANSWERS

Proportion	**Formula**

56. 20 mg : 1 mL :: 10 mg : x mL

  $20x = 10$

  $x = \dfrac{10}{20}$

  $x = 0.5$ mL

$\dfrac{10 \text{ mg}}{20 \text{ mg}} \times 1 \text{ mL} = 0.5 \text{ mL}$

57. 25 mg : 1 mL :: 5 mg : x mL

  $25x = 5$

  $x = \dfrac{5}{25}$

  $x = 0.2$ mL

$\dfrac{5 \text{ mg}}{25 \text{ mg}} \times 1 \text{ mL} = 0.2 \text{ mL}$

58. 125 mg : 1 mL :: 500 mg : x mL

  $125x = 500$

  $x = \dfrac{500}{125}$

  $x = 4$ mL

$\dfrac{500 \text{ mg}}{125 \text{ mg}} \times 1 \text{ mL} = 4 \text{ mL}$

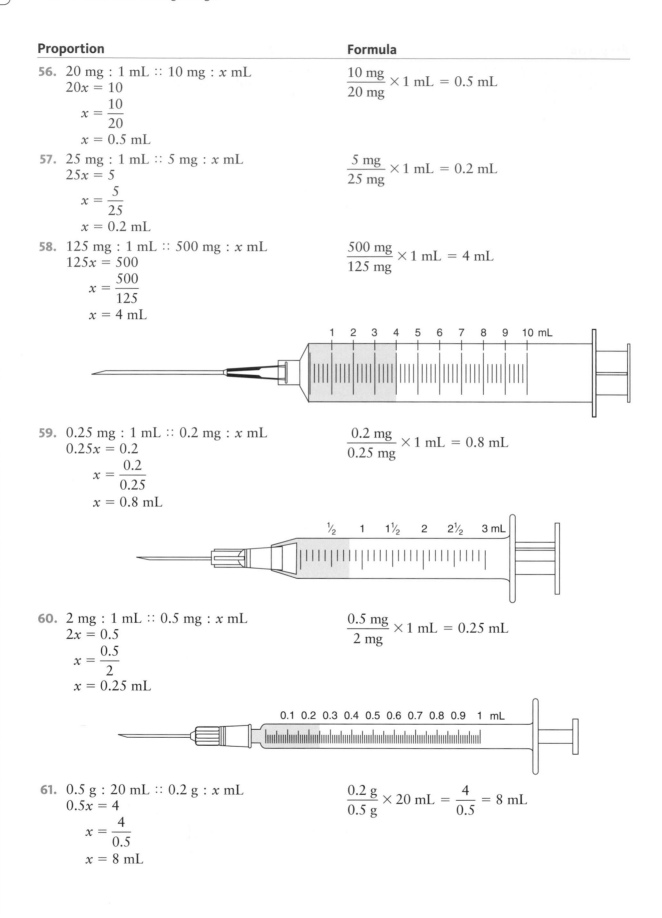

59. 0.25 mg : 1 mL :: 0.2 mg : x mL

  $0.25x = 0.2$

  $x = \dfrac{0.2}{0.25}$

  $x = 0.8$ mL

$\dfrac{0.2 \text{ mg}}{0.25 \text{ mg}} \times 1 \text{ mL} = 0.8 \text{ mL}$

60. 2 mg : 1 mL :: 0.5 mg : x mL

  $2x = 0.5$

  $x = \dfrac{0.5}{2}$

  $x = 0.25$ mL

$\dfrac{0.5 \text{ mg}}{2 \text{ mg}} \times 1 \text{ mL} = 0.25 \text{ mL}$

61. 0.5 g : 20 mL :: 0.2 g : x mL

  $0.5x = 4$

  $x = \dfrac{4}{0.5}$

  $x = 8$ mL

$\dfrac{0.2 \text{ g}}{0.5 \text{ g}} \times 20 \text{ mL} = \dfrac{4}{0.5} = 8 \text{ mL}$

ANSWERS

Proportion   **Formula**

62. 30 mg : 1 mL :: 15 mg : x mL

$30x = 15$

$x = \dfrac{15}{30}$

$x = 0.5$ mL

$\dfrac{15 \text{ mg}}{30 \text{ mg}} \times 1 \text{ mL} = 0.5 \text{ mL}$

63. 50 mg : 1 mL :: 100 mg : x mL

$50x = 100$

$x = \dfrac{100}{50}$

$x = 2$ mL

$\dfrac{100 \text{ mg}}{50 \text{ mg}} \times 1 \text{ mL} = 2 \text{ mL}$

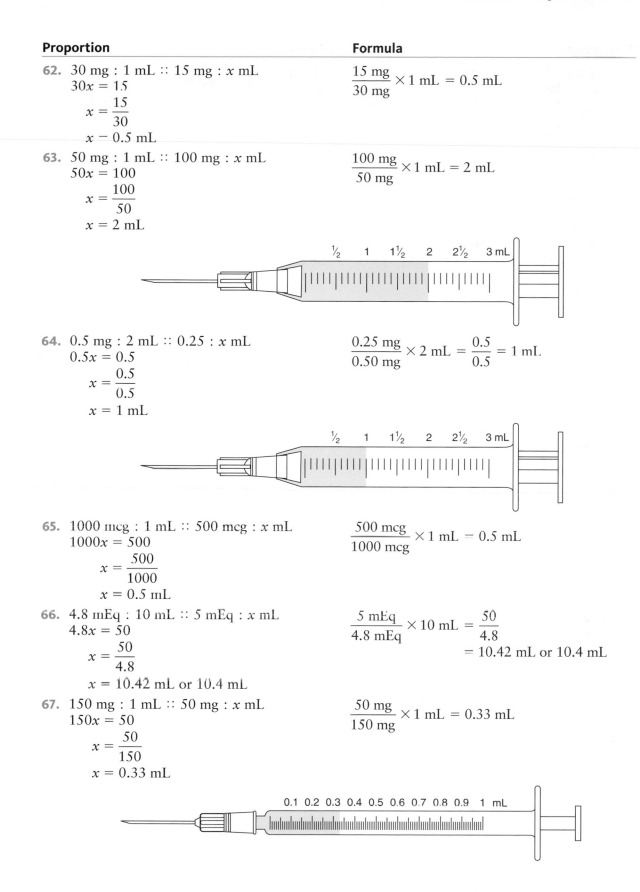

64. 0.5 mg : 2 mL :: 0.25 : x mL

$0.5x = 0.5$

$x = \dfrac{0.5}{0.5}$

$x = 1$ mL

$\dfrac{0.25 \text{ mg}}{0.50 \text{ mg}} \times 2 \text{ mL} = \dfrac{0.5}{0.5} = 1 \text{ mL}$

65. 1000 mcg : 1 mL :: 500 mcg : x mL

$1000x = 500$

$x = \dfrac{500}{1000}$

$x = 0.5$ mL

$\dfrac{500 \text{ mcg}}{1000 \text{ mcg}} \times 1 \text{ mL} = 0.5 \text{ mL}$

66. 4.8 mEq : 10 mL :: 5 mEq : x mL

$4.8x = 50$

$x = \dfrac{50}{4.8}$

$x = 10.42$ mL or 10.4 mL

$\dfrac{5 \text{ mEq}}{4.8 \text{ mEq}} \times 10 \text{ mL} = \dfrac{50}{4.8}$

$= 10.42 \text{ mL or } 10.4 \text{ mL}$

67. 150 mg : 1 mL :: 50 mg : x mL

$150x = 50$

$x = \dfrac{50}{150}$

$x = 0.33$ mL

$\dfrac{50 \text{ mg}}{150 \text{ mg}} \times 1 \text{ mL} = 0.33 \text{ mL}$

Copyright © 2016 by Mosby, an imprint of Elsevier Inc.

ANSWERS

Proportion	**Formula**

68. 0.4 mg : 1 mL :: 0.2 mg : x mL
$0.4x = 0.2$

$\quad x = \dfrac{0.2}{0.4}$

$\quad x = 0.5$ mL

$\dfrac{0.2 \text{ mg}}{0.4 \text{ mg}} \times 1 \text{ mL} = 0.5 \text{ mL}$

69. 80 mg : 2 mL :: 55 mg : x mL
$80x = 110$

$\quad x = \dfrac{110}{80}$

$\quad x = 1.38$ mL or 1.4 mL

$\dfrac{55 \text{ mg}}{80 \text{ mg}} \times 2 \text{ mL} = \dfrac{110}{80} = 1.38 \text{ mL or } 1.4 \text{ mL}$

70. 500 mg : 2 mL :: 600 mg : x mL
$500x = 1200$

$\quad x = \dfrac{1200}{500}$

$\quad x = 2.4$ mL

$\dfrac{600 \text{ mg}}{500 \text{ mg}} \times 2 \text{ mL} =$

$\dfrac{600}{\overset{}{\underset{250}{500}}} \times \dfrac{\overset{1}{\cancel{2}}}{1} = \dfrac{600}{250}$

$\quad\quad\quad x = 2.4 \text{ mL}$

71. 15 mg : 1 mL :: 6 mg : x mL
$15x = 6$

$\quad x = \dfrac{6}{15}$

$\quad x = 0.4$ mL

$\dfrac{6 \text{ mg}}{15 \text{ mg}} \times 1 \text{ mL} = 0.4 \text{ mL}$

72. 1000 mcg : 1 mL :: 1000 mcg : x mL
$1000x = 1000$

$\quad x = \dfrac{1000}{1000}$

$\quad x = 1$ mL

$\dfrac{1000 \text{ mcg}}{1000 \text{ mcg}} \times 1 \text{ mL} = 1 \text{ mL}$

73. 325 mg : 1 mL :: 800 mg : x mL
$325x = 800$

$\quad x = \dfrac{800}{325}$

$\quad x = 2.46$ mL or 2.5 mL

$\dfrac{800 \text{ mg}}{325 \text{ mg}} \times 1 \text{ mL} = 2.46 \text{ mL or } 2.5 \text{ mL}$

ANSWERS

Proportion	Formula
74. 50 mg : 1 mL :: 30 mg : x mL $50x = 30$ $x = \dfrac{30}{50}$ $x = 0.6$ mL	$\dfrac{30 \text{ mg}}{50 \text{ mg}} \times 1 \text{ mL} = 0.6 \text{ mL}$

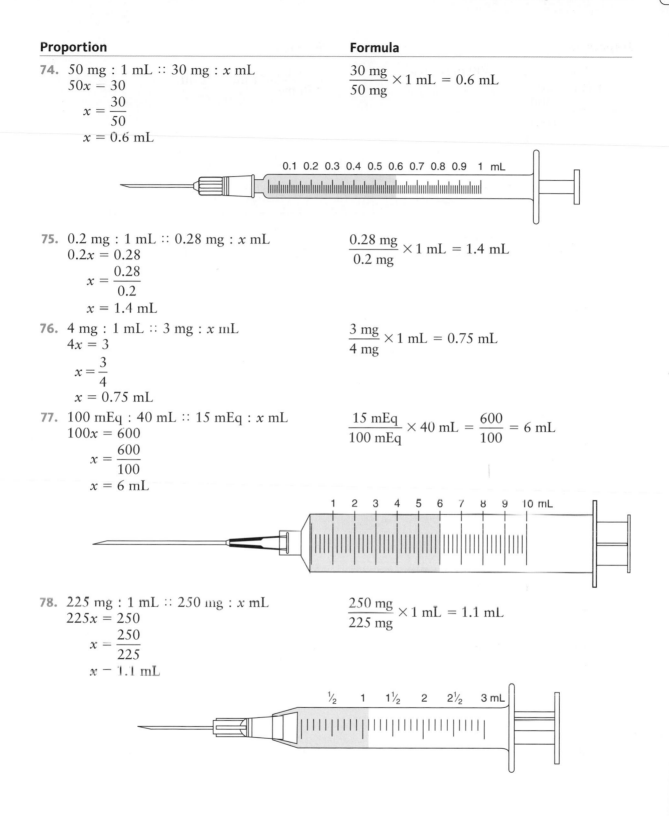

Proportion	Formula
75. 0.2 mg : 1 mL :: 0.28 mg : x mL $0.2x = 0.28$ $x = \dfrac{0.28}{0.2}$ $x = 1.4$ mL	$\dfrac{0.28 \text{ mg}}{0.2 \text{ mg}} \times 1 \text{ mL} = 1.4 \text{ mL}$
76. 4 mg : 1 mL :: 3 mg : x mL $4x = 3$ $x = \dfrac{3}{4}$ $x = 0.75$ mL	$\dfrac{3 \text{ mg}}{4 \text{ mg}} \times 1 \text{ mL} = 0.75 \text{ mL}$
77. 100 mEq : 40 mL :: 15 mEq : x mL $100x = 600$ $x = \dfrac{600}{100}$ $x = 6$ mL	$\dfrac{15 \text{ mEq}}{100 \text{ mEq}} \times 40 \text{ mL} = \dfrac{600}{100} = 6 \text{ mL}$
78. 225 mg : 1 mL :: 250 mg : x mL $225x = 250$ $x = \dfrac{250}{225}$ $x = 1.1$ mL	$\dfrac{250 \text{ mg}}{225 \text{ mg}} \times 1 \text{ mL} = 1.1 \text{ mL}$

ANSWERS

Proportion	Formula

79. 150 mg : 1 mL :: 300 mg : x mL
$150x = 300$
$x = \dfrac{300}{150}$
$x = 2$ mL

$\dfrac{300 \text{ mg}}{150 \text{ mg}} \times 1 \text{ mL} = 2 \text{ mL}$

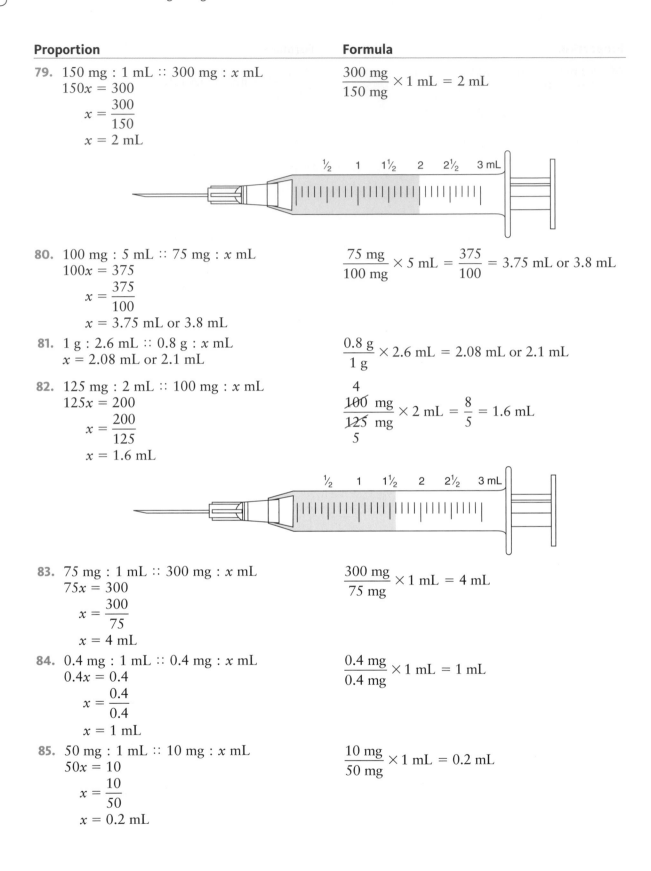

80. 100 mg : 5 mL :: 75 mg : x mL
$100x = 375$
$x = \dfrac{375}{100}$
$x = 3.75$ mL or 3.8 mL

$\dfrac{75 \text{ mg}}{100 \text{ mg}} \times 5 \text{ mL} = \dfrac{375}{100} = 3.75 \text{ mL or } 3.8 \text{ mL}$

81. 1 g : 2.6 mL :: 0.8 g : x mL
$x = 2.08$ mL or 2.1 mL

$\dfrac{0.8 \text{ g}}{1 \text{ g}} \times 2.6 \text{ mL} = 2.08 \text{ mL or } 2.1 \text{ mL}$

82. 125 mg : 2 mL :: 100 mg : x mL
$125x = 200$
$x = \dfrac{200}{125}$
$x = 1.6$ mL

$\dfrac{\overset{4}{\cancel{100}} \text{ mg}}{\underset{5}{\cancel{125}} \text{ mg}} \times 2 \text{ mL} = \dfrac{8}{5} = 1.6 \text{ mL}$

83. 75 mg : 1 mL :: 300 mg : x mL
$75x = 300$
$x = \dfrac{300}{75}$
$x = 4$ mL

$\dfrac{300 \text{ mg}}{75 \text{ mg}} \times 1 \text{ mL} = 4 \text{ mL}$

84. 0.4 mg : 1 mL :: 0.4 mg : x mL
$0.4x = 0.4$
$x = \dfrac{0.4}{0.4}$
$x = 1$ mL

$\dfrac{0.4 \text{ mg}}{0.4 \text{ mg}} \times 1 \text{ mL} = 1 \text{ mL}$

85. 50 mg : 1 mL :: 10 mg : x mL
$50x = 10$
$x = \dfrac{10}{50}$
$x = 0.2$ mL

$\dfrac{10 \text{ mg}}{50 \text{ mg}} \times 1 \text{ mL} = 0.2 \text{ mL}$

ANSWERS

Proportion	Formula

86. 10 mg : 1 mL :: 1 mg : x mL
$10x = 1$
$x = \dfrac{1}{10}$ or 0.1 mL

$\dfrac{1 \text{ mg}}{10 \text{ mg}} \times 1 \text{ mL} = 0.1 \text{ mL}$

87. 50 mg : 1 mL :: 50 mg : x mL
$50x = 50$
$x = \dfrac{50}{50}$
$x = 1$ mL

$\dfrac{50 \text{ mg}}{50 \text{ mg}} \times 1 \text{ mL} = 1 \text{ mL}$

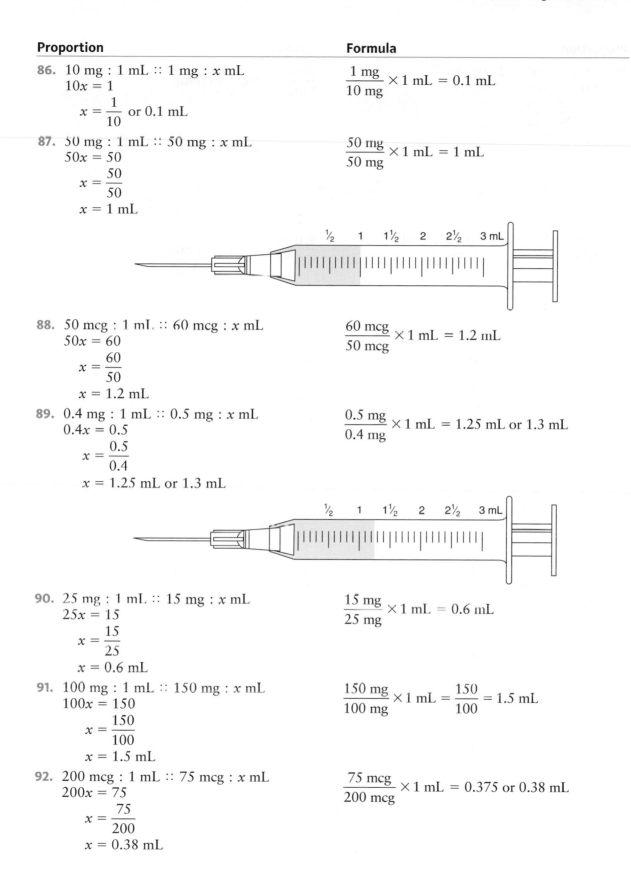

88. 50 mcg : 1 mL :: 60 mcg : x mL
$50x = 60$
$x = \dfrac{60}{50}$
$x = 1.2$ mL

$\dfrac{60 \text{ mcg}}{50 \text{ mcg}} \times 1 \text{ mL} = 1.2 \text{ mL}$

89. 0.4 mg : 1 mL :: 0.5 mg : x mL
$0.4x = 0.5$
$x = \dfrac{0.5}{0.4}$
$x = 1.25$ mL or 1.3 mL

$\dfrac{0.5 \text{ mg}}{0.4 \text{ mg}} \times 1 \text{ mL} = 1.25 \text{ mL or } 1.3 \text{ mL}$

90. 25 mg : 1 mL :: 15 mg : x mL
$25x = 15$
$x = \dfrac{15}{25}$
$x = 0.6$ mL

$\dfrac{15 \text{ mg}}{25 \text{ mg}} \times 1 \text{ mL} = 0.6 \text{ mL}$

91. 100 mg : 1 mL :: 150 mg : x mL
$100x = 150$
$x = \dfrac{150}{100}$
$x = 1.5$ mL

$\dfrac{150 \text{ mg}}{100 \text{ mg}} \times 1 \text{ mL} = \dfrac{150}{100} = 1.5 \text{ mL}$

92. 200 mcg : 1 mL :: 75 mcg : x mL
$200x = 75$
$x = \dfrac{75}{200}$
$x = 0.38$ mL

$\dfrac{75 \text{ mcg}}{200 \text{ mcg}} \times 1 \text{ mL} = 0.375 \text{ or } 0.38 \text{ mL}$

ANSWERS

Proportion   **Formula**

93. $5 \text{ mg} : 1 \text{ mL} :: 2 \text{ mg} : x \text{ mL}$
    $5x = 2$
    $x = \dfrac{2}{5}$
    $x = 0.4 \text{ mL}$

$\dfrac{2 \text{ mg}}{5 \text{ mg}} \times 1 \text{ mL} = 0.4 \text{ mL}$

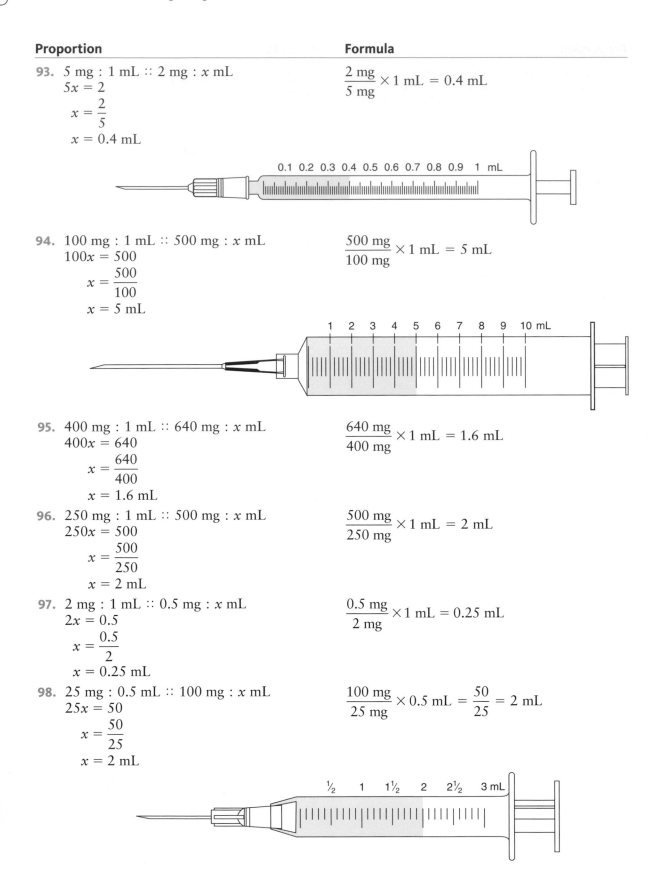

94. $100 \text{ mg} : 1 \text{ mL} :: 500 \text{ mg} : x \text{ mL}$
    $100x = 500$
    $x = \dfrac{500}{100}$
    $x = 5 \text{ mL}$

$\dfrac{500 \text{ mg}}{100 \text{ mg}} \times 1 \text{ mL} = 5 \text{ mL}$

95. $400 \text{ mg} : 1 \text{ mL} :: 640 \text{ mg} : x \text{ mL}$
    $400x = 640$
    $x = \dfrac{640}{400}$
    $x = 1.6 \text{ mL}$

$\dfrac{640 \text{ mg}}{400 \text{ mg}} \times 1 \text{ mL} = 1.6 \text{ mL}$

96. $250 \text{ mg} : 1 \text{ mL} :: 500 \text{ mg} : x \text{ mL}$
    $250x = 500$
    $x = \dfrac{500}{250}$
    $x = 2 \text{ mL}$

$\dfrac{500 \text{ mg}}{250 \text{ mg}} \times 1 \text{ mL} = 2 \text{ mL}$

97. $2 \text{ mg} : 1 \text{ mL} :: 0.5 \text{ mg} : x \text{ mL}$
    $2x = 0.5$
    $x = \dfrac{0.5}{2}$
    $x = 0.25 \text{ mL}$

$\dfrac{0.5 \text{ mg}}{2 \text{ mg}} \times 1 \text{ mL} = 0.25 \text{ mL}$

98. $25 \text{ mg} : 0.5 \text{ mL} :: 100 \text{ mg} : x \text{ mL}$
    $25x = 50$
    $x = \dfrac{50}{25}$
    $x = 2 \text{ mL}$

$\dfrac{100 \text{ mg}}{25 \text{ mg}} \times 0.5 \text{ mL} = \dfrac{50}{25} = 2 \text{ mL}$

ANSWERS

Proportion	Formula

99. $50 \text{ mg} : 1 \text{ mL} :: 10 \text{ mg} : x \text{ mL}$
$50x = 10$
$x = \dfrac{10}{50}$
$x = 0.2 \text{ mL}$

$\dfrac{10 \text{ mg}}{50 \text{ mg}} \times 1 \text{ mL} = 0.2 \text{ mL}$

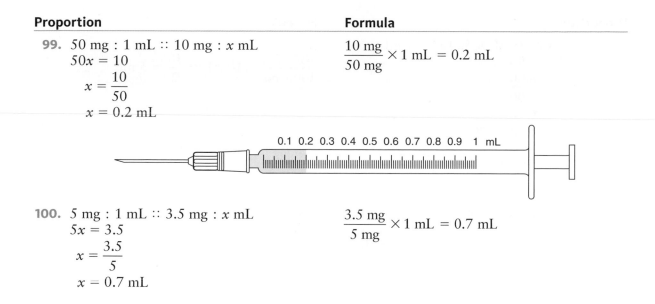

100. $5 \text{ mg} : 1 \text{ mL} :: 3.5 \text{ mg} : x \text{ mL}$
$5x = 3.5$
$x = \dfrac{3.5}{5}$
$x = 0.7 \text{ mL}$

$\dfrac{3.5 \text{ mg}}{5 \text{ mg}} \times 1 \text{ mL} = 0.7 \text{ mL}$

CHAPTER 12 Proportion/Formula Method—Posttest 1, pp. 307–311

Proportion	Formula

1. $50 \text{ mg} : 1 \text{ mL} :: 25 \text{ mg} : x \text{ mL}$
$50x = 25$
$x = \dfrac{25}{50}$
$x = 0.5 \text{ mL}$

$\dfrac{25 \text{ mg}}{50 \text{ mg}} \times 1 \text{ mL} = 0.5 \text{ mL}$

2. $50 \text{ mg} : 1 \text{ mL} :: 25 \text{ mg} : x \text{ mL}$
$50x = 25$
$x = \dfrac{25}{50}$
$x = 0.5 \text{ mL}$

$\dfrac{25 \text{ mg}}{50 \text{ mg}} \times 1 \text{ mL} = 0.5 \text{ mL}$

3. $15 \text{ mg} : 1 \text{ mL} :: 30 \text{ mg} : x \text{ mL}$
$15x = 30$
$x = \dfrac{30}{15}$
$x = 2 \text{ mL}$

$\dfrac{30 \text{ mg}}{15 \text{ mg}} \times 1 \text{ mL} = 2 \text{ mL}$

ANSWERS

Proportion	**Formula**

4. 1000 mg : 10 mL :: 500 mg : x mL

$1000x = 5000$

$x = \dfrac{5000}{1000}$

$x = 5$ mL

$$\dfrac{\overset{1}{\cancel{500}} \text{ mg}}{\underset{2}{\cancel{1000}} \text{ mg}} \times 10 \text{ mL} = \dfrac{10}{2} = 5 \text{ mL}$$

5. 100 mg : 2 mL :: 50 mg : x mL

$100x = 100$

$x = \dfrac{100}{100}$

$x = 1$ mL

$$\dfrac{50 \text{ mg}}{100 \text{ mg}} \times 2 \text{ mL} = \dfrac{100}{100} = 1 \text{ mL}$$

6. 2 mg : 1 mL :: 0.5 mg : x mL

$2x = 0.5$

$x = \dfrac{0.5}{2}$

$x = 0.25$ mL

$$\dfrac{0.5 \text{ mg}}{2 \text{ mg}} \times 1 \text{ mL} = 0.25 \text{ mL}$$

7. 30 mg : 1 mL :: 15 mg : x mL

$30x = 15$

$x = \dfrac{15}{30}$

$x = 0.5$ mL

$$\dfrac{15 \text{ mg}}{30 \text{ mg}} \times 1 \text{ mL} = 0.5 \text{ mL}$$

8. 0.4 mg : 1 mL :: 0.2 mg : x mL

$0.4x = 0.2$

$x = \dfrac{0.2}{0.4}$

$x = 0.5$ mL

$$\dfrac{0.2 \text{ mg}}{0.4 \text{ mg}} \times 1 \text{ mL} = 0.5 \text{ mL}$$

9. 25 mg : 1 mL :: 100 mg : x mL

$25x = 100$

$x = \dfrac{100}{25}$

$x = 4$ mL

$$\dfrac{100 \text{ mg}}{25 \text{ mg}} \times 1 \text{ mL} = 4 \text{ mL}$$

ANSWERS

Proportion	Formula

10. 5 mg : 1 mL :: 2 mg : x mL
$5x = 2$
$x = \dfrac{2}{5}$
$x = 0.4$ mL

$\dfrac{2 \text{ mg}}{5 \text{ mg}} \times 1 \text{ mL} = 0.4 \text{ mL}$

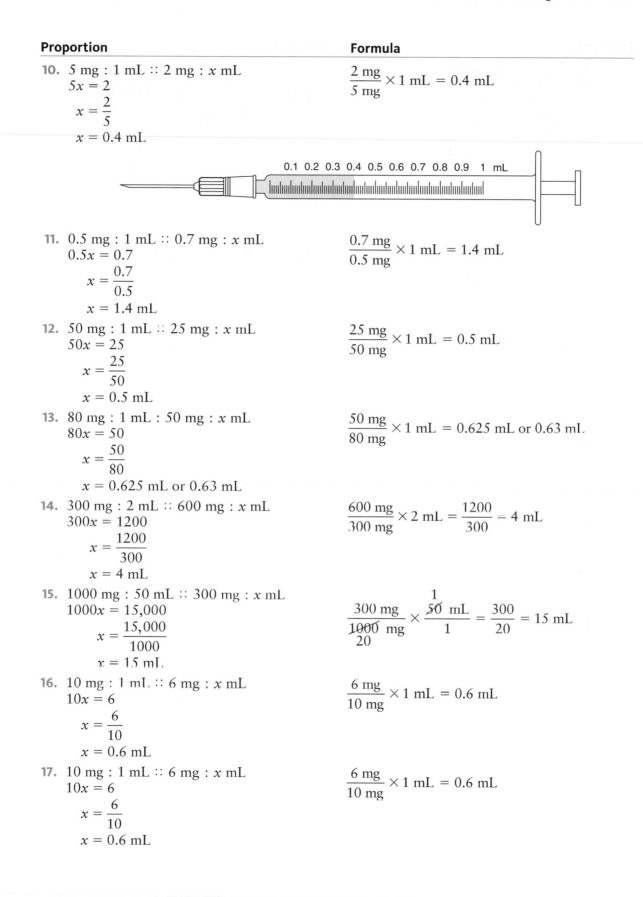

11. 0.5 mg : 1 mL :: 0.7 mg : x mL
$0.5x = 0.7$
$x = \dfrac{0.7}{0.5}$
$x = 1.4$ mL

$\dfrac{0.7 \text{ mg}}{0.5 \text{ mg}} \times 1 \text{ mL} = 1.4 \text{ mL}$

12. 50 mg : 1 mL :: 25 mg : x mL
$50x = 25$
$x = \dfrac{25}{50}$
$x = 0.5$ mL

$\dfrac{25 \text{ mg}}{50 \text{ mg}} \times 1 \text{ mL} = 0.5 \text{ mL}$

13. 80 mg : 1 mL : 50 mg : x mL
$80x = 50$
$x = \dfrac{50}{80}$
$x = 0.625$ mL or 0.63 mL

$\dfrac{50 \text{ mg}}{80 \text{ mg}} \times 1 \text{ mL} = 0.625 \text{ mL}$ or 0.63 mL

14. 300 mg : 2 mL :: 600 mg : x mL
$300x = 1200$
$x = \dfrac{1200}{300}$
$x = 4$ mL

$\dfrac{600 \text{ mg}}{300 \text{ mg}} \times 2 \text{ mL} = \dfrac{1200}{300} = 4 \text{ mL}$

15. 1000 mg : 50 mL :: 300 mg : x mL
$1000x = 15{,}000$
$x = \dfrac{15{,}000}{1000}$
$x = 15$ mL

$\dfrac{300 \text{ mg}}{\underset{20}{\cancel{1000}} \text{ mg}} \times \dfrac{\overset{1}{\cancel{50}} \text{ mL}}{1} = \dfrac{300}{20} = 15 \text{ mL}$

16. 10 mg : 1 mL :: 6 mg : x mL
$10x = 6$
$x = \dfrac{6}{10}$
$x = 0.6$ mL

$\dfrac{6 \text{ mg}}{10 \text{ mg}} \times 1 \text{ mL} = 0.6 \text{ mL}$

17. 10 mg : 1 mL :: 6 mg : x mL
$10x = 6$
$x = \dfrac{6}{10}$
$x = 0.6$ mL

$\dfrac{6 \text{ mg}}{10 \text{ mg}} \times 1 \text{ mL} = 0.6 \text{ mL}$

ANSWERS

Proportion	**Formula**

18. 40 mg : 4 mL :: 20 mg : x mL

$40x = 80$

$x = \dfrac{80}{40}$

$x = 2$ mL

$\dfrac{20 \text{ mg}}{40 \text{ mg}} \times 4 \text{ mL} =$

$\dfrac{20}{\overset{}{\underset{4}{40}}} \times \dfrac{\overset{1}{4}}{1} = \dfrac{20}{10}$

$\dfrac{20}{10} = 2$ mL

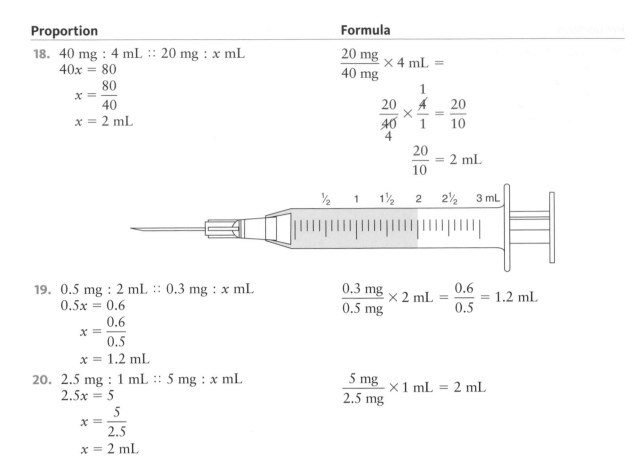

19. 0.5 mg : 2 mL :: 0.3 mg : x mL

$0.5x = 0.6$

$x = \dfrac{0.6}{0.5}$

$x = 1.2$ mL

$\dfrac{0.3 \text{ mg}}{0.5 \text{ mg}} \times 2 \text{ mL} = \dfrac{0.6}{0.5} = 1.2$ mL

20. 2.5 mg : 1 mL :: 5 mg : x mL

$2.5x = 5$

$x = \dfrac{5}{2.5}$

$x = 2$ mL

$\dfrac{5 \text{ mg}}{2.5 \text{ mg}} \times 1 \text{ mL} = 2$ mL

CHAPTER 12 Proportion/Formula Method—Posttest 2, pp. 313–318

Proportion	**Formula**

1. 4 mg : 1 mL :: 2 mg : x mL

$4x = 2$

$x = \dfrac{2}{4}$

$x = 0.5$ mL

$\dfrac{2 \text{ mg}}{4 \text{ mg}} \times 1 \text{ mL} = 0.5$ mL

2. 4 mg : 1 mL :: 2 mg : x mL

$4x = 2$

$x = \dfrac{2}{4}$

$x = 0.5$ mL

$\dfrac{2 \text{ mg}}{4 \text{ mg}} \times 1 \text{ mL} = 0.5$ mL

3. 500 mg : 10 mL :: 400 mg : x mL

$500x = 4000$

$x = \dfrac{4000}{500}$

$x = 8$ mL

$\dfrac{\overset{4}{400} \text{ mg}}{\underset{5}{500} \text{ mg}} \times 10 \text{ mL} = \dfrac{40}{5} = 8$ mL

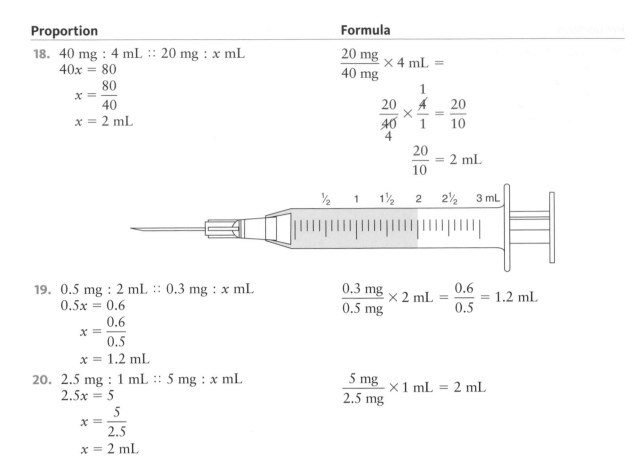

ANSWERS

Proportion	**Formula**

4. 5 mg : 1 mL :: 20 mg : x mL

$5x = 20$

$x = \dfrac{20}{5}$

$x = 4$ mL

$\dfrac{20 \text{ mg}}{5 \text{ mg}} \times 1 \text{ mL} = 4 \text{ mL}$

5. 30 mg : 1 mL :: 60 mg : x mL

$30x = 60$

$x = \dfrac{60}{30}$

$x = 2$ mL

$\dfrac{60 \text{ mg}}{30 \text{ mg}} \times 1 \text{ mL} = 2 \text{ mL}$

6. 100 mg : 1 mL :: 200 mg : x mL

$100x = 200$

$x = \dfrac{200}{100}$

$x = 2$ mL

$\dfrac{200 \text{ mg}}{100 \text{ mg}} \times 1 \text{ mL} = 2 \text{ mL}$

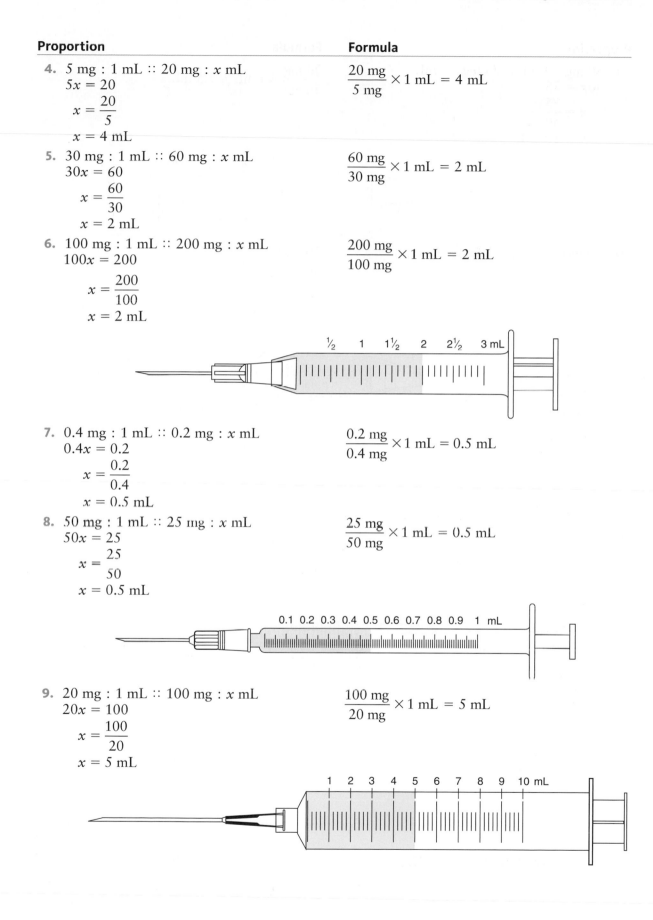

7. 0.4 mg : 1 mL :: 0.2 mg : x mL

$0.4x = 0.2$

$x = \dfrac{0.2}{0.4}$

$x = 0.5$ mL

$\dfrac{0.2 \text{ mg}}{0.4 \text{ mg}} \times 1 \text{ mL} = 0.5 \text{ mL}$

8. 50 mg : 1 mL :: 25 mg : x mL

$50x = 25$

$x = \dfrac{25}{50}$

$x = 0.5$ mL

$\dfrac{25 \text{ mg}}{50 \text{ mg}} \times 1 \text{ mL} = 0.5 \text{ mL}$

9. 20 mg : 1 mL :: 100 mg : x mL

$20x = 100$

$x = \dfrac{100}{20}$

$x = 5$ mL

$\dfrac{100 \text{ mg}}{20 \text{ mg}} \times 1 \text{ mL} = 5 \text{ mL}$

Proportion	**Formula**

10. 50 mg : 1 mL :: 75 mg : x mL
$50x = 75$
$x = \dfrac{75}{50}$
$x = 1.5$ mL

$\dfrac{75 \text{ mg}}{50 \text{ mg}} \times 1 \text{ mL} = 1.5 \text{ mL}$

11. 50 mcg : 1 mL :: 70 mcg : x mL
$50x = 70$
$x = \dfrac{70}{50}$
$x = 1.4$ mL

$\dfrac{70 \text{ mcg}}{50 \text{ mcg}} \times 1 \text{ mL} = 1.4 \text{ mL}$

12. 0.3 mg : 1 mL :: 0.4 mg : x mL
$0.3x = 0.4$
$x = \dfrac{0.4}{0.3}$
$x = 1.33$ mL or 1.3 mL

$\dfrac{0.4 \text{ mg}}{0.3 \text{ mg}} \times 1 \text{ mL} = 1.33 \text{ mL or } 1.3 \text{ mL}$

13. 1 g : 2.5 mL :: 2 g : x mL
$x = 5$ mL

$\dfrac{2 \text{ g}}{1 \text{ g}} \times 2.5 \text{ mL} = 5 \text{ mL}$

14. 40 mg : 1 mL :: 26 mg : x mL
$40x = 26$
$x = \dfrac{26}{40}$
$x = 0.65$ mL

$\dfrac{26 \text{ mg}}{40 \text{ mg}} \times 1 \text{ mL} = 0.65 \text{ mL}$

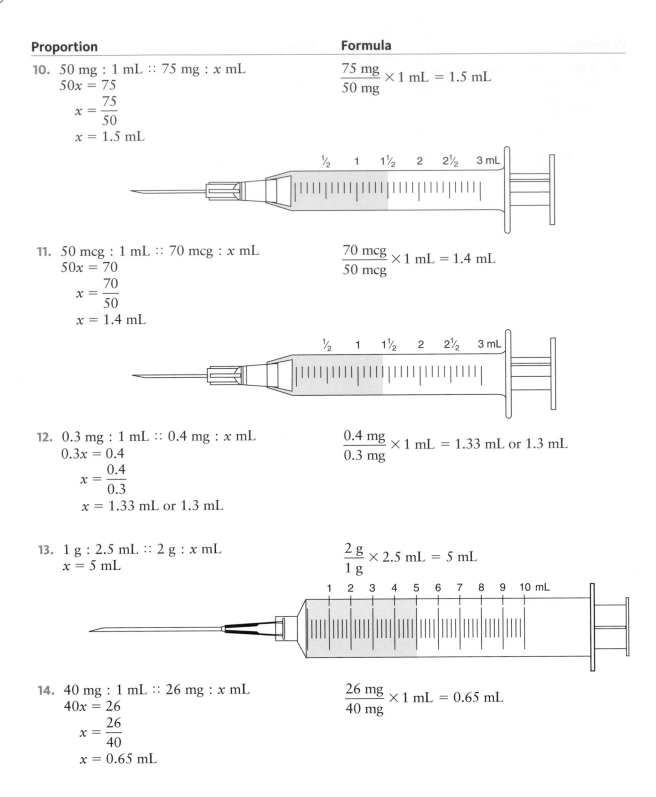

Proportion	Formula

15. 40 mg : 0.4 mL :: 85 mg : x mL

$40x = 34$

$x = \dfrac{34}{40}$

$x = 0.85$ mL

$\dfrac{85 \text{ mg}}{100 \text{ mg}} \times 1 \text{ mL} = 0.85 \text{ mL}$

16. 500 mcg : 2 mL :: 80 mcg : x mL

$500x = 160$

$x = \dfrac{160}{500}$

$x = 0.32$ mL

$\dfrac{80 \text{ mcg}}{500 \text{ mcg}} \times 2 \text{ mL} = \dfrac{160}{500} = 0.32 \text{ mL}$

17. 8 mg : 1 mL :: 4 mg : x mL

$8x = 4$

$x = \dfrac{4}{8}$

$x = 0.5$ mL

$\dfrac{4 \text{ mg}}{8 \text{ mg}} \times 1 \text{ mL} = 0.5 \text{ mL}$

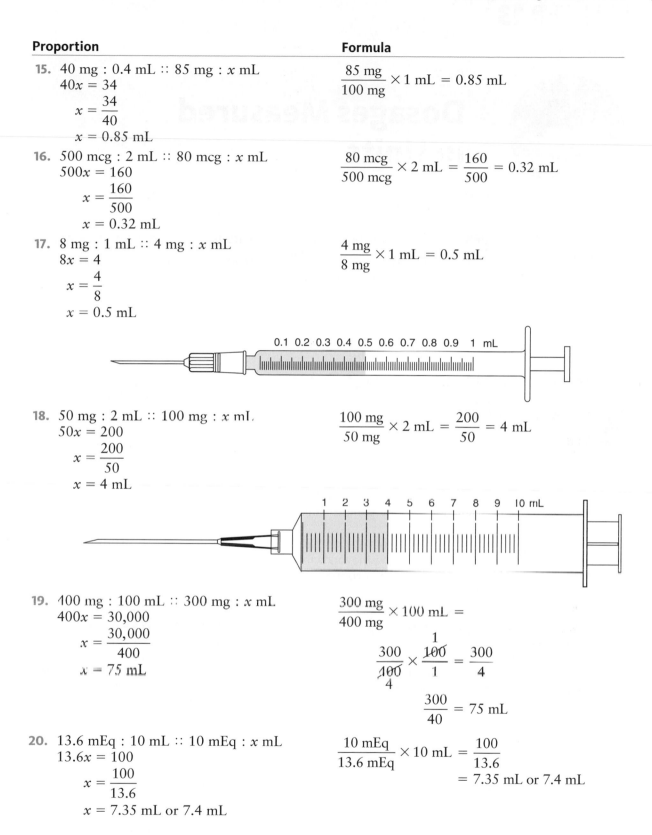

18. 50 mg : 2 mL :: 100 mg : x mL

$50x = 200$

$x = \dfrac{200}{50}$

$x = 4$ mL

$\dfrac{100 \text{ mg}}{50 \text{ mg}} \times 2 \text{ mL} = \dfrac{200}{50} = 4 \text{ mL}$

19. 400 mg : 100 mL :: 300 mg : x mL

$400x = 30,000$

$x = \dfrac{30,000}{400}$

$x = 75$ mL

$\dfrac{300 \text{ mg}}{400 \text{ mg}} \times 100 \text{ mL} =$

$\dfrac{300}{\overset{}{\underset{4}{100}}} \times \dfrac{\overset{1}{100}}{1} = \dfrac{300}{4}$

$\dfrac{300}{40} = 75 \text{ mL}$

20. 13.6 mEq : 10 mL :: 10 mEq : x mL

$13.6x = 100$

$x = \dfrac{100}{13.6}$

$x = 7.35 \text{ mL or } 7.4 \text{ mL}$

$\dfrac{10 \text{ mEq}}{13.6 \text{ mEq}} \times 10 \text{ mL} = \dfrac{100}{13.6}$

$= 7.35 \text{ mL or } 7.4 \text{ mL}$

ANSWERS

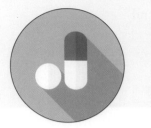

CHAPTER 13

Dosages Measured in Units

LEARNING OBJECTIVES

Upon completion of the materials provided in this chapter, you will be able to perform computations accurately by mastering the following mathematical concepts:

1 Solving problems involving drugs measured in unit dosages

2 Drawing a line through an insulin syringe to indicate the number of units desired

A unit is the amount of a drug needed to produce a given result. Various drugs are measured in units; the examples used in this chapter are among the more common drugs prescribed.

Drugs used in this chapter include:

Epogen—A drug that increases the production of red blood cells
Fragmin—An anticoagulant that prevents the clotting of blood
Heparin—An anticoagulant that inhibits clotting of the blood
Insulin—A hormone secreted by the pancreas that lowers blood glucose

Epogen is a drug that helps to combat the effects of anemia caused by chemotherapy or chronic renal failure. After administering the medicine, the nurse should monitor the patient's blood pressure and laboratory results on a routine basis.

Fragmin is used in the prevention of deep vein thrombosis after abdominal surgery, hip replacements, and unstable angina/non–Q wave myocardial infarction. It may also be used with patients who have restricted mobility during an acute illness. Fragmin may only be given by subcutaneous injections—never intramuscularly or intravenously. The patient's blood studies must be monitored on a routine basis during treatment with Fragmin.

Because heparin prolongs the time blood takes to clot, the dosage must be accurate. A larger dose may cause hemorrhage, and an insufficient dose may not have the desired result. After administering the drug, the nurse should observe the patient for signs of hemorrhage.

INSULIN

Insulin is used in the treatment of diabetes mellitus. Accuracy is important in the preparation of insulin. A higher dosage than needed may cause insulin shock. An insufficient amount of insulin may result in diabetic coma. Both conditions are extremely serious, and the nurse must be able to recognize the symptoms of each condition so that immediate treatment can be initiated to stabilize the patient. In many institutions, both insulin and heparin dosages are checked for accuracy by another nurse before the drug is administered to the patient. Figure 13-1 shows examples of different types of insulin.

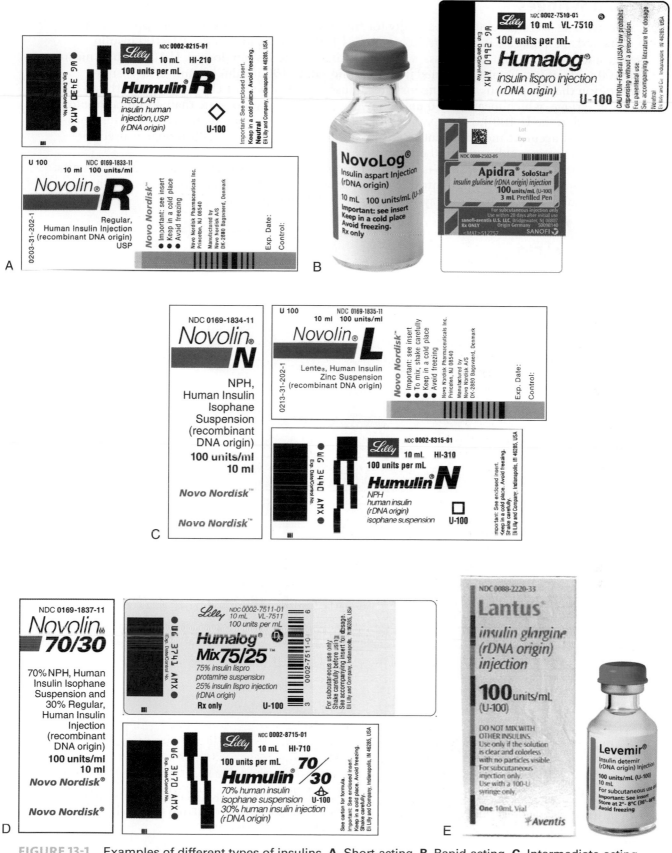

FIGURE 13-1 Examples of different types of insulins. **A,** Short-acting. **B,** Rapid-acting. **C,** Intermediate-acting. **D,** Intermediate- and rapid-acting mixture. **E,** Long-acting. (**B** and **E,** from Novo Nordisk Inc., Princeton, NJ.)

Insulin Syringes

Insulin syringes were developed specifically for the administration of insulin. They are calibrated in units and are available in 30 units, 50 units, and 100 units (Figure 13-2). A U-100 insulin syringe and U-100 insulin are necessary to ensure an accurate insulin dosage. U-100 insulin means that 100 units of insulin are contained in 1 mL of liquid. U-100 insulin is a universal insulin preparation that all persons requiring insulin can use. Another type of U-100 syringe is the U-100 Lo-Dose syringe, which measures 50 units; however, for accuracy, no more than 40 units should be measured in the U-100 Lo-Dose syringe. Because the doses are minute, the U-100 syringe provides the most accurate measurement of insulin dosages. The 30-unit U-100 syringe is used for insulin doses that equal less than 30 units.

IMPORTANT NOTE: Only insulin is measured and given in the syringes that are marked in units. Only regular insulin can be given intravenously. Heparin and other medication measured in units can be measured and given only in syringes marked in milliliters.

> **! ALERT**
>
> Only insulin is measured and given in insulin syringes.

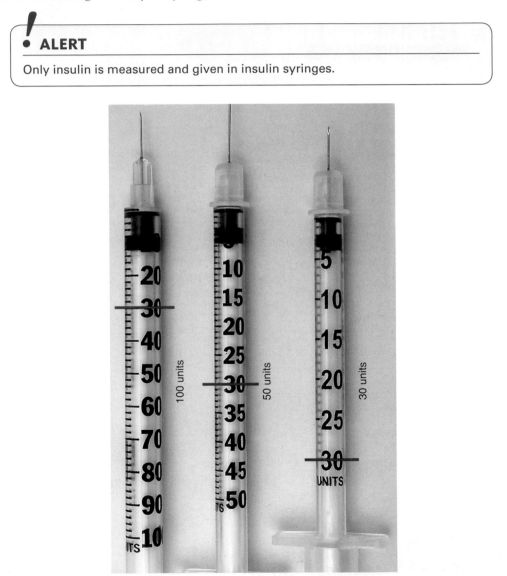

FIGURE 13-2   *Left to right:* 30 units measured on a 100-unit syringe (each calibration is 2 units), a 50-unit syringe (each calibration is 1 unit), and 30-unit syringe (each calibration is 1 unit). (From Macklin D, Chernecky C, Infortuna H: *Math for clinical practice,* ed 2, St Louis, 2011, Mosby.)

Insulin Pens

Insulin is also available in prefilled insulin pens. The insulin pens require a special needle to be attached. Each insulin pen contains a dial for choosing the desired number of units to be administered. For example, if 6 units of NovoLog insulin are desired, the dial on the NovoLog insulin pen would be turned to the Number 6. See Figure 13-3 for examples of insulin pens.

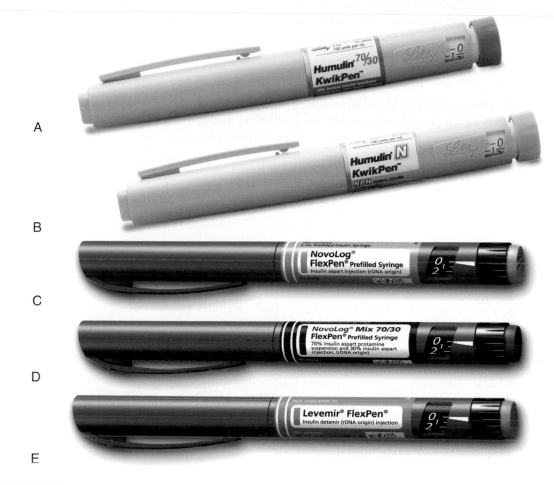

FIGURE 13-3 Prefilled insulin pens. **A,** Humulin 70/30 KwikPen™ short- and intermediate acting. **B,** Humulin KwikPen™ intermediate-acting. **C,** NovoLog® rapid-acting. **D,** NovoLog® 70/30 short- and intermediate-acting. **E,** Levemir® long-acting. (**A** and **B,** Copyright Eli Lilly and Company. All rights reserved. Used with permission. **C-E,** From Novo Nordisk Inc., Princeton, NJ.)

Dosages Measured in Units Involving Oral Medications

EXAMPLE: The physician orders mycostatin 400,000 units po four times a day. The drug is supplied as 100,000 units/mL after reconstitution. How many milliliters will the nurse administer?

Using the Dimensional Analysis Method

a. On the left side of the equation, place what you are solving for:

$$x \text{ mL} =$$

b. On the right side of the equation, place the available information related to the measurement or abbreviation that was placed on the left side. In this example, the measurement we are solving for is *mL*. This information is placed in the equation as part of a fraction; match the appropriate abbreviation. Remember that the abbreviation that matches the x quantity must be placed in the numerator.

$$x \text{ mL} = \frac{1 \text{ mL}}{100,000 \text{ units}}$$

c. Next, find the information that matches the measurement used in the denominator of the fraction you created. In this example, *units* is in the denominator, so 400,000 units is used.

$$x \text{ mL} = \frac{1 \text{ mL}}{100,000 \text{ units}} \times \frac{400,000 \text{ units}}{1}$$

d. Then cancel out the abbreviations on the right side of the equation. If you have set up the problem correctly, the remaining measurement should match the measurement on the left side of the equation. Now solve for x.

$$x \text{ mL} = \frac{1 \text{ mL}}{100,000 \ \cancel{\text{units}}} \times \frac{400,000 \ \cancel{\text{units}}}{1}$$

$$x \text{ mL} = \frac{400,000}{100,000}$$

$$x = 4 \text{ mL}$$

Using the Proportion Method

a. On the left side of the proportion, place what you know or have available. In this example, each milliliter contains 100,000 units. So the left side of the proportion would be

$$100,000 \text{ units} : 1 \text{ mL} ::$$

b. The right side of the proportion is determined by the physician's order and the abbreviations on the left side of the proportion. Only *two* different abbreviations may be used in a single proportion. The abbreviations must be in the same position on the right side as on the left side.

$$100,000 \text{ units} : 1 \text{ mL} :: 400,000 \text{ units} : \underline{\hspace{1cm}} \text{ mL}$$

We need to find the number of milliliters to be administered, so we use the symbol x to represent the unknown.

$$100,000 \text{ units} : 1 \text{ mL} :: 400,000 \text{ units} : x \text{ mL}$$

c. Rewrite the proportion without the abbreviations.

$$100,000 : 1 :: 400,000 : x$$

d. Solve for x.

$$100,000 : 1 :: 400,000 : x$$

$$100,000x = 400,000$$

$$x = \frac{400,000}{100,000}$$

$$x = 4$$

e. Label your answer as determined by the abbreviation placed next to x in the original proportion.

$$x = 4 \text{ mL}$$

The nurse would measure 4 mL to administer 400,000 units of mycostatin.

Dosages Measured in Units Involving Parenteral Medications

EXAMPLE: The physician orders heparin 4000 units subcutaneous q 8 h. How many milliliters will the nurse administer?

Using the Dimensional Analysis Method

a. On the left side of the equation, place what you are solving for:

$$x \text{ mL} =$$

b. On the right side of the equation, place the available information related to the measurement or abbreviation that was placed on the left side. In this example, the measurement we are solving for is *mL*. This information is placed in the equation as part of a fraction; match the appropriate abbreviation. Remember that the abbreviation that matches the x quantity must be placed in the numerator.

$$x \text{ mL} = \frac{1 \text{ mL}}{5000 \text{ units}}$$

c. Next, find the information that matches the measurement used in the denominator of the fraction you created. In this example, *units* is in the denominator, so 4000 units is used.

$$x \text{ mL} = \frac{1 \text{ mL}}{5000 \text{ units}} \times \frac{4000 \text{ units}}{1}$$

d. Then cancel out the abbreviations on the right side of the equation. If you have set up the problem correctly, the remaining measurement should match the measurement on the left side of the equation. Now solve for x.

$$x \text{ mL} = \frac{1 \text{ mL}}{5000 \text{ units}} \times \frac{4000 \text{ units}}{1}$$

$$x \text{ mL} = \frac{4000}{5000}$$

$$x = 0.8 \text{ mL}$$

Using the Proportion Method

a. 5000 units : 1 mL ::

b. 5000 units : 1 mL :: _____ units : _____ mL

N 0-168-1201-15   520201

HEPARIN SODIUM

INJECTION, USP

5,000 USP Units/mL

(Derived from Porcine Intestinal Mucosa)
For IV or SC Use
1 mL Multiple Dose Vial
Usual Dosage: See insert.
Fujisawa USA, Inc.
Deerfield, IL 60015-2548

40213F

LOT
EXP

5000 units : 1 mL :: 4000 units : x mL

c. $5000 : 1 :: 4000 : x$

d. $5000x = 4000$

$$x = \frac{4000}{5000}$$

$$x = 0.8$$

e. $x = 0.8$ mL

Therefore 0.8 mL of heparin would be the amount of each individual dose of heparin given q 8 h.

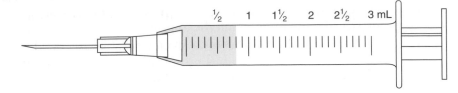

Insulin Given with a Lo-Dose Insulin Syringe

EXAMPLE: The physician orders Lantus U-100 insulin 36 units subcutaneous injection in AM. A U-100 Lo-Dose syringe is available. Shade the syringe to indicate the correct dose.

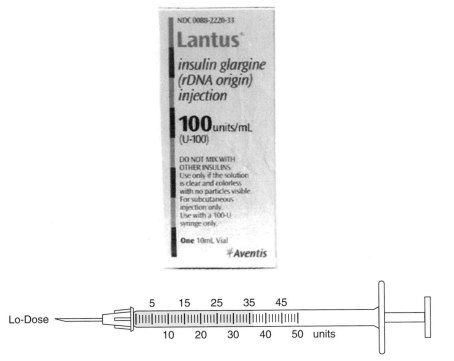

With a Lo-Dose insulin syringe, 36 units of U-100 insulin would be measured as indicated.

Mixed Insulin Administration

The physician may prescribe two types of insulin to be administered at the same time. As long as they are compatible, these insulins will be drawn up in the same syringe to avoid injecting the patient twice. The practice of mixing insulins is diminishing as the use of Lantus insulin increases.

Several guidelines apply to this type of administration:

1. Air equal to the amount of insulin being withdrawn should be injected into each vial. Do *not* touch the solution with the tip of the needle.
2. Using the same syringe, draw up the desired amount of insulin from the **regular** insulin bottle first.
3. Remove the syringe from the regular insulin bottle. Check the syringe for any air bubbles and remove them.
4. Using the same syringe, draw up the amount of cloudy insulin to the desired dose.
5. Hospitals usually require that you check your insulin dosages with another nurse before administration. Consult your hospital policy and procedures.

EXAMPLE 1: The physician orders Humulin Regular U-100 10 units plus Humulin NPH U-100 20 units subcutaneous now. The syringe is shaded in yellow to indicate the amount of Humulin regular insulin to be given, and in a different color to indicate the total dose.

The total amount of insulin is 30 units (10 units + 20 units = 30 units).

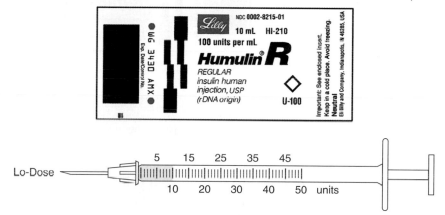

10 units of regular insulin is drawn up first; then 20 units of NPH insulin is drawn up.

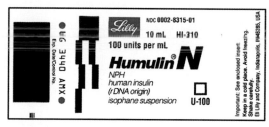

10 units of regular insulin + 20 units of NPH insulin = 30 units of insulin.

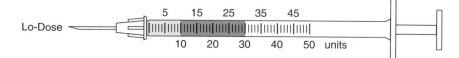

!

• **ALERT**

Some insulins such as Lantus should never be mixed. Be sure to always check whether an insulin can be mixed with another insulin.

EXAMPLE 2: The physician orders Humulin Lente U-100 46 units subcutaneous daily, plus regular Humulin U-100 20 units. A U-100 insulin syringe is available. The syringe is shaded in yellow to indicate the amount of Humulin regular insulin to be given, and in a different color to indicate the total dose.

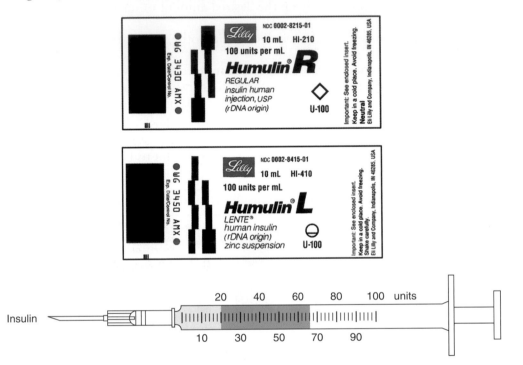

Complete the following work sheet, which provides for extensive practice in the calculation of dosages measured in units. Check your answers. If you have difficulties, go back and review the necessary material. When you feel ready to evaluate your learning, take the first posttest. Check your answers. An acceptable score as indicated on the posttest signifies that you have successfully completed this chapter. An unacceptable score signifies a need for further study before taking the second posttest.

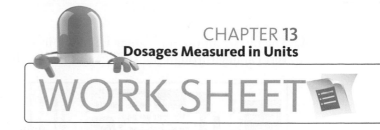
DIRECTIONS: The medication order is listed at the beginning of each problem. Calculate the doses. Show your work. Mark the syringe when provided to indicate the correct dose.

1. Mr. Curtis has Epogen 12,000 units subcutaneous injection three times a week to treat anemia related to chemotherapy. How many milliliters will you administer? __1.2 mL__

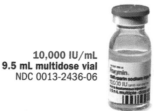

NDC 55513-283-01   Store at 2° to 8°C

EPOGEN®
EPOETIN ALFA
M 10
10,000 Units/mL (20,000 Units/2 mL) 2 mL Multidose Vial
Caution: Federal law prohibits dispensing without prescription
Dosage - See Package Insert
Amgen Inc. Thousand Oaks, CA 91320   U.S. License No. 1080

3112802   Lot   Exp.

$$\frac{12,000}{1} = \frac{1\,mL}{10,000} = \frac{12,000}{10,000} =$$

2. The physician orders Humalog U-100 insulin 10 units subcutaneous daily at 0800. Draw a vertical line through the syringe to indicate the amount of NPH insulin to be given.

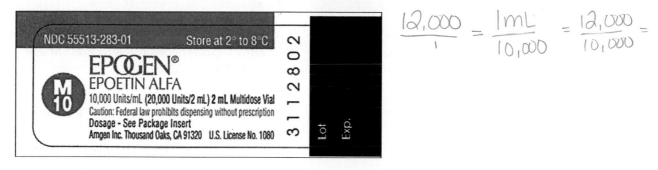

Lilly NDC 0002-7510-01
10 mL VL-7510
100 units per mL

Humalog®
insulin lispro injection
(rDNA origin)   **U-100**

CAUTION—Federal (USA) law prohibits dispensing without a prescription.
For parenteral use.
See accompanying literature for dosage
Eli Lilly and Co. Indianapolis, IN 46285, USA
Neutral

Lo-Dose

5   15   25   35   45
10   20   30   40   50 units

3. Following a right total hip replacement, Mr. Stephens has Fragmin 5000 international units by subcutaneous injection daily ordered. How many milliliters will the nurse administer? _____

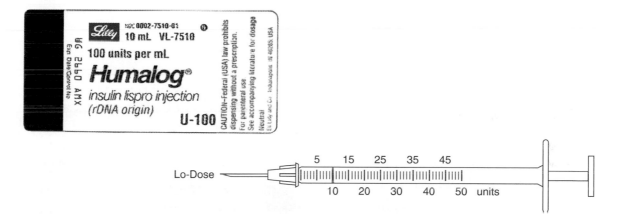

10,000 IU/mL
9.5 mL multidose vial
NDC 0013-2436-06

The product, as depicted in this label, is no longer available. This image was authorized for use by Pfizer, Inc. for educational purposes only.

4. The physician orders regular Humulin insulin 2 units subcutaneous daily at 1900. Draw a vertical line through the syringe to indicate the dose.

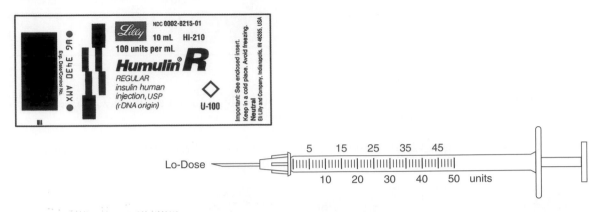

5. Your postoperative patient receives heparin 3000 units subcutaneous q 8 h to prevent deep vein thrombosis. How many milliliters will you administer? _____

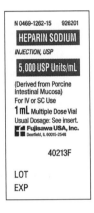

6. The physician orders Lente insulin 14 units, regular insulin 6 units subcutaneous every morning. Lente insulin U-100, regular insulin U-100, and a U-100 Lo-Dose syringe are supplied. Draw a vertical line through the syringe to indicate the amount of regular insulin to be given and a second line to indicate the total dose.

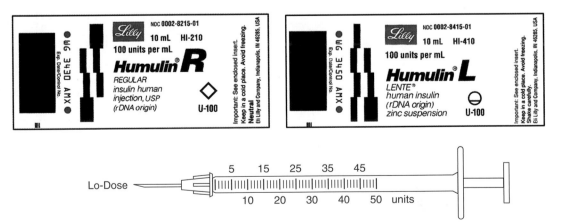

7. Mrs. Alvarez has Epogen 4500 units subcutaneous injection three times a week ordered for anemia caused by chronic renal failure. How many milliliters will you administer? (Round your final answer to the nearest hundredth.) _____

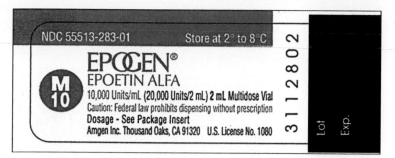

8. The physician orders Humulin regular insulin 18 units subcutaneous at 0700 daily. Draw a vertical line through the syringe to indicate the dose.

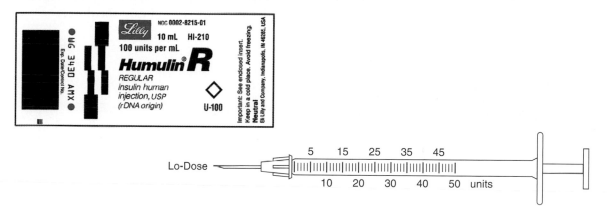

9. The physician orders Humulin 70/30 insulin 32 units subcutaneous tomorrow at 0745. Draw a vertical line through the syringe to indicate the dose.

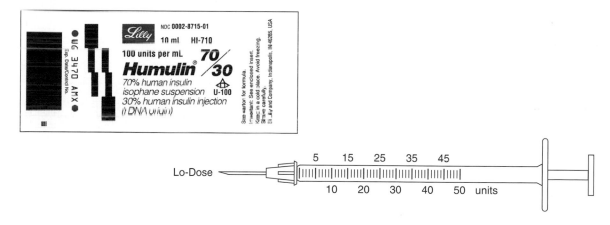

10. Your patient with a stapedectomy receives penicillin V 300,000 units po four times a day. The drug is supplied in oral solution 200,000 units/5 mL. How many milliliters will you administer? _____

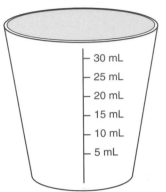

- 30 mL
- 25 mL
- 20 mL
- 15 mL
- 10 mL
- 5 mL

11. Your patient with insulin-dependent diabetes receives Humulin U Insulin 24 units subcutaneously every morning. Draw a vertical line through the syringe to indicate the dose.

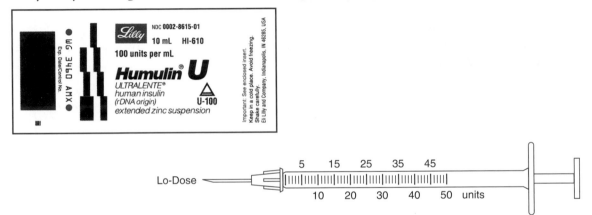

12. Your postoperative patient receives heparin 4000 units subcutaneous injection now. Draw a vertical line through the syringe to indicate the dose.

13. Your patient with a gastric pull-up receives penicillin G 200,000 units IM q 6 h. You have penicillin G 250,000 units/mL available. How many milliliters will you administer? _____ Draw a vertical line through the syringe to indicate the dose.

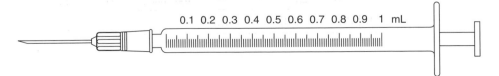

14. Mrs. Schroeder has orders for Fragmin 5500 international units by subcutaneous injection twice a day for system anticoagulation. You have Fragmin 10,000 international units/mL. How many milliliters will you administer? (Round your final answer to the nearest hundredth.) _____

15. The physician orders Humulin regular insulin 40 units and Humulin NPH 35 units every morning before breakfast. Draw a vertical line through the syringe to indicate the dosage for regular Humulin first; then draw a second line to indicate the total dose with the Humulin NPH.

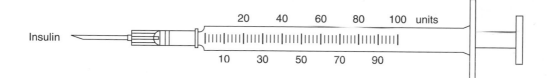

16. The physician orders heparin 2500 units subcutaneous q 12 h for your patient with a jejunostomy. How many milliliters will you administer? _____ Draw a vertical line through the syringe to indicate the dose.

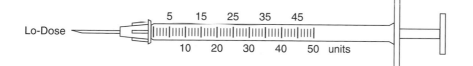

17. The physician orders 24 units Humulin U subcutaneous injection now. Draw a vertical line through the syringe to indicate the dose.

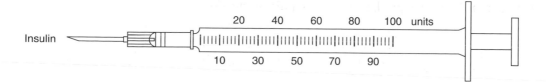

18. The physician orders Humulin 50/50 70 units subcutaneous injection. Draw a vertical line through the syringe to indicate the dose.

19. The physician orders 60 units Lantus U-100 subcutaneous injection daily at bedtime. Draw a vertical line through the syringe to indicate the dose.

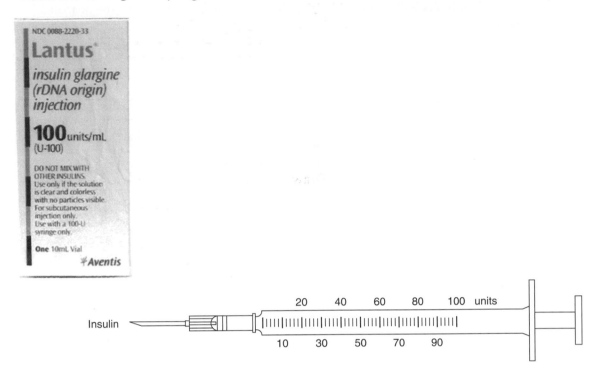

20. The physician orders 14 units NovoLog U-100 subcutaneous injection daily at bedtime. Draw a vertical line through the syringe to indicate the dose.

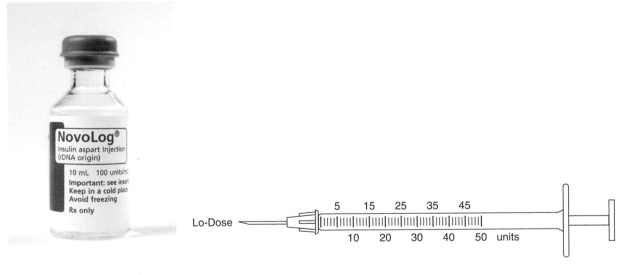

Used with permission from Novo Nordisk Inc.

ANSWERS ON PP. 382–384 AND 387–389.

√6/14 (MD)

NAME _____

DATE _____

ACCEPTABLE SCORE __14__

YOUR SCORE _____

DIRECTIONS: The medication order is listed at the beginning of each problem. Calculate the doses. Show your work. Mark the syringe when provided to indicate the correct dose.

1. The physician orders penicillin V 500,000 units po four times a day for your patient with a hysterectomy. Penicillin V pediatric suspension 400,000 units/5 mL is supplied. How many milliliters will you administer? __6.25__ Draw a vertical line through the syringe to indicate the dose.
ml

$$\frac{500,000u}{1} = \frac{5mL}{400,000u} =$$

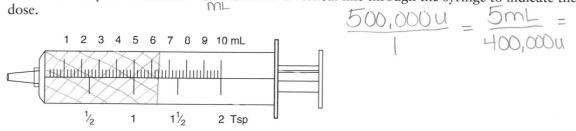

1 2 3 4 5 6 7 8 9 10 mL

½   1   1½   2 Tsp

2. The physician orders Lantus insulin 40 units subcutaneous daily. Draw a vertical line through the syringe to indicate the dose.

$$\frac{40u}{1} = \frac{1mL}{100u} = \frac{40}{100} = 0.4 \cdot 100 = 40u$$

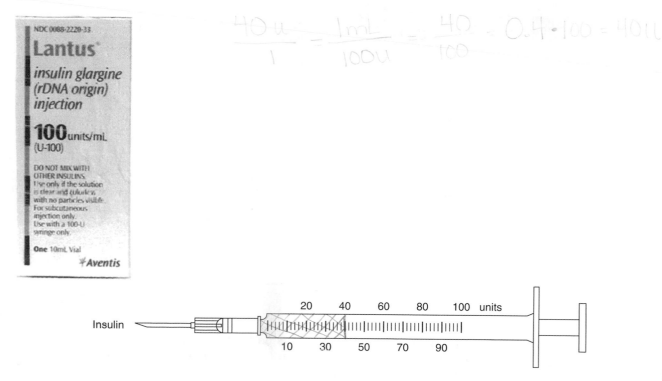

NDC 0088-2220-33

Lantus
*insulin glargine
(rDNA origin)
injection*

100 units/mL
(U-100)

DO NOT MIX WITH
OTHER INSULINS.
Use only if the solution
is clear and colorless,
with no particles visible.
For subcutaneous
injection only.
Use with a 100-U
syringe only.

One 10mL Vial

✝Aventis

20   40   60   80   100 units

Insulin

10   30   50   70   90

3. In preparation for his upcoming hip replacement surgery, Mr. Stone has Epogen 36,000 units subcutaneous injection once 3 weeks before his surgery. Epogen 40,000 units/mL is available. How many milliliters will the nurse administer? __0.9 mL__

$$\frac{36,000}{1} = \frac{1mL}{40,000} = \frac{36,000}{40,000}$$

4. The physician orders Humulin 50/50 insulin 6 units subcutaneous now. Draw a vertical line through the syringe to indicate the dose.

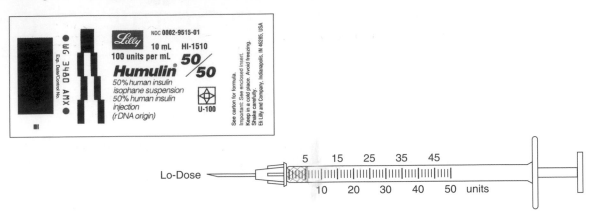

5. Your patient with insulin-dependent diabetes has orders for Humalog insulin 12 units subcutaneous four times a day. You have Humalog insulin U-100 and a U-100 syringe. Draw a vertical line through the syringe to indicate the dose.

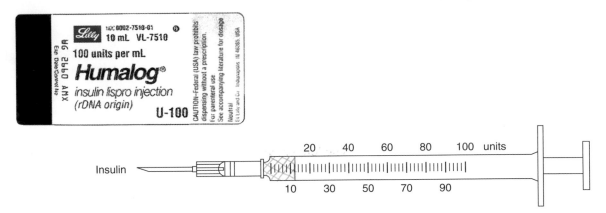

6. The physician orders Lente insulin 38 units, regular insulin 18 units subcutaneous daily. Lente U-100, regular insulin U-100, and a U-100 syringe are supplied. Draw a vertical line through the syringe to indicate the amount of regular insulin to be given and a second line to indicate the total dose.

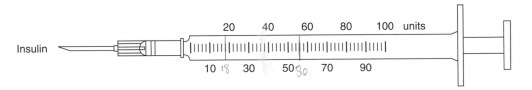

7. The physician orders penicillin V 300,000 units po four times a day for your patient with chronic otitis. The drug is supplied in oral solution 200,000 units/5 mL. How many milliliters will you administer? 7.5 mL

$$\frac{300,000}{1} = \frac{5\,mL}{200,000} = \frac{1,500,000}{200,000} =$$

8. Your patient with a sacral decubitus receives penicillin V 200,000 units po four times a day. You have penicillin V oral solution 400,000 units/5 mL. How many milliliters will you administer? _2.5 mL_

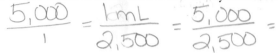

$$\frac{200,000}{1} = \frac{5 mL}{400,000} = \frac{1,000,000}{400,000} =$$

9. Your postoperative patient receives heparin 5000 units subcutaneous q 12 h. Heparin 2500 units/mL is available. How many milliliters will you administer? _2 mL_

$$\frac{5,000}{1} = \frac{1 mL}{2,500} = \frac{5,000}{2,500} =$$

10. Mrs. Tanaka has been admitted with unstable angina. The physician orders Fragmin 8700 international units subcutaneous injection q 12 h. How many milliliters will be administered? (Round your final answer to the nearest hundredth.) _0.87 mL_

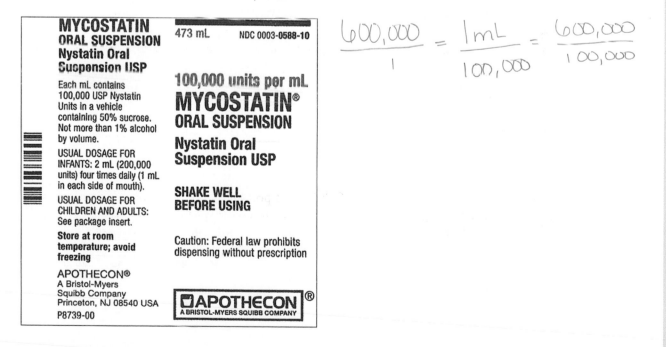

$$\frac{8,700}{1} = \frac{1 mL}{10,000} = \frac{8,700}{10,000} =$$

10,000 IU/mL
9.5 mL multidose vial
NDC 0013-2436-06

The product, as depicted in this label, is no longer available. This image was authorized for use by Pfizer, Inc. for educational purposes only.

11. Mrs. Daisy receives nystatin oral suspension 600,000 units po four times a day. How many milliliters will the nurse administer? _6 mL_

$$\frac{600,000}{1} = \frac{1 mL}{100,000} = \frac{600,000}{100,000} =$$

MYCOSTATIN
ORAL SUSPENSION
Nystatin Oral
Suspension USP

473 mL   NDC 0003-0588-10

Each mL contains 100,000 USP Nystatin Units in a vehicle containing 50% sucrose. Not more than 1% alcohol by volume.

USUAL DOSAGE FOR INFANTS: 2 mL (200,000 units) four times daily (1 mL in each side of mouth).

USUAL DOSAGE FOR CHILDREN AND ADULTS: See package insert.

Store at room temperature; avoid freezing

APOTHECON®
A Bristol-Myers Squibb Company
Princeton, NJ 08540 USA

P8739-00

100,000 units per mL
MYCOSTATIN®
ORAL SUSPENSION
Nystatin Oral
Suspension USP

SHAKE WELL BEFORE USING

Caution: Federal law prohibits dispensing without prescription

☐APOTHECON®
A BRISTOL-MYERS SQUIBB COMPANY

12. Ms. Sanders has Epogen 2200 units subcutaneous injection three times a week ordered for anemia caused by chronic renal failure. Epogen 3000 units/mL is available. How many milliliters will the patient receive for each dose? _0.73 mL_

$$\frac{2,200}{1} = \frac{1\,mL}{3,000} = \frac{2,200}{3,000} = 0.73$$

13. The physician orders 40 units Lantus U 100 subcutaneous injection daily at bedtime. Draw a vertical line through the syringe to indicate the dose.

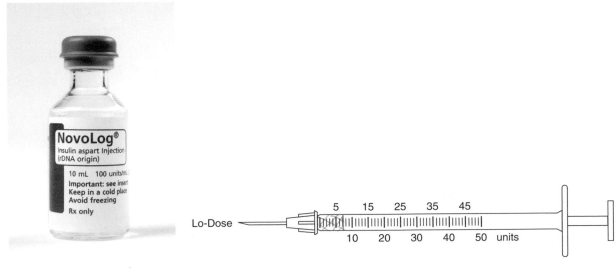

14. The physician orders 8 units NovoLog U-100 subcutaneous injection daily at bedtime. Draw a vertical line through the syringe to indicate the dose.

Used with permission from Novo Nordisk Inc.

15. The physician orders NPH insulin 12 units and regular insulin 8 units subcutaneous daily before breakfast and dinner. Draw a vertical line through the syringe to indicate the amount of regular insulin to be given and a second line to indicate the <u>total dose.</u>

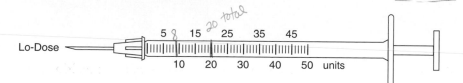

ANSWERS ON PP. 384–385 AND 390–391.

NAME _____

DATE _____

ACCEPTABLE SCORE __14__

YOUR SCORE _____

CHAPTER **13**
Dosages Measured in Units

POSTTEST 2

DIRECTIONS: The medication order is listed at the beginning of each problem. Calculate the doses. Show your work. Mark the syringe when provided to indicate the correct dose.

1. The physician orders regular insulin 10 units subcutaneous. Regular insulin U-100 and a U-100 Lo-Dose syringe are supplied. Draw a vertical line through the syringe to indicate the dose.

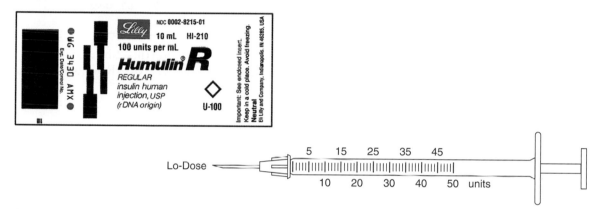

2. Mr. Blackwell has 14,000 units Epogen subcutaneous injection ordered three times a week for anemia related to his chemotherapy. How many milliliters will he receive each time? _____

3. Your patient with a septoplasty receives V-Cillin K 500,000 units po q 6 h. You have 200,000 units/5 mL available. How many milliliters will you administer? _____

4. The physician orders Novolin L insulin 28 units subcutaneous at 0745. Draw a vertical line through the syringe to indicate the dose of NPH insulin to be given.

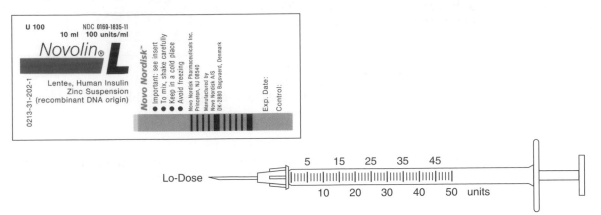

5. Mr. Noah has orders for Fragmin 2500 international units subcutaneous 2 hours before surgery for a total hip replacement. How many milliliters will he receive? (Round your final answer to the nearest hundredth.) _____

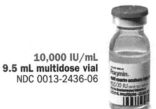

10,000 IU/mL
9.5 mL multidose vial
NDC 0013-2436-06

The product, as depicted in this label, is no longer available. This image was authorized for use by Pfizer, Inc. for educational purposes only.

6. The physician orders Humulin L Lente insulin 54 units subcutaneous. You have Lente insulin U-100 and a U-100 syringe. Draw a vertical line through the syringe to indicate the amount of Lente insulin to be given.

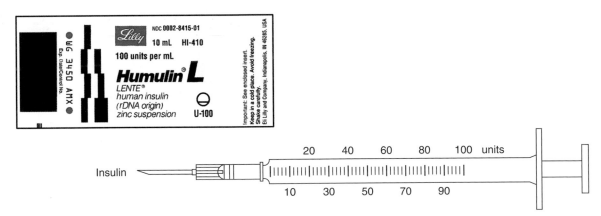

7. The physician orders NPH insulin 16 units and regular insulin 8 units subcutaneous daily at 0800. You have NPH insulin U-100, regular insulin U-100, and a U-100 Lo-Dose syringe. Draw a vertical line through the syringe to indicate the amount of regular insulin to be given and a second line to indicate the total dose.

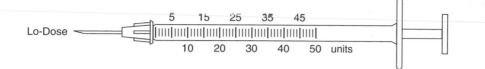

8. Your patient with chronic sinusitis receives penicillin V 300,000 units po four times a day. You have penicillin V oral solution 400,000 units/5 mL. How many milliliters will you administer? _____

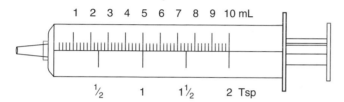

9. Your patient with insulin-dependent diabetes receives Lente insulin 25 units subcutaneous daily at 0800. Draw a vertical line through the syringe to indicate the amount of Lente insulin to be given.

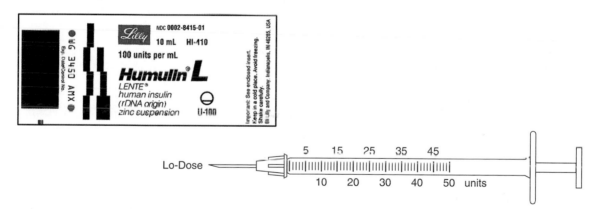

10. Mrs. Star has Epogen 16,000 units subcutaneous injection three times a week for anemia as a result of her chemotherapy. How many milliliters will you administer for each dose? _____

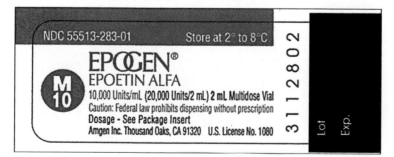

11. The physician orders 50 units Lantus U-100 subcutaneous injection daily at bedtime. Draw a vertical line through the syringe to indicate the dose.

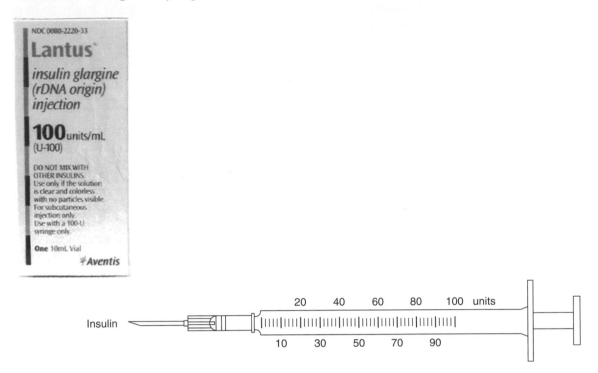

12. The physician orders 12 units NovoLog U-100 subcutaneous injection daily at bedtime. Draw a vertical line through the syringe to indicate the dose.

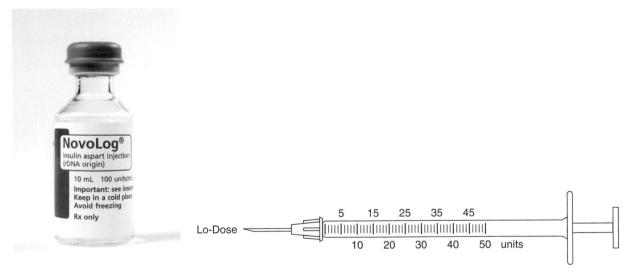

Used with permission from
Novo Nordisk Inc.

13. An order for Lovenox 20 mg subcutaneous q 12 h is received. Draw a vertical line through the syringe to indicate the milliliters to administer to the patient.

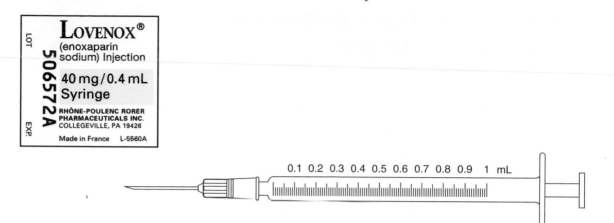

14. An order for Levimir 28 units subcutaneous daily is received. Draw a vertical line through the syringe to indicate the dose.

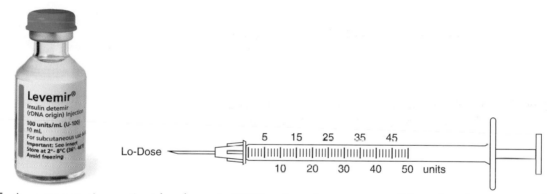

15. A postoperative patient has heparin 2500 units subcutaneous q 8 h ordered to prevent deep vein thrombosis. How many milliliters will the nurse administer?

NDC 63323-262-01 926201

HEPARIN SODIUM

INJECTION, USP

5,000 USP Units/mL

(Derived from Porcine
Intestinal Mucosa)
For IV or SC Use   Rx only
1 mL Multiple Dose Vial
Usual Dosage: See insert.
**American Pharmaceutical
Partners, Inc.**
Los Angeles, CA 90024

401810A

LOT
EXP

ANSWERS ON PP. 385–386 AND 392–393.

evolve   For additional practice problems, refer to the Advanced Calculations
section of *Drug Calculations Companion,* Version 5, on Evolve.

ANSWERS

CHAPTER 13 Dimensional Analysis—Work Sheet, pp. 365–370

1. $x \text{ mL} = \dfrac{1 \text{ mL}}{10{,}000 \text{ units}} \times \dfrac{12{,}000 \text{ units}}{1} = 1.2 \text{ mL}$

2. Lo-Dose

3. $x \text{ mL} = \dfrac{1 \text{ mL}}{10{,}000 \text{ IU}} \times \dfrac{5000 \text{ IU}}{1} = 0.5 \text{ mL}$

4. Lo-Dose

5. $x \text{ mL} = \dfrac{1 \text{ mL}}{5000 \text{ units}} \times \dfrac{3000 \text{ units}}{1} = 0.6 \text{ mL}$

6. Lo-Dose

7. $x \text{ mL} = \dfrac{1 \text{ mL}}{10{,}000 \text{ units}} \times \dfrac{4500 \text{ units}}{1} = 0.45 \text{ mL}$

8. Lo-Dose

9. Lo-Dose

10. $x \text{ mL} = \dfrac{5 \text{ mL}}{200{,}000 \text{ units}} \times \dfrac{300{,}000 \text{ units}}{1} = 7.5 \text{ mL}$

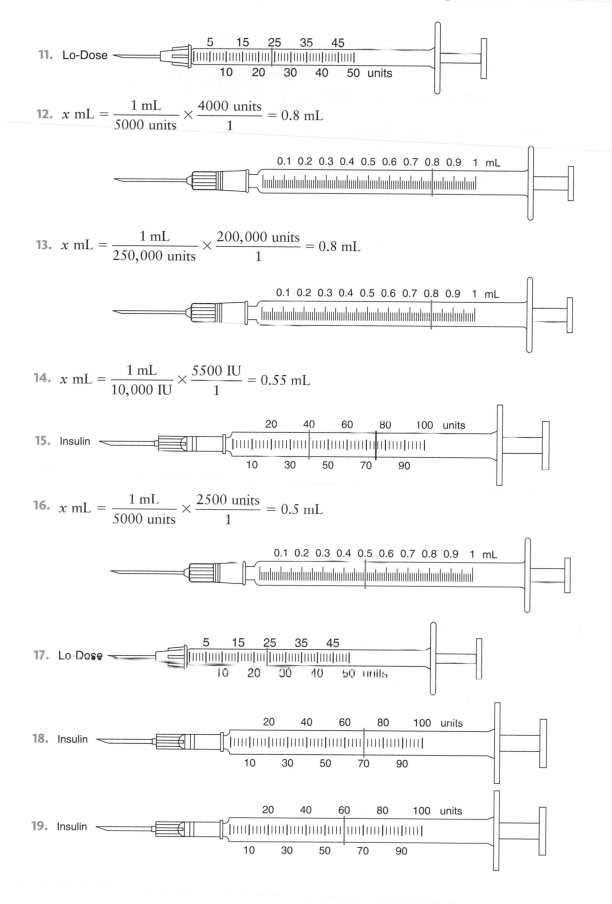

11. Lo-Dose

12. $x \text{ mL} = \dfrac{1 \text{ mL}}{5000 \text{ units}} \times \dfrac{4000 \text{ units}}{1} = 0.8 \text{ mL}$

13. $x \text{ mL} = \dfrac{1 \text{ mL}}{250{,}000 \text{ units}} \times \dfrac{200{,}000 \text{ units}}{1} = 0.8 \text{ mL}$

14. $x \text{ mL} = \dfrac{1 \text{ mL}}{10{,}000 \text{ IU}} \times \dfrac{5500 \text{ IU}}{1} = 0.55 \text{ mL}$

15. Insulin

16. $x \text{ mL} = \dfrac{1 \text{ mL}}{5000 \text{ units}} \times \dfrac{2500 \text{ units}}{1} = 0.5 \text{ mL}$

17. Lo-Dose

18. Insulin

19. Insulin

20. Lo-Dose

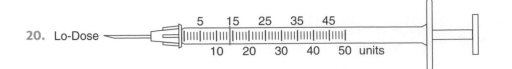

CHAPTER 13 Dimensional Analysis—Posttest 1, pp. 371–375

1. $x \text{ mL} = \dfrac{5 \text{ mL}}{400,000 \text{ units}} \times \dfrac{500,000 \text{ units}}{1} = 6.25, \ 6.3 \text{ mL}$

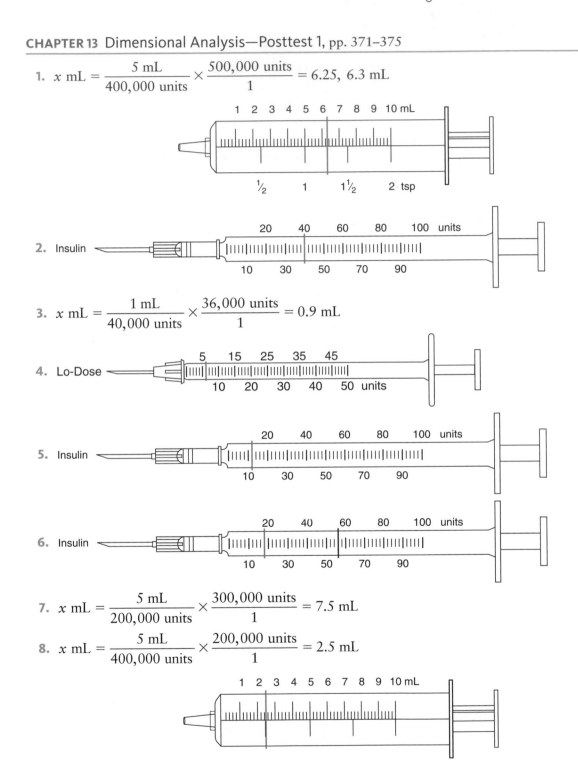

2. Insulin

3. $x \text{ mL} = \dfrac{1 \text{ mL}}{40,000 \text{ units}} \times \dfrac{36,000 \text{ units}}{1} = 0.9 \text{ mL}$

4. Lo-Dose

5. Insulin

6. Insulin

7. $x \text{ mL} = \dfrac{5 \text{ mL}}{200,000 \text{ units}} \times \dfrac{300,000 \text{ units}}{1} = 7.5 \text{ mL}$

8. $x \text{ mL} = \dfrac{5 \text{ mL}}{400,000 \text{ units}} \times \dfrac{200,000 \text{ units}}{1} = 2.5 \text{ mL}$

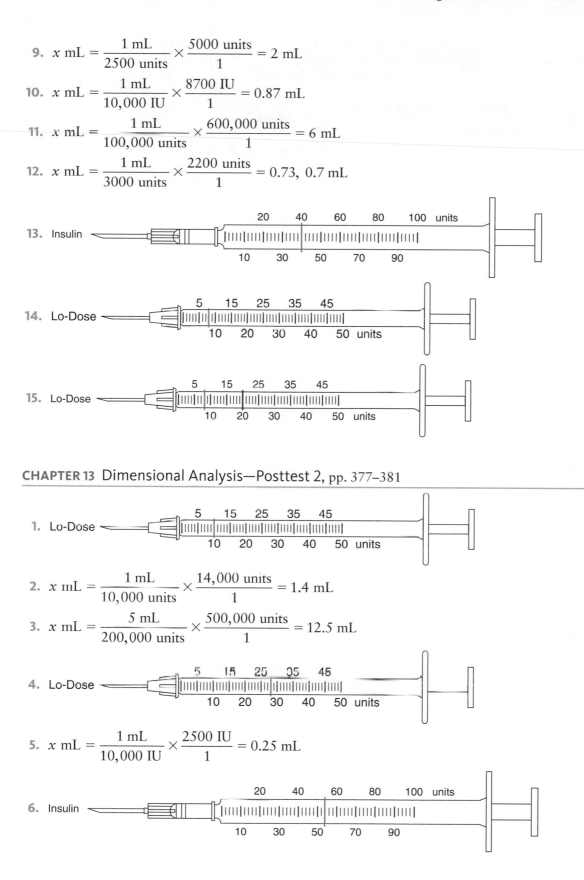

9. $x \text{ mL} = \dfrac{1 \text{ mL}}{2500 \text{ units}} \times \dfrac{5000 \text{ units}}{1} = 2 \text{ mL}$

10. $x \text{ mL} = \dfrac{1 \text{ mL}}{10,000 \text{ IU}} \times \dfrac{8700 \text{ IU}}{1} = 0.87 \text{ mL}$

11. $x \text{ mL} = \dfrac{1 \text{ mL}}{100,000 \text{ units}} \times \dfrac{600,000 \text{ units}}{1} = 6 \text{ mL}$

12. $x \text{ mL} = \dfrac{1 \text{ mL}}{3000 \text{ units}} \times \dfrac{2200 \text{ units}}{1} = 0.73, \ 0.7 \text{ mL}$

13. Insulin

14. Lo-Dose

15. Lo-Dose

CHAPTER 13 Dimensional Analysis—Posttest 2, pp. 377–381

1. Lo-Dose

2. $x \text{ mL} = \dfrac{1 \text{ mL}}{10,000 \text{ units}} \times \dfrac{14,000 \text{ units}}{1} = 1.4 \text{ mL}$

3. $x \text{ mL} = \dfrac{5 \text{ mL}}{200,000 \text{ units}} \times \dfrac{500,000 \text{ units}}{1} = 12.5 \text{ mL}$

4. Lo-Dose

5. $x \text{ mL} = \dfrac{1 \text{ mL}}{10,000 \text{ IU}} \times \dfrac{2500 \text{ IU}}{1} = 0.25 \text{ mL}$

6. Insulin

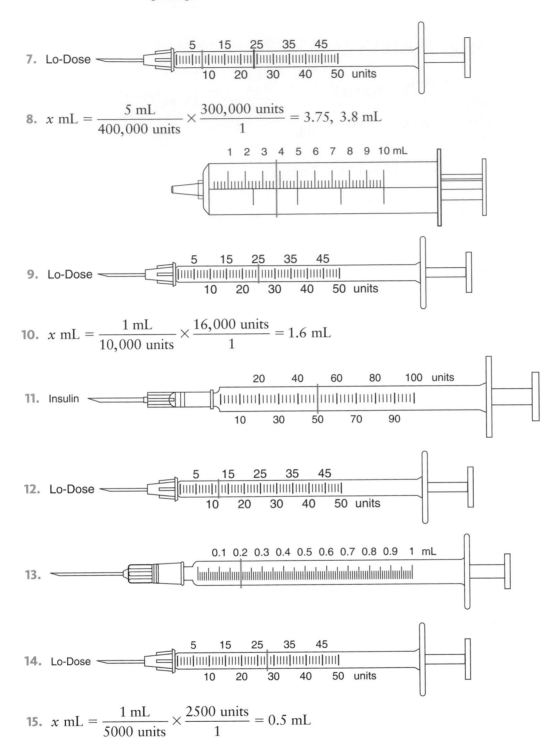

7. Lo-Dose

8. $x \text{ mL} = \dfrac{5 \text{ mL}}{400,000 \text{ units}} \times \dfrac{300,000 \text{ units}}{1} = 3.75, \ 3.8 \text{ mL}$

9. Lo-Dose

10. $x \text{ mL} = \dfrac{1 \text{ mL}}{10,000 \text{ units}} \times \dfrac{16,000 \text{ units}}{1} = 1.6 \text{ mL}$

11. Insulin

12. Lo-Dose

13.

14. Lo-Dose

15. $x \text{ mL} = \dfrac{1 \text{ mL}}{5000 \text{ units}} \times \dfrac{2500 \text{ units}}{1} = 0.5 \text{ mL}$

ANSWERS

CHAPTER 13 Proportion/Formula Method—Work Sheet, pp. 365–370

Proportion	Formula

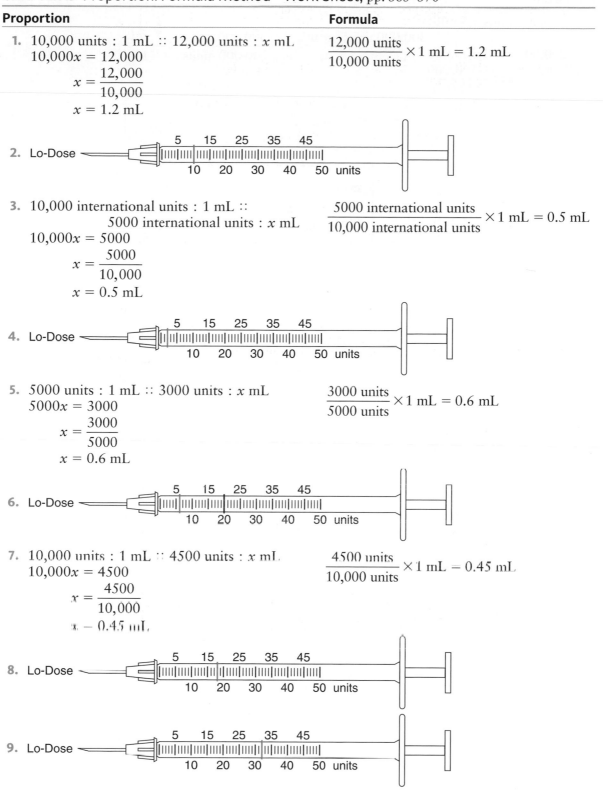

1. 10,000 units : 1 mL :: 12,000 units : x mL
   10,000x = 12,000
   $$x = \frac{12,000}{10,000}$$
   x = 1.2 mL

   $$\frac{12,000 \text{ units}}{10,000 \text{ units}} \times 1 \text{ mL} = 1.2 \text{ mL}$$

2. Lo-Dose

3. 10,000 international units : 1 mL ::
           5000 international units : x mL
   10,000x = 5000
   $$x = \frac{5000}{10,000}$$
   x = 0.5 mL

   $$\frac{5000 \text{ international units}}{10,000 \text{ international units}} \times 1 \text{ mL} = 0.5 \text{ mL}$$

4. Lo-Dose

5. 5000 units : 1 mL :: 3000 units : x mL
   5000x = 3000
   $$x = \frac{3000}{5000}$$
   x = 0.6 mL

   $$\frac{3000 \text{ units}}{5000 \text{ units}} \times 1 \text{ mL} = 0.6 \text{ mL}$$

6. Lo-Dose

7. 10,000 units : 1 mL :: 4500 units : x mL
   10,000x = 4500
   $$x = \frac{4500}{10,000}$$
   x = 0.45 mL

   $$\frac{4500 \text{ units}}{10,000 \text{ units}} \times 1 \text{ mL} = 0.45 \text{ mL}$$

8. Lo-Dose

9. Lo-Dose

Proportion	**Formula**

10. 200,000 units : 5 mL ::
$$300,000 \text{ units} : x \text{ mL}$$
$$200,000x = 1,500,000$$
$$x = \frac{1,500,000}{200,000}$$
$$x = 7.5 \text{ mL}$$

$$\frac{300,000 \text{ units}}{\overset{40,000}{\cancel{200,000}} \text{ units}} \times \frac{\overset{1}{\cancel{5}} \text{ mL}}{1} =$$
$$\frac{300,000}{40,000} = 7.5 \text{ mL}$$

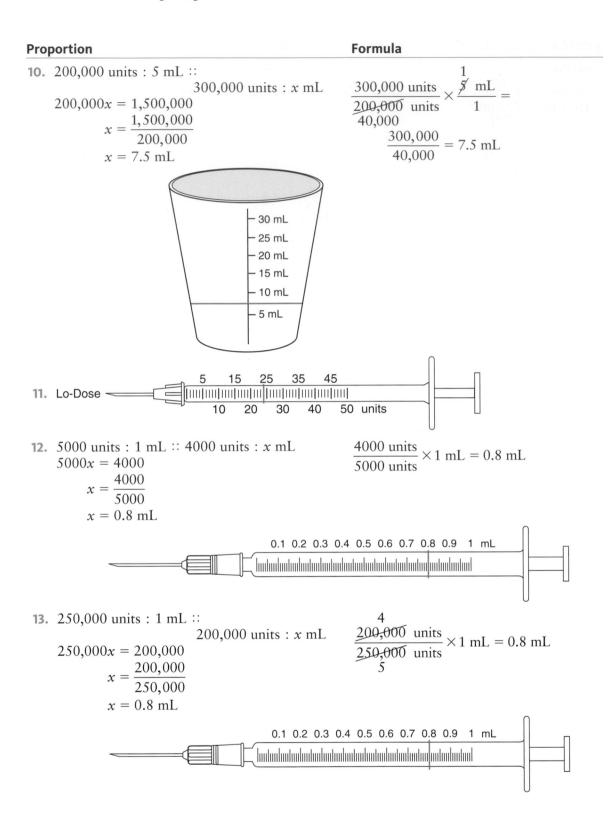

11. Lo-Dose

12. 5000 units : 1 mL :: 4000 units : x mL
$$5000x = 4000$$
$$x = \frac{4000}{5000}$$
$$x = 0.8 \text{ mL}$$

$$\frac{4000 \text{ units}}{5000 \text{ units}} \times 1 \text{ mL} = 0.8 \text{ mL}$$

13. 250,000 units : 1 mL ::
$$200,000 \text{ units} : x \text{ mL}$$
$$250,000x = 200,000$$
$$x = \frac{200,000}{250,000}$$
$$x = 0.8 \text{ mL}$$

$$\frac{\overset{4}{\cancel{200,000}} \text{ units}}{\underset{5}{\cancel{250,000}} \text{ units}} \times 1 \text{ mL} = 0.8 \text{ mL}$$

ANSWERS

Proportion	Formula

14. 10,000 international units : 1 mL ::
　　　　5500 international units : x mL
　　10,000x = 5500
　　　　$x = \dfrac{5500}{10,000}$
　　　　$x = 0.55$ mL

$\dfrac{5500 \text{ international units}}{10,000 \text{ international units}} \times 1 \text{ mL} = 0.55 \text{ mL}$

15. 40 units, then add the 35 for a total mark at 75.

16. 5000 units : 1 mL :: 2500 units : x mL
　　5000x = 2500
　　　$x = \dfrac{2500}{5000}$
　　　$x = 0.5$ mL

$\dfrac{2500 \text{ units}}{5000 \text{ units}} \times 1 \text{ mL} = 0.5 \text{ mL}$

17. Lo-Dose

18. Insulin

19. Insulin

20. Lo-Dose

CHAPTER 13 Proportion/Formula Method—Posttest 1, pp. 371–375

| Proportion | Formula |

1. 400,000 units : 5 mL ::
$$500,000 \text{ units} : x \text{ mL}$$
$$400,000x = 2,500,000$$
$$x = \frac{2,500,000}{400,000}$$
$$x = 6.25, 6.3 \text{ mL}$$

$$\frac{500,000 \text{ units}}{400,000 \text{ units}} \times 5 \text{ mL} =$$
$$\frac{25}{4} = 6.25, \; 6.3 \text{ mL}$$

2. Insulin

3. 40,000 units : 1 mL :: 36,000 units : x mL
$$40,000x = 36,000$$
$$x = \frac{36,000}{40,000}$$
$$x = 0.9 \text{ mL}$$

$$\frac{36,000 \text{ units}}{40,000 \text{ units}} \times 1 \text{ mL} = 0.9 \text{ mL}$$

4. Lo-Dose

5. Insulin

6. Insulin

7. 200,000 units : 5 mL ::
$$300,000 \text{ units} : x \text{ mL}$$
$$200,000x = 1,500,000$$
$$x = \frac{1,500,000}{200,000}$$
$$x = 7.5 \text{ mL}$$

$$\frac{300,000 \text{ units}}{200,000 \text{ units}} \times 5 \text{ mL} =$$
$$\frac{15}{2} = 7.5 \text{ mL}$$

ANSWERS

Proportion **Formula**

8. 400,000 units : 5 mL ::
   200,000 units : x mL

   $400,000x = 1,000,000$

   $x = \dfrac{1,000,000}{400,000}$

   $x = 2.5$ mL

   $\dfrac{200,000 \text{ units}}{400,000 \text{ units}} \times 5 \text{ mL} =$

   $\dfrac{1,000,000}{400,000} = 2.5$ mL

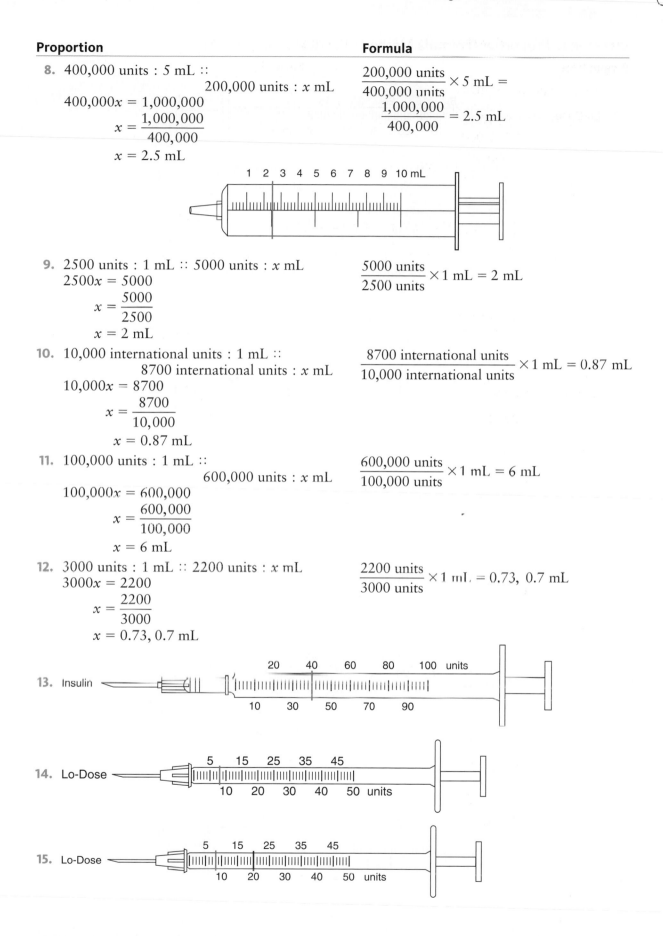

9. 2500 units : 1 mL :: 5000 units : x mL

   $2500x = 5000$

   $x = \dfrac{5000}{2500}$

   $x = 2$ mL

   $\dfrac{5000 \text{ units}}{2500 \text{ units}} \times 1 \text{ mL} = 2$ mL

10. 10,000 international units : 1 mL ::
    8700 international units : x mL

    $10,000x = 8700$

    $x = \dfrac{8700}{10,000}$

    $x = 0.87$ mL

    $\dfrac{8700 \text{ international units}}{10,000 \text{ international units}} \times 1 \text{ mL} = 0.87$ mL

11. 100,000 units : 1 mL ::
    600,000 units : x mL

    $100,000x = 600,000$

    $x = \dfrac{600,000}{100,000}$

    $x = 6$ mL

    $\dfrac{600,000 \text{ units}}{100,000 \text{ units}} \times 1 \text{ mL} = 6$ mL

12. 3000 units : 1 mL :: 2200 units : x mL

    $3000x = 2200$

    $x = \dfrac{2200}{3000}$

    $x = 0.73, 0.7$ mL

    $\dfrac{2200 \text{ units}}{3000 \text{ units}} \times 1 \text{ mL} = 0.73, 0.7$ mL

13. Insulin

14. Lo-Dose

15. Lo-Dose

ANSWERS

CHAPTER 13 Proportion/Formula Method—Posttest 2, pp. 377–381

Proportion	Formula

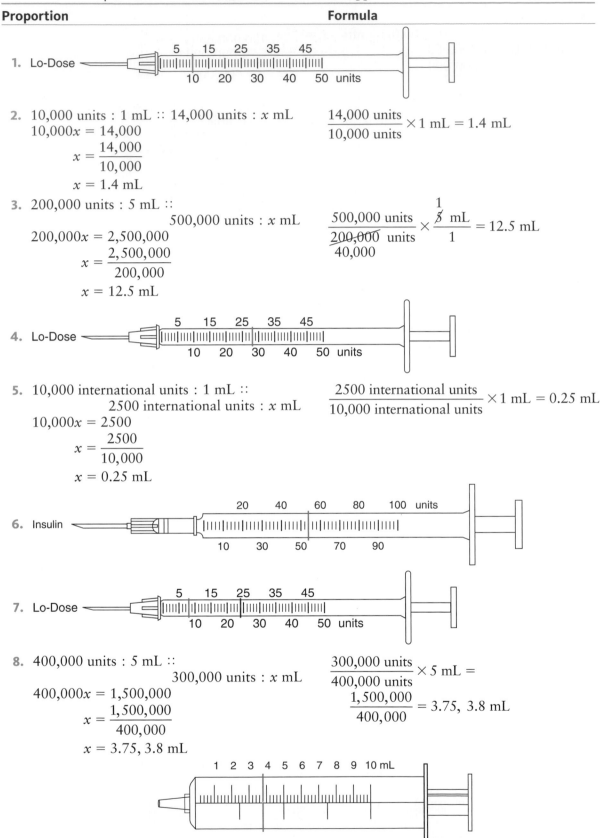

1. Lo-Dose

2. 10,000 units : 1 mL :: 14,000 units : x mL
   $10,000x = 14,000$
   $x = \dfrac{14,000}{10,000}$
   $x = 1.4$ mL

   $\dfrac{14,000 \text{ units}}{10,000 \text{ units}} \times 1 \text{ mL} = 1.4 \text{ mL}$

3. 200,000 units : 5 mL ::
              500,000 units : x mL
   $200,000x = 2,500,000$
   $x = \dfrac{2,500,000}{200,000}$
   $x = 12.5$ mL

   $\dfrac{500,000 \text{ units}}{\underset{40,000}{200,000} \text{ units}} \times \dfrac{\overset{1}{\cancel{5}} \text{ mL}}{1} = 12.5 \text{ mL}$

4. Lo-Dose

5. 10,000 international units : 1 mL ::
              2500 international units : x mL
   $10,000x = 2500$
   $x = \dfrac{2500}{10,000}$
   $x = 0.25$ mL

   $\dfrac{2500 \text{ international units}}{10,000 \text{ international units}} \times 1 \text{ mL} = 0.25 \text{ mL}$

6. Insulin

7. Lo-Dose

8. 400,000 units : 5 mL ::
              300,000 units : x mL
   $400,000x = 1,500,000$
   $x = \dfrac{1,500,000}{400,000}$
   $x = 3.75,\ 3.8$ mL

   $\dfrac{300,000 \text{ units}}{400,000 \text{ units}} \times 5 \text{ mL} =$
   $\dfrac{1,500,000}{400,000} = 3.75,\ 3.8 \text{ mL}$

Proportion   **Formula**

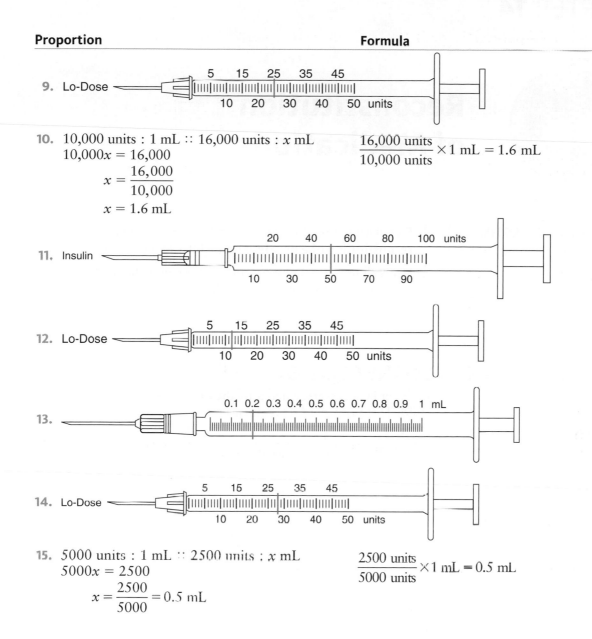

9. Lo-Dose

10. 10,000 units : 1 mL :: 16,000 units : x mL $\dfrac{16{,}000 \text{ units}}{10{,}000 \text{ units}} \times 1 \text{ mL} = 1.6 \text{ mL}$

    $10{,}000x = 16{,}000$

    $x = \dfrac{16{,}000}{10{,}000}$

    $x = 1.6 \text{ mL}$

11. Insulin

12. Lo-Dose

13.

14. Lo-Dose

15. 5000 units : 1 mL :: 2500 units : x mL $\dfrac{2500 \text{ units}}{5000 \text{ units}} \times 1 \text{ mL} = 0.5 \text{ mL}$

    $5000x = 2500$

    $x = \dfrac{2500}{5000} = 0.5 \text{ mL}$

ANSWERS

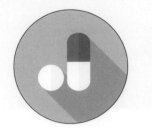
Reconstitution of Medications

LEARNING OBJECTIVES

Upon completion of the materials provided in this chapter, you will be able to perform computations accurately by mastering the following mathematical concepts:

1 Calculating drug dosage problems that first require reconstitution of a powdered drug into a liquid form

2 Using dimensional analysis, proportion, or formula methods to solve problems involving drugs measured in unit dosages

POWDER RECONSTITUTION

A drug in powdered form is necessary when a medication is unstable as a liquid form for a long period. This powdered drug must be reconstituted—dissolved with a sterile diluent—before administration. The diluents commonly used include sterile water, sterile normal saline solution, 5% dextrose solution (D_5W), and bacteriostatic normal saline.

> **! ALERT**
>
> Remember to always check the route of the administration for *all* reconstituted medications. Some will be oral and some will be parenteral.

Before reconstituting the medication, the nurse must follow several principles:

1. Carefully read the information and directions on the vial or package insert for reconstitution of the medication.

2. If no directions are available with the medication, consult the *Physicians' Desk Reference*, hospital drug formulary, pharmacology text, or hospital pharmacy.

3. Identify the type and amount of diluent and the route of administration.

4. Note the drug strength or concentration after reconstitution and circle or place this on the label, if not already written, when you use a multidose vial.

5. Note the length of time for which the medication is good once reconstituted and the directions for storage.

6. Be aware that the total reconstitution amount may be greater than the amount of diluent because of the volume of the powder.

7. After reconstitution of a multidose vial, place your initials, date of preparation, time of preparation, date of expiration, and time of expiration on the label.

In Figure 14-1, please review the steps required to reconstitute a medication.

> **! ● ALERT**
>
> A label must be placed on all multidose vials after reconstitution. The label must include the preparer's initials, the date and time of preparation, and the date and time of expiration.

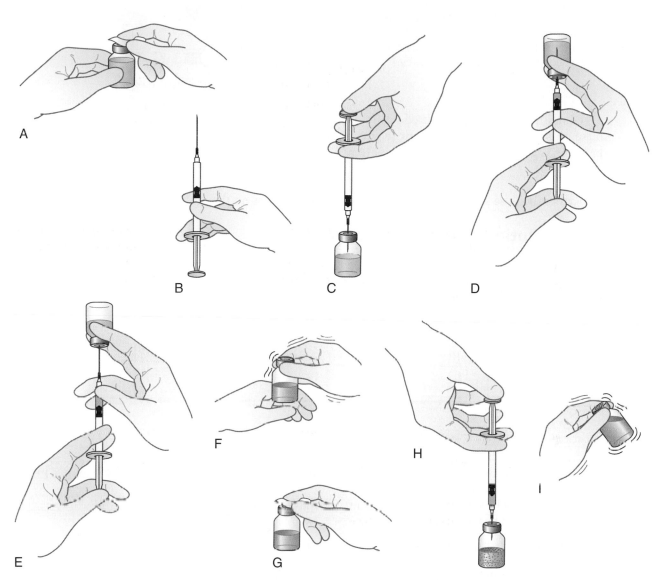

FIGURE 14-1   Removal of a volume of liquid from a vial: reconstitution of a powder. **A,** Cleanse the rubber diaphragm of the vial. **B,** Pull back on the plunger of the syringe to fill with an amount of air that is equal to the volume of the solution to be withdrawn. **C,** Insert the needle through the rubber diaphragm; inject the air with the vial sitting in a downward position. **D,** Withdraw the volume of diluent required to reconstitute the drug. **E,** Move the needle downward to facilitate the removal of all of the diluent. **F,** Tap the container with the powdered drug to break up the caked powder. **G,** Wipe the rubber diaphragm of the vial of the powdered drug with a new antiseptic alcohol wipe. **H,** Insert the needle with the diluent in the syringe into the rubber diaphragm, and inject the diluent into the powdered drug. **I,** Mix thoroughly to ensure that the powdered drug is dissolved before withdrawing the prescribed dose. **Note specific directions. Some medications should be rolled to mix—not shaken.** (From Clayton BD, Willihnganz M: *Basic pharmacology for nurses*, ed. 16, St Louis, 2013, Mosby.)

Medications may also be supplied in a Mix-O-Vial container. This container supplies both the powdered medication for reconstitution and the diluent. See Figure 14-2.

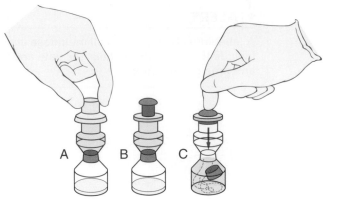

FIGURE 14-2 Using a Mix-O-Vial. **A,** Remove the plastic lid protector. **B,** The powdered drug is in the lower half; the diluent is in the upper half. **C,** Push firmly on the diaphragm plunger; downward pressure dislodges the divider between the two chambers. (From Clayton BD, Willihnganz M: *Basic pharmacology for nurses,* ed. 16, St Louis, 2013, Mosby.)

Penicillin can be administered orally or parenterally. Before administering penicillin, the nurse must confer with the patient regarding previous allergies to the drug. After administering the drug, the nurse must observe the patient for signs of an allergic reaction, as with any other medication.

Remember, the strength of the medication is dependent on the amount of diluent added.

Reconstitution of Oral Medication

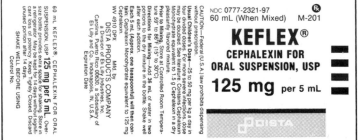

EXAMPLE:

a. What is the route of administration?   oral

b. What type of diluent can be used?   water

c. If 36 mL of diluent is added, what is the medication concentration?   125 mg per mL

d. The physician orders 75 mg po q 6 h. How many milliliters will you give for each dose?   3 mL

Dimensional Analysis

$$x \text{ mL} = \frac{5 \text{ mL}}{125 \text{ mg}} \times \frac{75 \text{ mg}}{1} = \frac{15}{5} = 3 \text{ mL}$$

Proportion Method

a. 125 mg : 5 mL ::

b. 125 mg : 5 mL :: _____ mg : _____ mL

c. 125 mg : 5 mL :: 75 mg : x mL

d. $125x = 375$

$$x = \frac{375}{125}$$

e. $x = 3$ mL

Reconstitution of Parenteral Medication

NDC 0049-0530-83
Buffered
Pfizerpen®
penicillin G potassium
For Injection
TWENTY MILLION UNITS **20**
FOR INTRAVENOUS INFUSION ONLY
CAUTION: Federal law prohibits dispensing without prescription.
ROeRIG *Pfizer*
A division of Pfizer Inc. N.Y., N.Y.10017

RECOMMENDED STORAGE IN DRY FORM
STORE BELOW 86°F (30°C)
Buffered with sodium citrate and citric acid to optimum pH.
AFTER RECONSTITUTION, SOLUTION SHOULD BE REFRIGERATED. DISCARD UNUSED SOLUTION AFTER 7 DAYS.
MADE IN U.S.A. 4

BULK PHARMACY PACKAGE
READ ACCOMPANYING PROFESSIONAL INFORMATION
USUAL DOSAGE
6 to 40 million units daily by intravenous infusion only
Approx. units per ml of solution

ml diluent added	units per ml
75 ml	250,000 u/ml
33 ml	500,000 u/ml
11.5 ml	1,000,000 u/ml

DATE/TIME PREPARED ____
BY ____

EXAMPLE:

a. What is the route of administration? — IV
b. What type of diluent can be used? — Check insert
c. How much diluent must be added? — 75 mL, 33 mL, or 11.3 mL
d. If 75 mL of diluent is added, what is the medication concentration? — 250,000 units/mL
e. How long will the medication maintain its potency after refrigeration? — 7 days
f. The physician orders 2,000,000 units IV q 4 h. How many milliliters will you give? Shade the syringe. — 8 mL

Dimensional Analysis

$$x \text{ mL} = \frac{1 \text{ mL}}{250,000 \text{ units}} \times \frac{2,000,000 \text{ units}}{1} = \frac{2,000,000}{250,000} = 8 \text{ mL}$$

Proportion Method

a. 250,000 units : 1 mL ::
b. 250,000 units : 1 mL :: ____ units : ____ mL
c. 250,000 units : 1 mL :: 2,000,000 units : x mL
d. $250,000x = 2,000,000$

$$x = \frac{2,000,000}{250,000}$$

$$x = 8$$

e. $x = 8$ mL

Formula

$$\frac{2,000,000}{250,000} \times 1 = 8 \text{ mL}$$

Once a medication has been reconstituted, you will solve the calculation dosage problems exactly as you have learned in previous chapters. The known strength, or what you have on hand, is just determined by the amount of diluent you added to the powdered medication.

Complete the following work sheet, which provides for extensive practice in the calculation of dosages measured in units. Check your answers. If you have difficulties, go back and review the necessary material. When you feel ready to evaluate your learning, take the first posttest. Check your answers. An acceptable score as indicated on the posttest signifies that you have successfully completed this chapter. An unacceptable score signifies a need for further study before taking the second posttest.

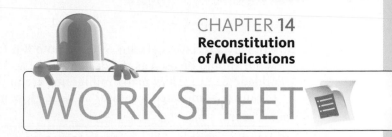

CHAPTER 14
Reconstitution of Medications

WORK SHEET

DIRECTIONS: Answer the questions. Calculate the doses. Show your work. Mark the medicine cup or syringe when provided to indicate the correct dose.

1. Your patient who has had a craniotomy has Ceclor suspension 250 mg po four times a day ordered. What should be used as the diluent? _____ How many milliliters of diluent should be added? _____ How many milligrams are in the bottle? _____ How many milliliters will you administer each dose? _____ How many doses are in the bottle? _____

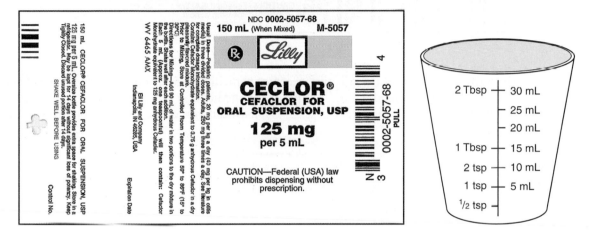

2. The physician has ordered Keflex 275 mg po q 6 h for Mr. Smith after his thyroidectomy. What should be used as the diluent? _____ How many milliliters of diluent should be added? _____ How many milligrams are in the bottle? _____ How many milliliters will the nurse administer per dose? _____ How many doses are in the bottle? _____

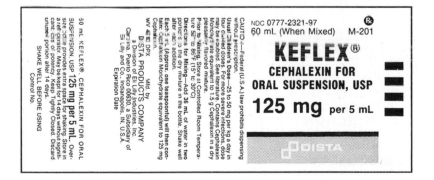

3. Mr. Davis receives cefaclor 600 mg po q 8 h for the treatment of acute bronchitis. What should be used as the diluent? _____ How many milliliters of diluent should be added? _____ How many milligrams are in the bottle? _____ How many milliliters will the nurse administer per dose? _____ How many doses are in the bottle? _____

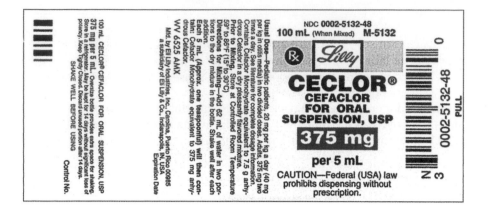

4. A patient with a temporal bone infection receives penicillin G 500,000 units IM q 6 h. How much diluent should be added? _____ What is the medication concentration? _____ How many milliliters will you administer? _____ What would you circle on the label to indicate concentration? _____

5. Your patient with a thoracotomy receives penicillin G 600,000 units IM twice a day. How much diluent should be added? _____ What is the medication concentration? _____ How many milliliters will you administer? _____ What is the best choice for the amount of dilution and why? _____

6. Mr. Rose has Pfizerpen 250,000 units IM now ordered. How many milliliters will the nurse administer if 8.2 mL of diluent is added? _____

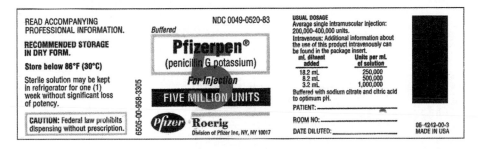

7. Mrs. Garden has penicillin G potassium 175,000 units IM now ordered. If 18.2 mL of diluent are added, how many milliliters will the nurse administer? _____

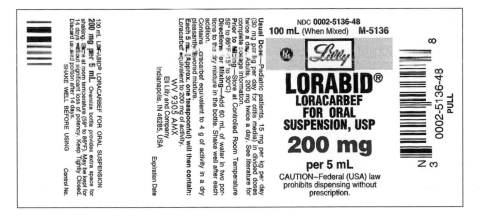

8. Lorabid 500 mg oral every 12 hours has been ordered for a patient with pneumonia. How much diluent will be added to the bottle? _____ What is the concentration after reconstitution? _____ How many milliliters will the nurse administer? _____

9. The physician orders oxacillin 250 mg IM every 6 hours for a patient with a skin infection. How much diluent will be added to the bottle? _____ What is the concentration after reconstitution? _____ How many milliliters will the nurse administer? _____

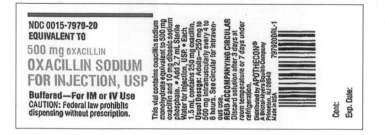

10. The physician orders Vancocin 500 mg oral every 12 hours for a patient with pseudomembranous colitis. How much diluent will be added to the bottle? _____ What is the concentration after reconstitution? _____ How many milliliters will the nurse administer? _____

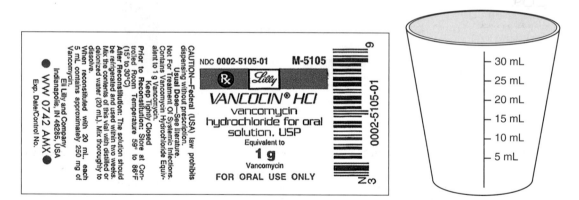

ANSWERS ON PP. 411–412 AND 414–416.

J MD 6/14

NAME _____

DATE _____

ACCEPTABLE SCORE ___**9**___

YOUR SCORE _____

DIRECTIONS: Answer the questions. Calculate the doses. Show your work. Mark the medicine cup or syringe when provided to indicate the correct dose.

1. Miss Kate has chronic sinusitis. Her physician orders amoxicillin 375 mg po q 8 h. What should be used as the diluent? *water* How many milliliters of diluent should be added? *105 mL* How many milligrams are in the bottle? *250* How many milliliters will you administer each dose? *7.5* How many doses are in the bottle? *20*

150/7.5 = 20

Amoxicillin for Oral Suspension, USP
250 mg per 5 mL
when reconstituted according to directions
Caution – Federal law prohibits dispensing without prescription.
150 mL bottle
N0047-2501-18 RECONSTITUTE w/105 mL WATER
WARNER CHILCOTT

SHAKE WELL BEFORE USING
Keep bottle tightly closed. Any unused portion must be discarded after 14 days. Refrigeration is preferable but not required. Be sure to take each dose prescribed by your physician. Keep this and all drugs out of the reach of children. This bottle will contain 150 mL when prepared for dispensing as directed. Extra space in the bottle allows for shaking.
2501G232

Dispensing Directions - Prepare suspension at time of dispensing. Shake bottle to loosen powder or break up the cake that may have formed. Add a total of **105 mL** water in 2 portions and shake well after each. This provides 150 mL of suspension. Each 5 mL contains amoxicillin trihydrate equivalent to 250 mg amoxicillin. **Usual Dosage – Patients weighing less than 20kg (44 lb):** 20mg / kg / day in divided doses every eight hours. **Patients weighing 20 kg or more:** 250 mg every eight hours. See package insert. Bottle contains amoxicillin trihydrate equivalent to 7.5 g amoxicillin. **Store below 30°C (86°F). Protect from moisture** Manufactured for: **WARNER CHILCOTT LABS** Div of Warner-Lambert Co · 1990 Morris Plains, NJ 07950 USA By: Clonmel Chemicals Co. Ltd Clonmel, Republic of Ireland 2501J031

$$\frac{375}{1} = \frac{5mL}{250} = \frac{1875}{250} = 7.5\ per\ dose$$

2. The physician has ordered Amoxil suspension 250 po mg q 6 h. What should be used as the diluent? *water* How many milliliters of diluent should be added? *78 mL* How many milligrams are in the bottle? *125* How many milliliters will the nurse administer per dose? *10* How many doses are in the bottle? *12.5*

$$\frac{250}{1} = \frac{5mL}{125} = \frac{1250}{125} =$$

10 per dose

AMOXIL® 125mg/5mL
125mg/5mL NDC 0029-6008-23
AMOXIL® AMOXICILLIN FOR ORAL SUSPENSION
100mL (when reconstituted)

Directions for mixing: Tap bottle until all powder flows freely. Add approximately 1/3 total amount of water for reconstitution (total=78 mL); shake vigorously to wet powder. Add remaining water; again shake vigorously. Each 5 mL (1 teaspoonful) will contain amoxicillin trihydrate equivalent to 125 mg amoxicillin. **Usual Adult Dosage:** 250 to 500 mg every 8 hours. **Usual Child Dosage:** 20 to 40 mg/kg/day in divided doses every 8 hours, depending on age, weight and infection severity. See accompanying prescribing information.
Keep tightly closed. Shake well before using. Refrigeration preferable but not required. Discard suspension after 14 days.

Net contents: Equivalent to 2.5 grams amoxicillin. Store dry powder at room temperature. SmithKline Beecham Pharmaceuticals Philadelphia, PA 19101
NSN 6505-01-153-3862
Rx only
3 0029-6008-23 1
LOT EXP.
SB SmithKline Beecham
9405793-F

3. Mrs. Hall has acute bronchitis and has cefaclor 450 mg po q 12 h ordered. What should be used as the diluent? _Water_ How many milliliters of diluent should be added? _62_ How many milligrams are in the bottle? _375_ How many milliliters will the nurse administer per dose? _6_ How many doses are in the bottle? _62.5_

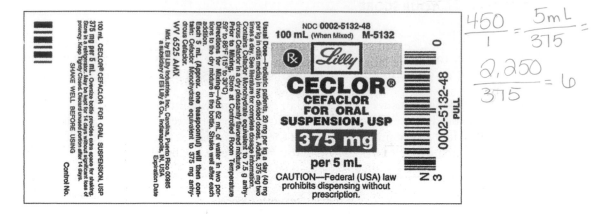

$$\frac{450}{1} = \frac{5\,mL}{375} =$$

$$\frac{2,250}{375} = 6$$

4. The physician orders penicillin G potassium 3,000,000 units IV q 6 h for your patient with an ethmoidectomy. What is the medication concentration if 11.5 mL of diluent is added? _1,000,000 u/mL_ How many milliliters will you administer? _3 mL_

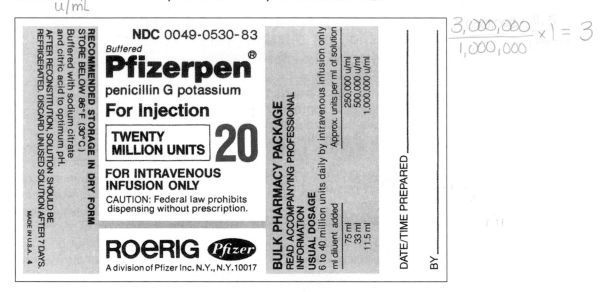

$$\frac{3,000,000}{1,000,000} \times 1 = 3$$

5. Mr. Cory has orders for Pfizerpen 600,000 units IM q 6 h for a serious pneumococcal infection. Select the most appropriate dilution. How many milliliters of diluent will you add? _6.8_ How many milliliters will you administer? _6.2 mL_

6. The physician orders Pfizerpen 1.2 million units IV in a single dose today. What is the medication concentration if 11.5 mL of diluent is added? 1,000,000 How many milliliters will the nurse administer? 1.2

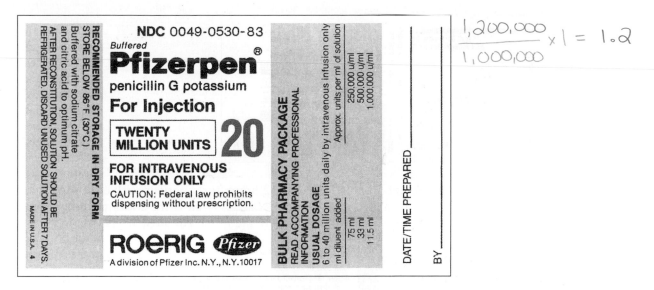

$$\frac{1,200,000}{1,000,000} \times 1 = 1.2$$

7. Mrs. Daisy receives nystatin oral suspension 600,000 units po four times a day. How many milliliters will the nurse administer? 6 mL

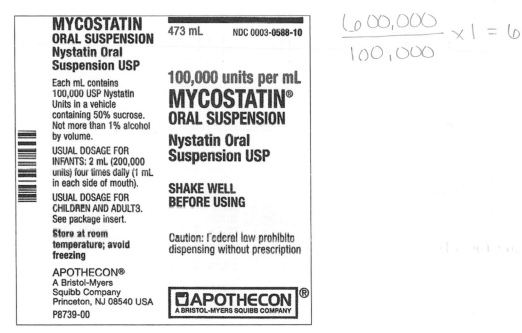

$$\frac{600,000}{100,000} \times 1 = 6$$

8. The physician orders ampicillin 500 mg IM every 6 hours for a patient with pneumonia. How much diluent will be added to the bottle? 3.5 What is the concentration after reconstitution? 250 How many milliliters will the nurse administer? 2mL

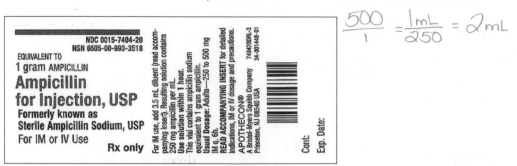

$$\frac{500}{1} = \frac{1\,mL}{250} = 2\,mL$$

9. The physician orders Ancef 500 mg IM every 12 hours for a patient with cellulitis. How much diluent will be added to the bottle? 2.5 What is the concentration after reconstitution? 330 mg How many milliliters will the nurse administer? 1.5mL

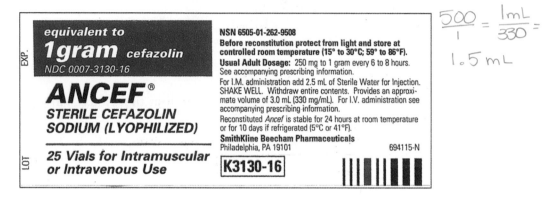

$$\frac{500}{1} = \frac{1\,mL}{330} = 1.5\,mL$$

10. Vancocin 1000 mg oral every 6 hours has been ordered for a patient with colitis. How much diluent will be added to the bottle? 20mL What is the concentration after reconstitution? 250 mg How many milliliters will the nurse administer? 20 ml

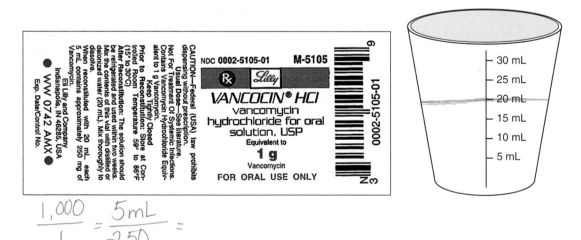

$$\frac{1,000}{1} = \frac{5\,mL}{250} =$$

ANSWERS ON PP. 412–413 AND 416–418.

NAME _____

DATE _____

ACCEPTABLE SCORE ___**9**___

YOUR SCORE _____

POSTTEST 2

DIRECTIONS: Answer the questions. Calculate the doses. Show your work. Mark the medicine cup or syringe when provided to indicate the correct dose.

1. The physician orders Keflin 400 mg IV q 6 h for your patient with an infection. Add 10 mL of 0.9% sodium chloride for diluent. How many milligrams are in the vial? _____ How many milliliters will you administer? _____ How many doses are in the vial? _____

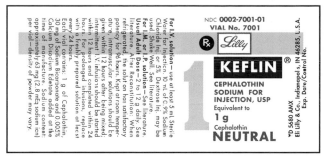

2. Your patient with an infection receives ampicillin 500 mg IV q 12 h. How many milliliters of diluent should be added? _____ How many milligrams are in the vial? _____ How many milliliters will you administer for each dose? _____ How many doses are in the vial? _____

3. The physician orders penicillin G potassium 1.2 million units IV q 4 h for your patient after dental extraction. You have a vial containing 1,000,000 units/mL. How many milliliters will you prepare? _____

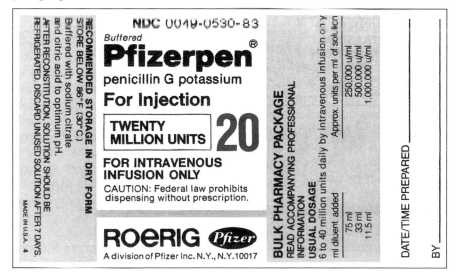

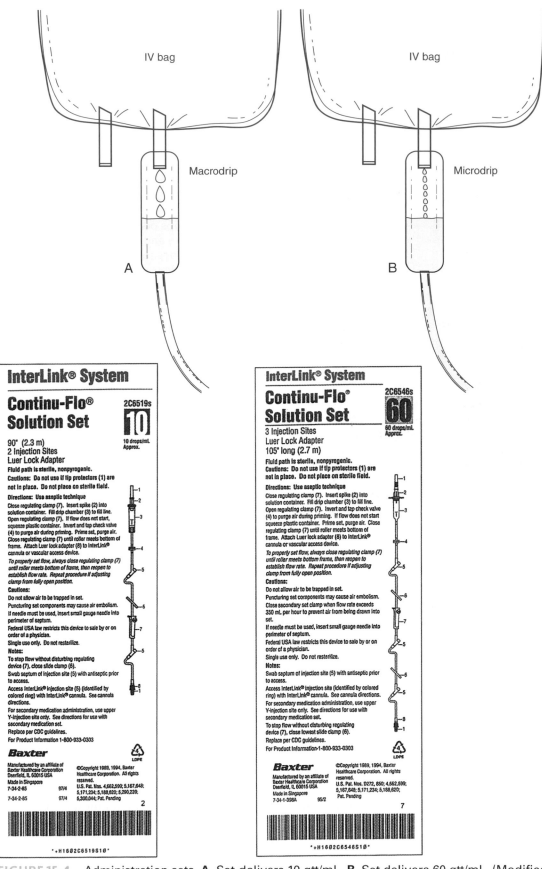

FIGURE 15-4 Administration sets. **A,** Set delivers 10 gtt/mL. **B,** Set delivers 60 gtt/mL. (Modified from Morris DG: *Calculate with confidence,* ed 5, St Louis, 2010, Mosby.)

Copyright © 2016 by Mosby, an imprint of Elsevier Inc.

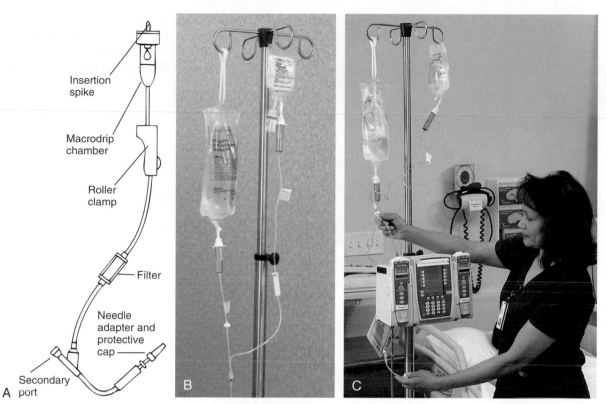

FIGURE 15-5   **A,** Infusion set. **B,** Gravity-flow IVPB. The IVPB is elevated above the existing IV solution, allowing it to infuse by gravity. **C,** IVPB infusion using an IV controller. (**A** from Clayton BD, Willihnganz M: *Basic pharmacology for nurses,* ed 16, St Louis, 2013, Mosby. **B** from Lilley LL, Collins SR, Snyder JS: *Pharmacology and nursing process,* ed 7, St Louis, 2014, Mosby. **C** from Perry AG, Potter PA, Ostendorf WR: *Clinical nursing skills and techniques,* ed 8, St Louis, 2014, Mosby.)

If the physician does not include an infusion time or rate, it is the nurse's responsibility to follow the manufacturer's guidelines. The hospital pharmacy and drug books such as the *Hospital Formulary* and *Intravenous Medications: A Handbook for Nurses and Health Professionals,* published by Mosby, are known resources for fluid rates. The nurse should always refer to recommended fluid limits and rates before IVPB administration.

It is usually the nurse's responsibility to regulate and maintain the infusion flow rate. It is the nurse's goal to ensure that the IV flow is regular. If the rate is irregular, too much or too little fluid may be infused. This may lead to complications such as fluid overload, dehydration, or medication overdose. Sometimes the flow rate must be adjusted because of interruptions caused by needle placement, condition of the vein, infiltration, or by a patient leaving the unit for a procedure.

The nurse must be able to determine the number of drops per minute (gtt/min) the patient must receive for the infusion to be completed within the specified time.

When the volume, time, or length of the infusion, and the constant drop factor are known, dimensional analysis or a simple formula can be used to calculate the desired drops per minute (gtt/min).

Calculating the Infusion of IV Fluids and Medications by Gravity: Dimensional Analysis Method

EXAMPLE 1: Hespan 500 mL is ordered to be infused over 3 hours. The drop factor is 15 gtt/mL. How many drops per minute should be given to infuse the total amount of Hespan over 3 hours?

a. On the left side of the equation, place what you are solving for:

$$\frac{x \text{ gtt}}{\text{min}} =$$

b. On the right side of the equation, place the available information related to the measurement or abbreviation that was placed on the left side. In this example the measurement we are solving for is *gtt/min*. We will deal with the numerator portion of our answer first, the *gtt*. This information is placed in the equation as a fraction, with the numerators matching.

$$\frac{x \text{ gtt}}{\text{min}} = \frac{15 \text{ gtt}}{1 \text{ mL}}$$

c. Next, find the information that matches the measurement used in the denominator of the fraction you created. In this example, *mL* is in the denominator, so Hespan 500 mL over 3 hours is used. Continue this process until all of the denominators except for *minute* can be canceled.

$$\frac{x \text{ gtt}}{\text{min}} = \frac{15 \text{ gtt}}{1 \text{ mL}} \times \frac{500 \text{ mL}}{3 \text{ h}} \times \frac{1 \text{ h}}{60 \text{ min}}$$

d. Then cancel out the abbreviations on the right side of the equation. If you have set up the problem correctly, the remaining measurements should match the measurements on the left side of the equation. Now solve for *x*.

$$\frac{x \text{ gtt}}{\text{min}} = \frac{15 \text{ gtt}}{1 \text{ mL}} \times \frac{500 \text{ mL}}{3 \text{ h}} \times \frac{1 \text{ h}}{60 \text{ min}}$$

$$\frac{x \text{ gtt}}{\text{min}} = \frac{15 \times 500}{3 \times 60}$$

$$x = 41.6 \text{ rounded to } 42 \text{ gtt/min}$$

Therefore the nurse will regulate the IV to drip at 42 drops/min, and the 500 mL of Hespan will be infused over 3 hours (Figure 15-3). Because the nurse cannot count a fraction of a drop, drops per minute are always rounded to the nearest whole number.

EXAMPLE 2: The physician orders cefuroxime 1 g in 50 mL of normal saline solution (NS) to be infused over 30 minutes. The tubing drop factor is 60 gtt/mL. How many drops per minute should be given to infuse the total amount of cefuroxime over 30 minutes?

a. On the left side of the equation, place what you are solving for:

$$\frac{x \text{ gtt}}{\text{min}} =$$

b. On the right side of the equation, place the available information related to the measurement or abbreviation that was placed on the left side. In this example the measurement we are solving for is *gtt/min*. We will deal with the numerator portion of our answer first, the *gtt*. This information is placed in the equation as a fraction, with the numerators matching.

$$\frac{x \text{ gtt}}{\text{min}} = \frac{60 \text{ gtt}}{1 \text{ mL}}$$

c. Next, find the information that matches the measurement used in the denominator of the fraction you created. In this example, *mL* is in the denominator, so cefuroxime 50 mL over 30 minutes is used.

$$\frac{x \text{ gtt}}{\text{min}} = \frac{60 \text{ gtt}}{1 \text{ mL}} \times \frac{50 \text{ mL}}{30 \text{ min}}$$

d. Then cancel out the abbreviations on the right side of the equation. If you have set up the problem correctly, the remaining measurements should match the measurements on the left side of the equation. Now solve for x.

$$\frac{x \text{ gtt}}{\text{min}} = \frac{60 \text{ gtt}}{1 \text{ mL}} \times \frac{50 \text{ mL}}{30 \text{ min}}$$

$$\frac{x \text{ gtt}}{\text{min}} = \frac{60 \times 50}{30}$$

$$x = 100 \text{ gtt/min}$$

Therefore the nurse will regulate the IV to drip at 100 drops/min, and the 50 mL of cefuroxime will be infused over 30 minutes.

Calculating the Infusion of IV Fluids and Medications by Gravity: Formula Method

EXAMPLE 1: Hespan 500 mL is ordered to be infused over 3 hours. The drop factor is 15 gtt/mL. How many drops per minute should be given to infuse the total amount of Hespan over 3 hours?

$$\text{The formula: } \frac{\text{Total volume to be infused}}{\text{Total amount of time in minutes}} \times \text{Drop factor} = x \text{ gtt/min}$$

a. Convert total hours to minutes.

1 h : 60 min :: 3 h : x min

$x = 180$

Therefore 3 hours equals 180 minutes.

b. Calculate gtt/min.

This calculation depends on the drop factor of the tubing being used. Remember, this information is found on the package. For the problems in this work text, the drop factor is indicated. The drop factor for this problem is 15.

$$\text{(Formula setup)} \quad \frac{500 \text{ mL}}{180 \text{ min}} \times \frac{15 \text{ gtt/mL}}{} = x \text{ gtt/min}$$

$$\text{(Cancel)} \quad \frac{500 \text{ mL}}{\underset{12}{\cancel{180} \text{ min}}} \times \frac{\overset{1}{\cancel{15}} \text{ gtt/ mL}}{} = x \text{ gtt/min}$$

$$\text{(Calculate)} \quad \frac{500}{12 \text{ min}} \times \frac{1 \text{ gtt}}{} = \frac{500}{12} = 41.6 \text{ rounded to } 42 \text{ gtt/min}$$

Therefore the nurse will regulate the IV to drip at 42 drops/min, and the 500 mL of Hespan will be infused over 3 hours (see Figure 15-3). Because the nurse cannot count a fraction of a drop, drops per minute are always rounded to a whole number.

> **! ● ALERT**
>
> When administering an IV fluid or medication by gravity, the nurse solves for gtt/min.

EXAMPLE 2: The physician orders cefuroxime 1 g in 50 mL of normal saline solution (NS) to be infused over 30 minutes. The tubing drop factor is 60 gtt/mL. How many drops per minute should be given to infuse the total amount of cefuroxime over 30 minutes?

$$\text{The formula: } \frac{\text{Total volume to be infused}}{\text{Total amount of time in minutes}} \times \text{Drop factor} = x \text{ gtt/min}$$

Calculate gtt/min.

$$\text{(Formula setup)} \quad \frac{50 \text{ mL}}{30 \text{ min}} \times \frac{60 \text{ gtt/mL}}{} = x \text{ gtt/min}$$

$$\text{(Cancel)} \quad \frac{50 \text{ mL}}{\cancel{30} \text{ min}} \times \frac{\overset{2}{\cancel{60}} \text{ gtt/mL}}{} = x \text{ gtt/min}$$

$$\text{(Calculate)} \quad \frac{50}{1} \times 2 = 100 \text{ gtt/min}$$

Therefore the nurse will regulate the IVPB to drip at 100 gtt/min, and the cefuroxime will be infused over 30 minutes.

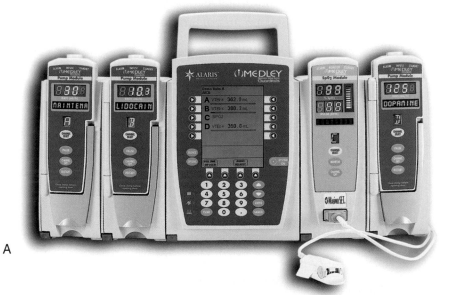

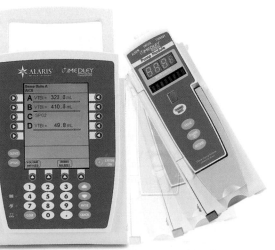

FIGURE 15-6   A, Medley™ Medication Safety System. **B,** Example of the Medley™ pump module attached to the Medley programming module. (From ALARIS Medical Systems, Inc., San Diego, CA.)

INFUSION OF IV FLUIDS AND MEDICATIONS BY AN IV PUMP

IV flow rates are often controlled by an electronic device or pump. The IV pumps are programmed to deliver a set amount of fluid per hour. Safety for the patient is an advantage of electronic IV pumps. The pumps are used for patients in regular medical-surgical units, critical care areas, pediatrics, the operating room, and ambulatory care settings.

Many electronic pumps are on the market today. These vary from simple one-channel models to four multichannel pumps. Many of the newer models actually calculate flow rates and automatically start infusions at a later time. Convenience, safety, accuracy, and time-saving options are driving forces in the innovations currently available.

Some examples of equipment are pictured in Figures 15-6 and 15-7; in Figure 15-6 the Medley Medication Safety System and the Medley pump module (attached to the programming module) are shown. In Figure 15-7 the Medley Medication Safety System is being used on a patient in a critical care setting. Each company offers tubing for use with its pumps.

Newer IV pumps, as pictured in Figure 15-6, contain software that allows each facility to program safeguard information for medications into the IV pump. If a health care professional programs a rate, dose, or duration that is considered to be unsafe, a visual or audible alert will occur. The safeguards are determined by the facility to prevent IV medication errors. In some situations the health care professional will be required to infuse medications using an IV pump. Whether the medication is an electrolyte replacement, an antiinfective agent, or another type of medication to be infused by IVPB, the health care professional needs to calculate the rate, in milliliters per hour, for which the IV pump should be programmed.

! ALERT

When administering a medication or IV fluid by an IV pump, the nurse solves for mL/h.

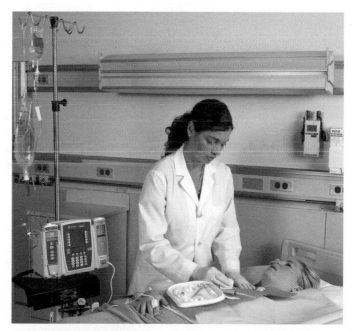

FIGURE 15-7   Medley™ Medication Safety System being used on a patient in a critical care setting. (From ALARIS Medical Systems, Inc., San Diego, CA.)

Calculating the Infusion of IV Fluids and Medications by a Pump: Dimensional Analysis Method

EXAMPLE 1: Infuse 1000 mL of lactated Ringer's solution (LR) over 12 hours. How many mL/h should the IV pump be programmed for?

a. On the left side of the equation, place what you are solving for:

$$\frac{x \text{ mL}}{h} =$$

b. On the right side of the equation, place the available information related to the measurement or abbreviation that was placed on the left side. In this example the measurement we are solving for is *mL/h*. We will deal with the numerator portion of our answer first, the *mL*. This information is placed in the equation as a fraction, with the numerators matching.

$$\frac{x \text{ mL}}{h} = \frac{1000 \text{ mL}}{12 \text{ h}}$$

c. Now solve for *x*.

$$\frac{x \text{ mL}}{h} = \frac{1000 \text{ mL}}{12 \text{ h}}$$

$$\frac{x \text{ mL}}{h} = \frac{1000}{12}$$

$$x = 83.3 \text{ or } 83 \text{ mL/h}$$

Therefore the nurse will program the IV pump for 83 mL/h and the 1000 mL of LR will be infused over 12 hours.

EXAMPLE 2: The physician orders Kefzol 1 g dissolved in 50 mL of D5W to be infused over 30 minutes. The IVPB may be given using an IV pump. How many milliliters per hour should the IV pump be programmed for to infuse the Kefzol over 30 minutes?

a. On the left side of the equation, place what you are solving for:

$$\frac{x \text{ mL}}{h} =$$

b. On the right side of the equation, place the available information related to the measurement or abbreviation that was placed on the left side of the equation. In this example, the measurement we are solving for is *mL/h*. We will deal with the numerator portion of our answer first, the *mL*. This information is placed in the equation as a fraction, with the numerators matching.

$$\frac{x \text{ mL}}{h} = \frac{50 \text{ mL}}{30 \text{ min}}$$

c. Next, find the information that matches the measurement used in the denominator of the fraction you created. In this example, *min* is in the denominator, so 60 minutes over 1 hour is used.

$$\frac{x \text{ mL}}{h} = \frac{50 \text{ mL}}{30 \text{ min}} \times \frac{60 \text{ min}}{1 \text{ h}}$$

d. Then cancel out the abbreviations on the right side of the equation. If you have set up the problem correctly, the remaining measurements should match the measurements on the left side of the equation. Now solve for x.

$$\frac{x \text{ mL}}{h} = \frac{50 \text{ mL}}{30 \text{ min}} \times \frac{60 \text{ min}}{1 \text{ h}}$$

$$\frac{x \text{ mL}}{h} = \frac{50 \times 60}{30}$$

$$x = 100 \text{ mL/h}$$

Therefore the nurse will program the IV pump for 100 mL/h, and the Kefzol will be infused over 30 minutes.

EXAMPLE 3: Dilute potassium 40 mEq in 250 mL of D5W and administer IV now. The facility's policy states to infuse potassium at a rate of 10 mEq/h. How many milliliters per hour should the IV pump be programmed for to infuse the potassium at a rate of 10 mEq/h?

a. On the left side of the equation, place what you are solving for:

$$\frac{x \text{ mL}}{h} =$$

b. On the right side of the equation, place the available information related to the measurement or abbreviation that was placed on the left side of the equation. In this example, the measurement we are solving for is mL/h. We will deal with the numerator portion of our answer first, the mL. This information is placed in the equation as a fraction, with the numerators matching.

$$\frac{x \text{ mL}}{h} = \frac{250 \text{ mL}}{40 \text{ mEq}}$$

c. Next, find the information that matches the measurement used in the denominator of the fraction you created. In this example, mEq is in the denominator, so the policy of 10 mEq/h is used.

$$\frac{x \text{ mL}}{h} = \frac{250 \text{ mL}}{40 \text{ mEq}} \times \frac{10 \text{ mEq}}{1 \text{ h}}$$

d. Then cancel out the abbreviations on the right side of the equation. If you have set up the problem correctly, the remaining measurements should match the measurements on the left side of the equation. Now solve for x.

$$\frac{x \text{ mL}}{h} = \frac{250 \text{ mL}}{40 \text{ mEq}} \times \frac{10 \text{ mEq}}{1 \text{ h}}$$

$$\frac{x \text{ mL}}{h} = \frac{250 \times 10}{40}$$

$$x = 62.5 \text{ or } 63 \text{ mL/h}$$

Therefore the nurse will program the IV pump for 63 mL/h, and the 40 mEq of potassium will infuse per the hospital policy.

Calculating the Infusion of IV Fluids and Medications by a Pump: Formula Method

In many facilities IV fluids are infused using an IV pump. IV pumps are programmed to infuse IV fluids by milliliters per hour (mL/h).

$$\text{The formula:} \quad \frac{\text{Total volume in milliliters}}{\text{Total time in hours}} = x \text{ mL/h}$$

EXAMPLE 1: Infuse 1000 mL of lactated Ringer's solution (LR) over 12 hours. How many mL/h should the IV pump be programmed for?

Calculate mL/h.

$$\text{(Formula setup)} \quad \frac{1000 \text{ mL}}{12 \text{ h}} = 83.3 \text{ or } 83 \text{ mL/h}$$

Therefore the nurse will program the IV pump for 83 mL/h, and the 1000 mL of LR will be infused over 12 hours.

EXAMPLE 2: The physician orders Kefzol 1 g dissolved in 50 mL of D_5W to be infused over 30 minutes. The IVPB may be given using an IV pump. How many milliliters per hour should the IV pump be programmed for to infuse the Kefzol over 30 minutes?

a. Convert minutes to hours.

1 h : 60 min :: x h : 30 min

$60x = 30$

$$x = \frac{30}{60} = 0.5 \text{ h}$$

b. Calculate mL/h.

$$\text{(Formula setup)} \quad \frac{50 \text{ mL}}{0.5 \text{ h}} = 100 \text{ mL/h}$$

EXAMPLE 3: Dilute potassium 40 mEq in 250 mL of D_5W and administer IV now. The facility's policy states to infuse potassium at a rate of 10 mEq/h. How many milliliters per hour should the IV pump be programmed for to infuse the potassium at a rate of 10 mEq/h?

Using the ratio-proportion method:

Calculate mL/h.

(Formula setup)   40 mEq : 250 mL :: 10 mEq : x mL

(Calculate) $40x = 2500$

$$x = \frac{2500}{40}$$

$x = 62.5$ or 63 mL

Therefore the nurse will program the IV pump for 63 mL/h, and the potassium will be infused at 10 mEq/h as stated in the facility's policy. (NOTE: Follow your facility's policy when you calculate the rate for any electrolyte replacement.)

Using the $\dfrac{D}{A} \times Q = x$ mL/h method:

Calculate mL/h.

(Formula setup) $\quad \dfrac{10 \text{ mEq}}{40 \text{ mEq}} \times 250 \text{ mL} = x \text{ mL}$

(Cancel) $\quad \dfrac{\overset{1}{\cancel{10}} \ \cancel{\text{mEq}}}{\underset{4}{\cancel{40}} \ \cancel{\text{mEq}}} \times 250 \text{ mL} = x \text{ mL}$

(Calculate) $\quad \dfrac{1}{4} \times 250 \text{ mL} = \dfrac{250}{4} = 62.5 \text{ or } 63 \text{ mL/h}$

SALINE AND HEPARIN LOCKS

Saline and heparin locks are commonly used in a variety of health care settings. A saline lock is an IV catheter that is inserted into a peripheral vein. It may be used for medications or fluids, usually on an intermittent basis. The use of a saline lock prevents the patient from having to endure numerous venipunctures. Also, when fluid is not being infused, the patient enjoys greater freedom of movement. Each institution will have its own policy concerning the use and care of saline locks. The locks may be flushed with 2 to 3 mL of normal saline solution (Figures 15-8 and 15-9). Central line ports that are not being used for fluid or medication administration are heparin locks. The locks will be flushed with a heparin flush solution of 10 units of heparin per 1 mL. This practice is called *heparinization,* and it prevents clotting of the heparin lock. Because of concerns regarding heparin overdose errors and heparin-induced thrombocytopenia (HIT), the routine use of heparin flushes is decreasing.

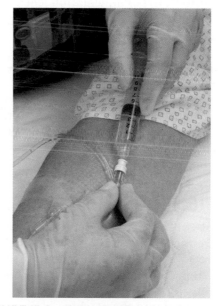

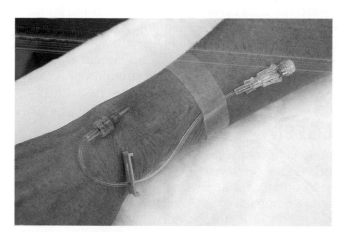

FIGURE 15-8   Example of a saline lock. (From Perry AG, Potter PA, Ostendorf WR: *Clinical nursing skills and techniques,* ed 8, St Louis, 2014, Mosby.)

FIGURE 15-9   Example of a needleless system used within an intravenous line. (From Perry AG, Potter PA, Ostendorf WR: *Clinical nursing skills and techniques,* ed 8, St Louis, 2014, Mosby.)

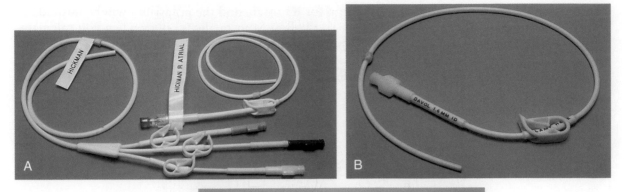

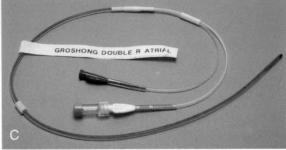

FIGURE 15-10   **A,** Hickman catheter. **B,** Broviac catheter. **C,** Groshong catheter. (From Clayton BD, Willihnganz M: *Basic pharmacology for nurses,* ed 16, St Louis, 2013, Mosby.)

CENTRAL VENOUS CATHETERS

Occasionally, a patient will need a central venous catheter. Central venous catheters are indwelling, semipermanent central lines that are inserted into the right atrium of the heart via the cephalic, subclavian, or jugular vein (Figure 15-10).

This type of catheter may be required for clients who need frequent venipuncture, long-term IV infusions, hyperalimentation, chemotherapy, intermittent blood transfusions, or antibiotics. These catheters may be referred to as *triple-lumen catheters, Hickman lines, or peripherally inserted central catheters (PICCs).*

Central venous catheter management involves flushing the catheter with 5 to 10 mL of normal saline when the catheter access is routinely capped or clamped after blood draws. Please consult your institution's procedure or policy guidelines about central venous line flushes. If continuous fluids are ordered, these fluids **must** be regulated via an infusion pump. All central venous catheter management must be done under the supervision of a registered nurse.

The central venous catheter site must be assessed regularly. The catheter site should always remain sterile under an occlusive dressing that is changed according to the institution's procedure regarding central venous catheters.

PATIENT-CONTROLLED ANALGESIA

Patient-controlled analgesia (PCA) or a PCA pump involves patients giving themselves an IV narcotic by pressing a button. This IV narcotic is given at intervals via an infusion pump (Figure 15-11). Only a registered nurse can be accountable for dispensing analgesia to be given in this manner. In addition, only a registered nurse can administer a PCA loading dose. For safety, most institutions now require that two registered nurses verify the PCA drug, dosage, and rate programmed into the machine.

Several considerations are crucial in the administration of PCA. IV narcotics may cause depressed respirations, hypotension, sedation, dizziness, and nausea or vomiting in the patient.

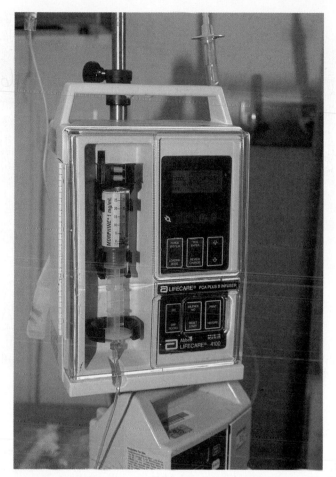

FIGURE 15-11   Patient-controlled analgesia infusion pump. (Elkin MK, Perry PA, Potter AG: *Nursing interventions and clinical skills,* ed 5, St Louis, 2012, Mosby.)

The patient must be able to understand and comply with instructions and must have a desire to use the PCA because *only* the patient can press the button to dispense the dose. The materials needed for infusion include a PCA pump, PCA tubing, a PCA pump key, a narcotic injector vial, and maintenance IV fluids through which the IV narcotic will be infused.

> **EXAMPLE 1:** The physician orders morphine sulfate 1 mg every 10 minutes to a maximum of 30 mg in 4 hours. Morphine concentration is 1 mg/mL per 30-mL injector vial. What is the pump setting?
>
> 1 mg/10 min; 4-hour limit is 30 mg

> **EXAMPLE 2:** The physician orders hydromorphone 0.2 mg every 15 minutes to a maximum of 2 mg in 4 hours. Hydromorphone concentration is 1 mg/mL per 30-mL injector vial. What is the pump setting?
>
> 0.2 mg/15 min; 4-hour limit is 2 mg

Complete the following work sheet, which provides for practice in the calculation of IV solutions and IVPB by either the IV pump or gravity. Check your answers. If you have difficulties, go back and review the necessary material. When you feel ready to evaluate your learning, take the first posttest. Check your answers. An acceptable score as indicated on the posttest signifies that you have successfully completed the chapter. An unacceptable score signifies a need for further study before taking the second posttest.

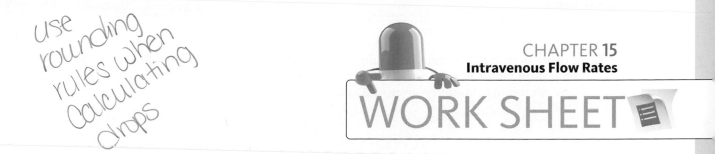

use rounding rules when calculating drops

WORK SHEET

DIRECTIONS: The IV fluid or medication order is listed in each problem. Calculate the IV flow rates using the appropriate formula. Show your work. Follow your instructor's rules on rounding final answers.

1. The physician orders 500 mL of dextran to be infused over 24 hours. How many milliliters per hour should the IV pump be programmed for? 21.8 mL

$$\frac{X\,mL}{h} = \frac{500\,mL}{24\,h} = 20.8\,mL$$

2. A patient with genital herpes has an order for acyclovir 400 mg IVPB q 8 h. The acyclovir is dissolved in 100 mL 0.9% NS and is to be infused over 1 hour. How many milliliters per hour should the IV pump be programmed for? 100 mL

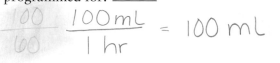

$$\frac{100}{60} \quad \frac{100\,mL}{1\,hr} = 100\,mL$$

3. Amikacin 80 mg is ordered IVPB q 12 h. The amikacin is dissolved in 100 mL D_5W and is to be infused over 30 minutes. With a tubing drop factor of 15 gtt/mL, how many drops per minute should be given? 50

$$\frac{X\,gtt}{min} = \frac{15\,gtt}{1\,mL} \times \frac{100\,mL}{30\,min} \times \frac{15\,gtt/mL}{60\,min} = 50\,drops \quad \frac{1,500}{1,800} \quad \frac{1500}{1800}$$

4. The physician orders 3000 mL of total parenteral nutrition (TPN) to be infused from 1900 to 0700. How many milliliters per hour should the IV pump be programmed for? 250 mL

$$\frac{X\,mL}{h} = \frac{3,000\,mL}{12\,hr} = 250\,mL$$

5. Mr. McCane, who has peptic ulcer disease, has Pepcid 20 mg in 100 mL D_5W ordered q 12 h. The Pepcid is to be infused over 30 minutes. With a tubing drop factor of 10 gtt/mL, how many drops per minute should be given? 33.3

$$\frac{100\,mL}{30\,min} \times 10\,gtt/mL = 33.3\,drops$$

6. A malnourished patient has an order for 500 mL of Intralipid 10% to be infused over 6 hours. How many milliliters per hour should the IV pump be programmed for? 83.3 mL

$$\frac{X\,mL}{h} = \frac{500\,mL}{6\,h} = 83.3\,mL$$

7. An order is received to infuse penicillin G 4,000,000 units in 100 mL of D_5W q 12 h. The tubing drop factor is 10 gtt/mL. The penicillin should be infused over 60 minutes. How many drops per minute should be given? 16.76

$$\frac{100mL}{60\ min} \times 10\ gtt/mL = 16\ drops$$

8. Mrs. Ruiz has hypokalemia. The physician orders potassium 60 mEq in 250 mL of D_5W. The facility's policy states to infuse the potassium at 20 mEq/h. How many milliliters per hour should the IV pump be programmed for? 83.3mL

$$\frac{250\ mL}{60\ min} \times 20 = 83.mL$$

9. A postoperative patient has Kefzol 1 g ordered q 8 h. The Kefzol is dissolved in 50 mL of D_5W and is to be infused over 30 minutes. The tubing drop factor is 60 gtt/mL. How many drops per minute should be given? 100

$$\frac{50mL}{30\ min} \times 60\ gtt/mL = 100\ drops$$

10. A postoperative patient has an order for 1000 mL of LR over 10 hours. How many milliliters per hour should the IV pump be programmed for? 100 mL

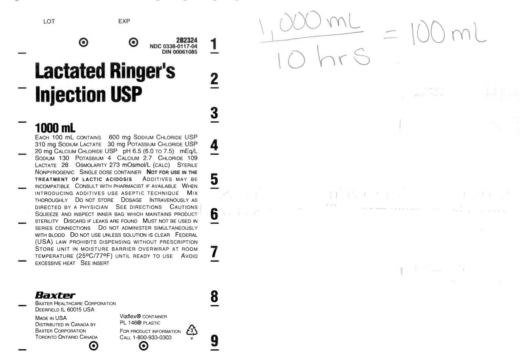

$$\frac{1,000\ mL}{10\ hrs} = 100\ mL$$

11. Mrs. England has sepsis and has an order for Kefzol 1 g in 50 mL of D_5W IVPB over 15 minutes. The drop factor is 60 gtt/mL. How many drops per minute should be given? 200

$$\frac{50\ mL}{15\ min} \times 60\ gtt/mL = 200\ drops$$

12. A patient with a methicillin-resistant *Staphylococcus aureus* infection has Cipro 400 mg in 200 mL D$_5$W ordered. The pharmacy recommends that the Cipro be infused at a rate of 200 mg/h with an IV pump. How many milliliters per hour should the IV pump be programmed for? _____

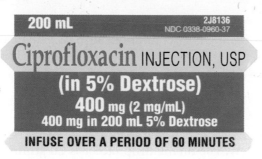

200 mL   2J8136
                NDC 0338-0960-37

Ciprofloxacin INJECTION, USP
(in 5% Dextrose)
400 mg (2 mg/mL)
400 mg in 200 mL 5% Dextrose
INFUSE OVER A PERIOD OF 60 MINUTES

13. A patient with anuria has an order for 1000 mL of 0.9% NS to be infused over 1 hour. The tubing drop factor is 10 gtt/mL. How many drops per minute should be given? _167_

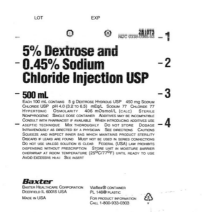

$$\frac{1,000\ mL}{60\ min} \times 10 = 167$$

0.9% Sodium
Chloride
Injection USP

1000 mL
Each 100 mL contains   900 mg Sodium Chloride USP
pH 5.0 (4.5 to 7.0) mEq/L Sodium 154 Chloride 154
Osmolarity   308 mOsmol/L (calc)   Sterile
Nonpyrogenic Single dose container Additives may be
incompatible Consult with pharmacist if available When
introducing additives use aseptic technique   Mix
thoroughly Do not store   Dispense Intravenously as
directed by a physician   See directions   Cautions
Squeeze and inspect inner bag which maintains product
sterility Discard if leaks are found   Must not be used
in series connections   Do not use unless solution is
clear   Federal (USA) law prohibits dispensing without
prescription Store unit in moisture barrier overwrap at
room temperature (25ºC/77ºF) until ready to use Avoid
excessive heat See insert

Baxter
Baxter Healthcare Corporation
Deerfield IL 60015 USA
Made in USA   Viaflex® container
Distributed in Canada by   PL 146® plastic
Baxter Corporation   For product information
Toronto Ontario Canada   Call 1-800-933-0303

NDC 0338-0049-04
DIN 00060208   2B1324

14. After his operation Mr. Chambers has an order for 500 mL of D$_5$W 0.45 NS to be infused over 4 hours. How many milliliters per hour should the IV pump be programmed for? _____

5% Dextrose and
0.45% Sodium
Chloride Injection USP

500 mL
Each 100 mL contains   5 g Dextrose Hydrous USP   450 mg Sodium
Chloride USP pH 4.0 (3.2 to 6.5) mEq/L Sodium 77 Chloride 77
Hypertonic Osmolarity   406 mOsmol/L (calc)   Sterile
Nonpyrogenic Single dose container Additives may be incompatible
Consult with pharmacist if available When introducing additives use
aseptic technique   Mix thoroughly   Do not store   Dosage
Intravenously as directed by a physician   See directions   Cautions
Squeeze and inspect inner bag which maintains product sterility
Discard if leaks are found   Must not be used in series connections
Do not use unless solution is clear   Federal (USA) law prohibits
dispensing without prescription   Store unit in moisture barrier
overwrap at room temperature (25ºC/77ºF) until ready to use
Avoid excessive heat See insert

Baxter
Baxter Healthcare Corporation   Viaflex® container
Deerfield IL 60015 USA   PL 146® plastic
Made in USA   For product information
                                Call 1-800-933-0303

NDC 0338-

15. After a total hip replacement, a patient has an order for Toradol 60 mg IVPB q 6 h over 15 minutes. The Toradol is diluted in 25 mL of D$_5$W. The tubing drop factor is 15 gtt/mL. How many drops per minute should be given? __25__

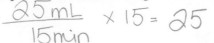

$$\frac{25\,mL}{15\,min} \times 15 = 25$$

16. A terminal patient has an order for Dilaudid at 0.5 mg/h by continuous drip. Given a bag with a concentration of 20 mg Dilaudid in 100 mL of D$_5$W, how many milliliters per hour should the IV pump be programmed for? __100 mL__

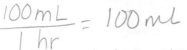

$$\frac{100\,mL}{1\,hr} = 100\,mL$$

17. A patient with peptic ulcer disease has an order for Pepcid 20 mg IVPB q 12 h over 15 minutes. The Pepcid is diluted in 25 mL of D$_5$W. The tubing drop factor is 20 gtt/mL. How many drops per minute should be given? _____

18. Mr. Russell, who has alcoholism, has an order for magnesium sulfate 2 g in 100 mL of D$_5$W. The pharmacy recommends that the magnesium be infused at a rate of 1 g/h with an IV pump. How many milliliters per hour should the IV pump be programmed for? _____

19. A patient with aplastic anemia has an order for 1 unit of packed red blood cells (250 mL) to be infused. The facility's policy states to infuse the blood over 4 hours. The tubing drop factor is 20 gtt/mL. How many drops per minute should be given? _____

20. Ms. Tung has an order for Ofirmev 1000 mg in 100 mL of normal saline over 15 minutes for pain. How many milliliters per hour should be given? _____

21. A patient with hypokalemia has an order for 40 mEq of potassium to be infused intravenously now. The potassium is diluted in 200 mL of D$_5$W. The facility's policy states to infuse IV potassium at a rate of 10 mEq/h. How many milliliters per hour should the IV pump be programmed for? __50 mL__

$$\frac{10\,mL}{40\,min} \times 200 = 50\,mL$$

22. A patient with Crohn's disease has an order for TPN from 2200 to 0800. The total volume of the TPN bag is 1350 mL. How many milliliters per hour should the IV pump be programmed for? _____

23. Mr. Goldberg, who has hypomagnesemia, receives an order for magnesium sulfate 2 g in 50 mL D$_5$W IV. The pharmacist recommends that the magnesium be infused at 1 g/h. How many milliliters per hour should the IV pump be programmed for? _____

24. An immunosuppressed patient with herpes simplex virus 1 has acyclovir 700 mg in 200 mL of D$_5$W ordered to infuse over 1 hour. How many milliliters per hour should the IV pump be programmed for? _____

25. A patient with anasarca has albumin 25% 100 mL ordered over 30 minutes. The tubing drop factor is 20 gtt/mL. How many drops per minute should be given? _____

NDC 0053-7680-33   25%

Albuminar®-25
Albumin (Human)
USP 25%

100 mL

For Intravenous
Administration Only.

26. After the patient in question 25 receives her albumin, the physician orders Lasix 100 mg in 50 mL of D$_5$W to be given over 30 minutes. How many milliliters per hour should the IV pump be set for? _____

27. A patient with multiple antibiotic allergies has a urinary tract infection. Amikacin 250 mg IVPB q 8 h is ordered over 1 hour. The amikacin is dissolved in 200 mL of D$_5$W. The drop factor is 20 gtt/mL. How many drops per minute should be given? _____

28. After an operation Mrs. Avery is hemorrhaging and has Amicar 8 g over 8 hours ordered. The Amicar is diluted in 500 mL of 0.9% NS. How many milliliters per hour should the IV pump be set for? _____

29. A patient with rapid atrial flutter has an order for Cardizem at 5 mg/h. The Cardizem concentration is 200 mg in 250 mL of 0.9% NS. How many milliliters per hour should the IV pump be set for? _____

30. A malnourished patient has folic acid 1 mg in 50 mL of 0.9% NS ordered to infuse over 30 minutes. An IV pump is not available. The nurse chooses a tubing with a 60 gtt/mL drop factor. How many drops per minute should be given? _____

31. Vancomycin 1250 mg in 250 mL of D$_5$W is ordered to infuse over 2 hours. How many milliliters per hour should the IV pump be set for? _____

32. A patient has a blood urea nitrogen level of 52 with oliguria and a blood pressure of 90/50 mm Hg. The physician orders 1000 mL of 0.9% NS to be infused over 10 hours. How many milliliters per hour should the IV pump infuse? _____

33. Using the Parkland formula, the fluid requirements for a patient with severe burns reveal that 9600 mL should be infused over 8 hours. How many milliliters per hour should the IV pump be set for? _____

34. Mr. Cortez has IV immunoglobulin G (IgG) 100 mL ordered over 3 hours. How many milliliters per hour should the IV pump be set for? _____

35. A patient with rapid atrial fibrillation has an order for diltiazem at 20 mg/h. The diltiazem concentration is 100 mg in 100 mL of 0.9% NS. How many milliliters per hour should the IV pump be set for? _____

36. A STAT dose of Zosyn 3.375 mg in 100 mL of 0.9% NS is ordered to be given over 15 minutes. How many milliliters per hour should the nurse program the IV pump for? _____

37. A patient with a vancomycin-resistant enterococci (VRE) has Zyvox 600 mg intravenously ordered over 2 hours every 12 hours. How many milliliters per hour should the nurse program the IV pump for? _____

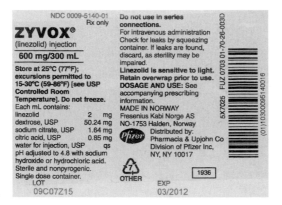

ANSWERS ON PP. 451 AND 453–455.

NAME _____

DATE _____

ACCEPTABLE SCORE __14__

YOUR SCORE _____

POSTTEST 1

DIRECTIONS: The IV fluid order is listed in the problem. Calculate the appropriate infusion rate for each problem. Show your work. Follow your instructor's rules on rounding final answers.

1. A patient with hypotension has an order for 500 mL of Plasmanate to be infused over 2 hours. How many milliliters per hour should the IV pump be programmed for? _____

2. An order is received to infuse amphotericin B 240 mg in 500 mL D_5W over 4 hours. How many milliliters per hour should the IV pump be programmed for? _____

3. An NPO patient has an order for 0.9% NS at 120 mL/h. The drop factor is 12 gtt/mL. How many drops per minute should be given? __24__

$$\frac{120}{60} \times 12 = 24 \text{ gtts}$$

LOT   EXP

⊙   ⊙   2B1324
NDC 0338-0049-04   **1**
DIN 00060208

0.9% Sodium   **2**
Chloride
Injection USP   **3**

                                        4

1000 mL
Each 100 ml contains 900 mg Sodium Chloride USP
pH 5.0 (4.5 to 7.0)   mEq/L Sodium 154 Chloride 154   **5**
Osmolarity   308 mOsmol/L (calc)   Sterile
Nonpyrogenic Single dose container Additives may be
incompatible Consult with pharmacist if available When
introducing additives use aseptic technique   Mix
thoroughly Do not store Dosage Intravenously as   **6**
directed by a physician   See directions   Cautions
Squeeze and inspect inner bag which maintains product
sterility   Discard if leaks are found Must not be used
in series connections Do not use unless solution is
clear   Federal (USA) law prohibits dispensing without   **7**
prescription Store unit in moisture barrier overwrap at
room temperature (25°C/77°F) until ready to use   Avoid
excessive heat See insert

Baxter
Baxter Healthcare Corporation
Deerfield IL 60015 USA   **8**
Made in USA   Viaflex® container
Distributed in Canada by   1 L HUB FLUID
Baxter Corporation   Fur health professionals
Toronto Ontario Canada   Call 1 800 033 0303   **9**

⊙   ⊙

4. After a burn injury Mr. Warren is to receive 500 mL of blood plasma over 4 hours. The tubing drop factor is 15 gtt/mL. How many drops per minute should be given? _____

5. A postpartum patient is to receive 1500 mL of LR over the next 8 hours. How many milliliters per hour should the IV pump be programmed for? _____

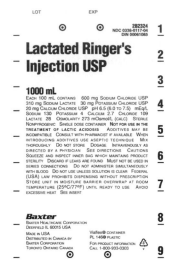

6. A patient is admitted with pernicious anemia. The physician orders a unit of packed red blood cells (250 mL) to be infused over 3 hours. The tubing drop factor is 12 gtt/mL. How many drops per minute should be given? _____

7. Ms. Chandar has an order for 1000 mL of LR over 12 hours. The tubing drop factor is 15 gtt/mL. How many drops per minute should be given? _____

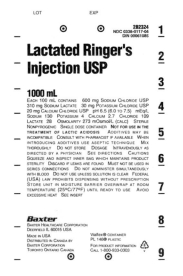

8. A patient with hypomagnesemia has an order for infusion of magnesium sulfate 2 g diluted in 50 mL D$_5$W. Policy states that the magnesium be infused at a rate of 1 g/h. How many milliliters per hour should the IV pump be programmed for? _____

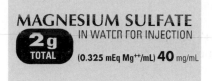

MAGNESIUM SULFATE
IN WATER FOR INJECTION
2g TOTAL (0.325 mEq Mg^{++}/mL) **40** mg/mL

9. Mr. Simpson has an order for NS to be infused at 150 mL/h after a transesophageal echocardiogram. The tubing drop factor is 60 gtt/mL. How many drops per minute should be given? _____

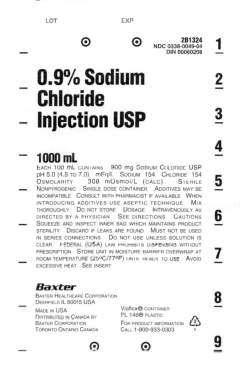

10. A patient has an order for 2500 mL of TPN to be infused over 24 hours. How many milliliters per hour should the IV pump be programmed for? _____

11. A patient with hypokalemia and hypophosphatemia has an order for potassium phosphate 30 milliosmole in 200 mL of 0.9% NS IV. The facility's policy states to infuse the potassium phosphate at 10 mOsm/h. How many milliliters per hour should the IV pump be programmed for? _____

12. A postoperative patient has an order for ceftazidime 1 g in 25 mL of D_5W over 15 minutes. The tubing drop factor is 60 gtt/mL. How many drops per minute should be given? _____

13. Mr. Anderson has metastatic cancer. The physician orders morphine sulfate 15 mg/h IV. Given a bag with a concentration of 100 mg of morphine sulfate in 200 mL of D_5W, how many milliliters per hour should the IV pump be programmed for? _____

14. A patient with a methicillin-resistant *S. aureus* infection has an order for vancomycin 1.5 g in 200 mL of D_5W IVPB q 12 h. The physician orders the vancomycin to be infused over 4 hours. How many milliliters per hour should the IV pump be programmed for? _____

15. Mrs. Marx, who has sepsis, has an order for Timentin 3.1 g in 100 mL of D_5W IVPB over 1 hour. The drop factor is 60 gtt/mL. How many drops per minute should be given?

ANSWERS ON PP. 452 AND 455–456.

NAME _____

DATE _____

ACCEPTABLE SCORE __14__

YOUR SCORE _____

htw ✓6/21

POSTTEST 2

DIRECTIONS: The IV fluid order is listed in each problem. Calculate the appropriate infusion rate for each problem. Show your work. Follow your instructor's rules on rounding final answers.

1. A patient with poor wound healing has ascorbic acid 300 mg in 200 mL of 0.9% NS ordered to be infused over 6 hours. How many milliliters per hour should the IV pump be programmed for? 33 mL

$$\frac{mL}{hr} = \frac{200 \, mL}{6 \, hr} = 33 \, mL$$

2. Avelox 400 mg daily IVPB is ordered for Mrs. Graham, who has osteomyelitis. The Avelox is to be infused over 60 minutes. The tubing drop factor is 10 gtt/mL. How many drops per minute should be given? 42 gtt

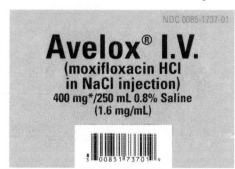

NDC 0085-1737-01

Avelox® I.V.
(moxifloxacin HCl
in NaCl injection)
400 mg*/250 mL 0.8% Saline
(1.6 mg/mL)

INFUSE OVER A PERIOD OF 60 MINUTES

$$\frac{250 \, mL}{60 \, min} \times 10 \, gtt/mL = 42$$

3. A patient with iron-deficiency anemia has an order for iron dextran 100 mg in 200 mL of 0.9% NS over 6 hours. How many milliliters per hour should the IV pump be programmed for? 33 mL

$$\frac{200 \, mL}{6 \, hrs} = 33$$

4. Your patient with a gastrointestinal bleed has an order for 1 unit of whole blood (500 mL) to be given over 3 hours. The tubing drop factor is 15 gtt/mL. How many drops per minute should be given? 42 gtt

$$\frac{500 \, mL}{180 \, min} \times 15 \, gtt/mL = 42$$

5. Mr. Sanchez has hypotension and receives an order for 1000 mL of 0.9% NS over 6 hours. The tubing drop factor is 10 gtt/mL. How many drops per minute should be given? 28 gtt

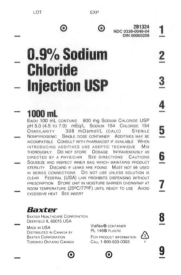

$$\frac{1000\,mL}{360\,min} \times 10\,gtt/mL = 28$$

6. An order for a patient with hypocalcemia states to infuse 1 g of calcium chloride 10% over 30 minutes. The calcium chloride is diluted in 50 mL of 0.9% NS. How many milliliters per hour should the IV pump be programmed for? 100 mL

$$\frac{50\,mL}{0.50\,hr} = 100$$

7. A terminal patient has morphine sulfate ordered at 8 mg/h. The medication concentration is morphine 100 mg diluted in 100 mL of D_5W. How many milliliters per hour should the IV pump be programmed for? 8 mL

$$\frac{8\,mg}{100\,mg} \times 100 = 8$$

8. Mrs. Watkins, who has undergone hip replacement, has an order for Toradol 30 mg q 6 h. The Toradol is diluted in 50 mL of 0.9% NS and is to be infused over 15 minutes. The tubing drop factor is 60 gtt/mL. How many drops per minute should be given? 200 gtt

$$\frac{50\,mL}{15\,min} \times 60\,gtt/mL = 200$$

9. A patient with severe nausea and vomiting has a one-time order for Zofran 8 mg IVPB over 15 minutes. The Zofran is diluted in 50 mL of D_5W. The tubing drop factor is 15 gtt/mL. How many drops per minute should be given? 50 gtt

$$\frac{50\,mL}{15\,min} \times 15\,gtt/mL = 50$$

10. A postoperative patient has an order for 1000 mL of LR over 6 hours. How many milliliters per hour should the IV pump be programmed for? 167 mL

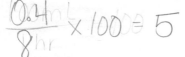

$$\frac{1000\,mL}{6\,hr} = 167$$

11. Mr. Nakamura experiences bradypnea after intrathecal administration of anesthesia. An order for Narcan 0.4 mg/h is written. Given a bag with a concentration of 8 mg in 100 mL of 0.9% NS, how many milliliters per hour should the IV pump be programmed for? 5 mL

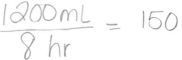

$$\frac{0.4\,ml}{8\,hr} \times 1000 = 5$$

12. A patient with a total gastrectomy has TPN ordered to be infused from 2200 to 0600. The total volume of the TPN bag is 1200 mL. How many milliliters per hour should the IV pump be programmed for? 150 mL

$$\frac{1200\,mL}{8\,hr} = 150$$

13. A postoperative patient has an order for Kefzol 1 g in 25 mL of D_5W over 15 minutes. The medication will be infused with an IV pump. How many milliliters per hour should the IV pump be programmed for? 100 mL

$$\frac{25\,mL}{0.25\,hr} = 100\,mL$$

14. Ms. Pailey has oliguria and receives an order for 1000 mL of 0.9% NS over 3 hours. The tubing drop factor is 10 gtt/mL. How many drops per minute should be given? _56 gtt_

LOT   EXP

⊙   ⊙   2B1324
                 NDC 0338-0049-04
                 DIN 00060208   **1**

0.9% Sodium   **2**
Chloride
Injection USP   **3**

                                  4
1000 mL
EACH 100 mL CONTAINS   900 mg SODIUM CHLORIDE USP
pH 5.0 (4.5 TO 7.0)   mEq/L   SODIUM 154   CHLORIDE 154   **5**
OSMOLARITY   308 mOsmol/L (CALC)   STERILE
NONPYROGENIC   SINGLE DOSE CONTAINER ADDITIVES MAY BE
INCOMPATIBLE CONSULT WITH PHARMACIST IF AVAILABLE   WHEN
INTRODUCING ADDITIVES USE ASEPTIC TECHNIQUE   MIX   **6**
THOROUGHLY   DO NOT STORE   DOSAGE   INTRAVENOUSLY AS
DIRECTED BY A PHYSICIAN   SEE DIRECTIONS   CAUTIONS
SQUEEZE AND INSPECT INNER BAG WHICH MAINTAINS PRODUCT
STERILITY   DISCARD IF LEAKS ARE FOUND   MUST NOT BE USED
IN SERIES CONNECTIONS   DO NOT USE UNLESS SOLUTION IS   **7**
CLEAR   FEDERAL (USA) LAW PROHIBITS DISPENSING WITHOUT
PRESCRIPTION   STORE UNIT IN MOISTURE BARRIER OVERWRAP AT
ROOM TEMPERATURE (25ºC/77ºF) UNTIL READY TO USE   AVOID
EXCESSIVE HEAT   SEE INSERT

Baxter
BAXTER HEALTHCARE CORPORATION
DEERFIELD IL 60015 USA   **8**
MADE IN USA   Viaflex® CONTAINER
DISTRIBUTED IN CANADA BY   PL 146® PLASTIC
BAXTER CORPORATION   FOR PRODUCT INFORMATION
TORONTO ONTARIO CANADA   CALL 1-800-933-0303   **9**

⊙   ⊙

$$\frac{1000\,mL}{180\,min} \times 10\,gtt/mL =$$

$$556$$

15. An NPO patient has an order for 500 mL of D_5W 0.45% NS over 6 hours. How many milliliters per hour should the IV pump be programmed for?

LOT   EXP

⊙   ⊙   2B1073
                 NDC 0338-0085-03   **1**

5% Dextrose and
0.45% Sodium   **2**
Chloride Injection USP

500 mL   **3**
EACH 100 mL CONTAINS   5 g DEXTROSE HYDROUS USP   450 mg SODIUM
CHLORIDE USP pH 4.0 (3.2 TO 6.5) mEq/L SODIUM 77 CHLORIDE 77
HYPERTONIC   OSMOLARITY   406 mOsmol/L (CALC)   STERILE
NONPYROGENIC SINGLE DOSE CONTAINER   ADDITIVES MAY BE INCOMPATIBLE
CONSULT WITH PHARMACIST IF AVAILABLE   WHEN INTRODUCING ADDITIVES USE   **4**
ASEPTIC TECHNIQUE   MIX THOROUGHLY   DO NOT STORE   DOSAGE
INTRAVENOUSLY AS DIRECTED BY A PHYSICIAN   SEE DIRECTIONS   CAUTIONS
SQUEEZE AND INSPECT INNER BAG WHICH MAINTAINS PRODUCT STERILITY
DISCARD IF LEAKS ARE FOUND   MUST NOT BE USED IN SERIES CONNECTIONS
DO NOT USE UNLESS SOLUTION IS CLEAR   FEDERAL (USA) LAW PROHIBITS
DISPENSING WITHOUT PRESCRIPTION   STORE UNIT IN MOISTURE BARRIER
OVERWRAP AT ROOM TEMPERATURE (25ºC/77ºF) UNTIL READY TO USE
AVOID EXCESSIVE HEAT   SEE INSERT

Baxter
BAXTER HEALTHCARE CORPORATION   Viaflex® CONTAINER
DEERFIELD IL 60015 USA   PL 146® PLASTIC
MADE IN USA   FOR PRODUCT INFORMATION
                                CALL 1-800-933-0303

$$\frac{500\,mL}{6\,hrs} = 83\,ml$$

ANSWERS ON PP. 452 AND 457–458.

evolve   For additional practice problems, refer to the Intravenous Calculations section of *Drug Calculations Companion,* Version 5, on Evolve.

ANSWERS

CHAPTER 15 Dimensional Analysis—Work Sheet, pp. 437–442

1. $\dfrac{x \text{ mL}}{\text{h}} = \dfrac{500 \text{ mL}}{24 \text{ h}} = 20.8 \text{ or } 21 \text{ mL/h}$

2. $\dfrac{x \text{ mL}}{\text{h}} = \dfrac{100 \text{ mL}}{1 \text{ h}} = 100 \text{ mL/h}$

3. $\dfrac{x \text{ gtt}}{\text{min}} = \dfrac{15 \text{ gtt}}{1 \text{ mL}} \times \dfrac{100 \text{ mL}}{30 \text{ min}} = 50 \text{ gtt/min}$

4. $\dfrac{x \text{ mL}}{\text{h}} = \dfrac{3000 \text{ mL}}{12 \text{ h}} = 250 \text{ mL/h}$

5. $\dfrac{x \text{ gtt}}{\text{min}} = \dfrac{10 \text{ gtt}}{1 \text{ mL}} \times \dfrac{100 \text{ mL}}{30 \text{ min}}$
   $= 33.3 \text{ rounded to } 33 \text{ gtt/min}$

6. $\dfrac{x \text{ mL}}{\text{h}} = \dfrac{500 \text{ mL}}{6 \text{ h}} = 83.3 \text{ or } 83 \text{ mL/h}$

7. $\dfrac{x \text{ gtt}}{\text{min}} = \dfrac{10 \text{ gtt}}{1 \text{ mL}} \times \dfrac{100 \text{ mL}}{60 \text{ min}}$
   $= 16.6 \text{ rounded to } 17 \text{ gtt/min}$

8. $\dfrac{x \text{ mL}}{\text{h}} = \dfrac{250 \text{ mL}}{60 \text{ mEq}} \times \dfrac{20 \text{ mEq}}{1 \text{ h}}$
   $= 83.3 \text{ or } 83 \text{ mL/h}$

9. $\dfrac{x \text{ gtt}}{\text{min}} = \dfrac{60 \text{ gtt}}{1 \text{ mL}} \times \dfrac{50 \text{ mL}}{30 \text{ min}} = 100 \text{ gtt/min}$

10. $\dfrac{x \text{ mL}}{\text{h}} = \dfrac{1000 \text{ mL}}{10 \text{ h}} = 100 \text{ mL/h}$

11. $\dfrac{x \text{ gtt}}{\text{min}} = \dfrac{60 \text{ gtt}}{1 \text{ mL}} \times \dfrac{50 \text{ mL}}{15 \text{ min}} = 200 \text{ gtt/min}$

12. $\dfrac{x \text{ mL}}{\text{h}} = \dfrac{200 \text{ mL}}{400 \text{ mg}} \times \dfrac{200 \text{ mg}}{1 \text{ h}} = 100 \text{ mL/h}$

13. $\dfrac{x \text{ gtt}}{\text{min}} = \dfrac{10 \text{ gtt}}{1 \text{ mL}} \times \dfrac{1000 \text{ mL}}{1 \text{ h}} \times \dfrac{1 \text{ h}}{60 \text{ min}}$
    $= 166.6 \text{ rounded to } 167 \text{ gtt/min}$

14. $\dfrac{x \text{ mL}}{\text{h}} = \dfrac{500 \text{ mL}}{4 \text{ h}} = 125 \text{ mL/h}$

15. $\dfrac{x \text{ gtt}}{\text{min}} = \dfrac{15 \text{ gtt}}{1 \text{ mL}} \times \dfrac{25 \text{ mL}}{15 \text{ min}} = 25 \text{ gtt/min}$

16. $\dfrac{x \text{ mL}}{\text{h}} = \dfrac{100 \text{ mL}}{20 \text{ mg}} \times \dfrac{0.5 \text{ mg}}{1 \text{ h}}$
    $= 2.5 \text{ or } 3 \text{ mL/h}$

17. $\dfrac{x \text{ gtt}}{\text{min}} = \dfrac{20 \text{ gtt}}{1 \text{ mL}} \times \dfrac{25 \text{ mL}}{15 \text{ min}}$
    $= 33.3 \text{ rounded to } 33 \text{ gtt/min}$

18. $\dfrac{x \text{ mL}}{\text{h}} = \dfrac{100 \text{ mL}}{2 \text{ g}} \times \dfrac{1 \text{ g}}{1 \text{ h}} = 50 \text{ mL/h}$

19. $\dfrac{x \text{ gtt}}{\text{min}} = \dfrac{20 \text{ gtt}}{1 \text{ mL}} \times \dfrac{250 \text{ mL}}{4 \text{ h}} \times \dfrac{1 \text{ h}}{60 \text{ min}}$
    $= 20.8 \text{ rounded to } 21 \text{ gtt/min}$

20. $\dfrac{x \text{ mL}}{\text{h}} = \dfrac{100 \text{ mL}}{15 \text{ min}} \times \dfrac{60 \text{ min}}{1 \text{ h}} = 400 \text{ mL/h}$

21. $\dfrac{x \text{ mL}}{\text{h}} = \dfrac{200 \text{ mL}}{40 \text{ mEq}} \times \dfrac{10 \text{ mEq}}{1 \text{ h}} = 50 \text{ mL/h}$

22. $\dfrac{x \text{ mL}}{\text{h}} = \dfrac{1350 \text{ mL}}{10 \text{ h}} = 135 \text{ mL/h}$

23. $\dfrac{x \text{ mL}}{\text{h}} = \dfrac{50 \text{ mL}}{2 \text{ g}} \times \dfrac{1 \text{ g}}{1 \text{ h}} = 25 \text{ mL/h}$

24. $\dfrac{x \text{ mL}}{\text{h}} = \dfrac{200 \text{ mL}}{1 \text{ h}} = 200 \text{ mL/h}$

25. $\dfrac{x \text{ gtt}}{\text{min}} = \dfrac{20 \text{ gtt}}{1 \text{ mL}} \times \dfrac{100 \text{ mL}}{30 \text{ min}}$
    $= 66.6 \text{ rounded to } 67 \text{ gtt/min}$

26. $\dfrac{x \text{ mL}}{\text{h}} = \dfrac{50 \text{ mL}}{30 \text{ min}} \times \dfrac{60 \text{ min}}{1 \text{ h}} = 100 \text{ mL/h}$

27. $\dfrac{x \text{ gtt}}{\text{min}} = \dfrac{20 \text{ gtt}}{1 \text{ mL}} \times \dfrac{200 \text{ mL}}{1 \text{ h}} \times \dfrac{1 \text{ h}}{60 \text{ min}}$
    $= 66.6 \text{ rounded to } 67 \text{ gtt/min}$

28. $\dfrac{x \text{ mL}}{\text{h}} = \dfrac{500 \text{ mL}}{8 \text{ h}} = 62.5 \text{ or } 63 \text{ mL/h}$

29. $\dfrac{x \text{ mL}}{\text{h}} = \dfrac{250 \text{ mL}}{200 \text{ mg}} \times \dfrac{5 \text{ mg}}{1 \text{ h}} = 6.3 \text{ or } 6 \text{ mL/h}$

30. $\dfrac{x \text{ gtt}}{\text{min}} = \dfrac{60 \text{ gtt}}{1 \text{ mL}} \times \dfrac{50 \text{ mL}}{30 \text{ min}} = 100 \text{ gtt/min}$

31. $\dfrac{x \text{ mL}}{\text{h}} = \dfrac{250 \text{ mL}}{2 \text{ h}} = 125 \text{ mL/h}$

32. $\dfrac{x \text{ mL}}{\text{h}} = \dfrac{1000 \text{ mL}}{10 \text{ h}} = 100 \text{ mL/h}$

33. $\dfrac{x \text{ mL}}{\text{h}} = \dfrac{9600 \text{ mL}}{8 \text{ h}} = 1200 \text{ mL/h}$

34. $\dfrac{x \text{ mL}}{\text{h}} = \dfrac{100 \text{ mL}}{3 \text{ h}} = 33.3 \text{ or } 33 \text{ mL/h}$

35. $\dfrac{x \text{ mL}}{\text{h}} = \dfrac{100 \text{ mL}}{100 \text{ mg}} \times \dfrac{20 \text{ mg}}{1 \text{ h}} = 20 \text{ mL/h}$

36. $\dfrac{x \text{ mL}}{\text{h}} = \dfrac{100 \text{ mL}}{15 \text{ min}} \times \dfrac{60 \text{ min}}{1 \text{ h}} = 400 \text{ mL/h}$

37. $\dfrac{x \text{ mL}}{\text{h}} = \dfrac{300 \text{ mL}}{2 \text{ h}} = 150 \text{ mL/h}$

CHAPTER 15 Dimensional Analysis—Posttest 1, pp. 443–446

1. $\dfrac{x \text{ mL}}{\text{h}} = \dfrac{500 \text{ mL}}{2 \text{ h}} = 250 \text{ mL/h}$

2. $\dfrac{x \text{ mL}}{\text{h}} = \dfrac{500 \text{ mL}}{4 \text{ h}} = 125 \text{ mL/h}$

3. $\dfrac{x \text{ gtt}}{\text{min}} = \dfrac{12 \text{ gtt}}{1 \text{ mL}} \times \dfrac{120 \text{ mL}}{1 \text{ h}} \times \dfrac{1 \text{ h}}{60 \text{ min}}$
$= 24 \text{ gtt/min}$

4. $\dfrac{x \text{ gtt}}{\text{min}} = \dfrac{15 \text{ gtt}}{1 \text{ mL}} \times \dfrac{500 \text{ mL}}{4 \text{ h}} \times \dfrac{1 \text{ h}}{60 \text{ min}}$
$= 31.2 \text{ rounded to } 31 \text{ gtt/min}$

5. $\dfrac{x \text{ mL}}{\text{h}} = \dfrac{1500 \text{ mL}}{8 \text{ h}} = 187.5 \text{ or } 188 \text{ mL/h}$

6. $\dfrac{x \text{ gtt}}{\text{min}} = \dfrac{12 \text{ gtt}}{1 \text{ mL}} \times \dfrac{250 \text{ mL}}{3 \text{ h}} \times \dfrac{1 \text{ h}}{60 \text{ min}}$
$= 16.6 \text{ rounded to } 17 \text{ gtt/min}$

7. $\dfrac{x \text{ gtt}}{\text{min}} = \dfrac{15 \text{ gtt}}{1 \text{ mL}} \times \dfrac{1000 \text{ mL}}{12 \text{ h}} \times \dfrac{1 \text{ h}}{60 \text{ min}}$
$= 20.8 \text{ rounded to } 21 \text{ gtt/min}$

8. $\dfrac{x \text{ mL}}{\text{h}} = \dfrac{50 \text{ mL}}{2 \text{ g}} \times \dfrac{1 \text{ g}}{1 \text{ h}} = 25 \text{ mL/h}$

9. $\dfrac{x \text{ gtt}}{\text{min}} = \dfrac{60 \text{ gtt}}{1 \text{ mL}} \times \dfrac{150 \text{ mL}}{1 \text{ h}} \times \dfrac{1 \text{ h}}{60 \text{ min}}$
$= 150 \text{ gtt/min}$

10. $\dfrac{x \text{ mL}}{\text{h}} = \dfrac{2500 \text{ mL}}{24 \text{ h}} = 104.1 \text{ or } 104 \text{ mL/h}$

11. $\dfrac{x \text{ mL}}{\text{h}} = \dfrac{200 \text{ mL}}{30 \text{ mOsm}} \times \dfrac{10 \text{ mOsm}}{1 \text{ h}}$
$= 66.7 \text{ or } 67 \text{ mL/h}$

12. $\dfrac{x \text{ gtt}}{\text{min}} = \dfrac{60 \text{ gtt}}{1 \text{ mL}} \times \dfrac{25 \text{ mL}}{15 \text{ min}} = 100 \text{ gtt/min}$

13. $\dfrac{x \text{ mL}}{\text{h}} = \dfrac{200 \text{ mL}}{100 \text{ mg}} \times \dfrac{15 \text{ mg}}{1 \text{ h}} = 30 \text{ mL/h}$

14. $\dfrac{x \text{ mL}}{\text{h}} = \dfrac{200 \text{ mL}}{4 \text{ h}} = 50 \text{ mL/h}$

15. $\dfrac{x \text{ gtt}}{\text{min}} = \dfrac{60 \text{ gtt}}{1 \text{ mL}} \times \dfrac{100 \text{ mL}}{1 \text{ h}} \times \dfrac{1 \text{ h}}{60 \text{ min}}$
$= 100 \text{ gtt/min}$

CHAPTER 15 Dimensional Analysis—Posttest 2, pp. 447–450

1. $\dfrac{x \text{ mL}}{\text{h}} = \dfrac{200 \text{ mL}}{6 \text{ h}} = 33.3 \text{ or } 33 \text{ mL/h}$

2. $\dfrac{x \text{ gtt}}{\text{min}} = \dfrac{10 \text{ gtt}}{1 \text{ mL}} \times \dfrac{250 \text{ mL}}{60 \text{ min}}$
$= 41.6 \text{ rounded to } 42 \text{ gtt/min}$

3. $\dfrac{x \text{ mL}}{\text{h}} = \dfrac{200 \text{ mL}}{6 \text{ h}} = 33.3 \text{ or } 33 \text{ mL/h}$

4. $\dfrac{x \text{ gtt}}{\text{min}} = \dfrac{15 \text{ gtt}}{1 \text{ mL}} \times \dfrac{500 \text{ mL}}{3 \text{ h}} \times \dfrac{1 \text{ h}}{60 \text{ min}}$
$= 41.6 \text{ rounded to } 42 \text{ gtt/min}$

5. $\dfrac{x \text{ gtt}}{\text{min}} = \dfrac{10 \text{ gtt}}{1 \text{ mL}} \times \dfrac{1000 \text{ mL}}{6 \text{ h}} \times \dfrac{1 \text{ h}}{60 \text{ min}}$
$= 27.7 \text{ rounded to } 28 \text{ gtt/min}$

6. $\dfrac{x \text{ mL}}{\text{h}} = \dfrac{50 \text{ mL}}{30 \text{ min}} \times \dfrac{60 \text{ min}}{1 \text{ h}} = 100 \text{ mL/h}$

7. $\dfrac{x \text{ mL}}{\text{h}} = \dfrac{100 \text{ mL}}{100 \text{ mg}} \times \dfrac{8 \text{ mg}}{1 \text{ h}} = 8 \text{ mL/h}$

8. $\dfrac{x \text{ gtt}}{\text{min}} = \dfrac{60 \text{ gtt}}{1 \text{ mL}} \times \dfrac{50 \text{ mL}}{15 \text{ min}} = 200 \text{ gtt/min}$

9. $\dfrac{x \text{ gtt}}{\text{min}} = \dfrac{15 \text{ gtt}}{1 \text{ mL}} \times \dfrac{50 \text{ mL}}{15 \text{ min}} = 50 \text{ gtt/min}$

10. $\dfrac{x \text{ mL}}{\text{h}} = \dfrac{1000 \text{ mL}}{6 \text{ h}} = 166.7 \text{ or } 167 \text{ mL/h}$

11. $\dfrac{x \text{ mL}}{\text{h}} = \dfrac{100 \text{ mL}}{8 \text{ mg}} \times \dfrac{0.4 \text{ mg}}{1 \text{ h}} = 5 \text{ mL/h}$

12. $\dfrac{x \text{ mL}}{\text{h}} = \dfrac{1200 \text{ mL}}{8 \text{ h}} = 150 \text{ mL/h}$

13. $\dfrac{x \text{ mL}}{\text{h}} = \dfrac{25 \text{ mL}}{15 \text{ min}} \times \dfrac{60 \text{ min}}{1 \text{ h}} = 100 \text{ mL/h}$

14. $\dfrac{x \text{ gtt}}{\text{min}} = \dfrac{10 \text{ gtt}}{1 \text{ mL}} \times \dfrac{1000 \text{ mL}}{3 \text{ h}} \times \dfrac{1 \text{ h}}{60 \text{ min}}$
$= 55.5 \text{ rounded to } 56 \text{ gtt/min}$

15. $\dfrac{x \text{ mL}}{\text{h}} = \dfrac{500 \text{ mL}}{6 \text{ h}} = 83.3 \text{ or } 83 \text{ mL/h}$

CHAPTER 15 Proportion/Formula Method—Work Sheet, pp. 437–442

Proportion	Formula

1.

$$\frac{500\ \text{mL}}{24\ \text{h}} = 20.8 \text{ or } 21 \text{ mL/h}$$

2.

$$\frac{100\ \text{mL}}{1\ \text{h}} = 100 \text{ mL/h}$$

3.

$$\frac{100\ \text{mL}}{\overset{}{\underset{2}{\cancel{30}}}\ \text{min}} \times \overset{1}{\cancel{15}} \text{ gtt/mL} = \frac{100}{2} = 50 \text{ gtt/min}$$

4.

$$\frac{3000\ \text{mL}}{12\ \text{h}} = 250 \text{ mL/h}$$

5.

$$\frac{100\ \text{mL}}{\underset{3}{\cancel{30}}\ \text{min}} \times \overset{1}{\cancel{10}} \text{ gtt/mL} = \frac{100}{3}$$

$$= 33.3 \text{ rounded to } 33 \text{ gtt/min}$$

6.

$$\frac{500\ \text{mL}}{6\ \text{h}} = 83.3 \text{ or } 83 \text{ mL/h}$$

7.

$$\frac{100\ \text{mL}}{\underset{6}{\cancel{60}}\ \text{min}} \times \overset{1}{\cancel{10}} \text{ gtt/mL} = \frac{100}{6}$$

$$= 16.6 \text{ rounded to } 17 \text{ gtt/min}$$

8. $60 \text{ mEq} : 250 \text{ mL} :: 20 \text{ mEq} : x \text{ mL}$
$60x = 5000$
$x = \dfrac{5000}{60}$
$x = 83.3 \text{ or } 83 \text{ mL/h}$

$$\frac{\overset{1}{\cancel{20}}\ \text{mEq}}{\underset{3}{\cancel{60}}\ \text{mEq}} \times 250 \text{ mL} =$$

$$\frac{500}{6} = 83.3 \text{ mL or } 83 \text{ mL/h}$$

9.

$$\frac{50\ \text{mL}}{\underset{1}{\cancel{30}}\ \text{min}} \times \overset{2}{\cancel{60}} \text{ gtt/mL} = \frac{100}{1} = 100 \text{ gtt/min}$$

10.

$$\frac{1000\ \text{mL}}{10\ \text{h}} = 100 \text{ mL/h}$$

11.

$$\frac{50\ \text{mL}}{\underset{1}{\cancel{15}}\ \text{min}} \times \overset{4}{\cancel{60}} \text{ gtt/mL} = 200 \text{ gtt/min}$$

12. $400 \text{ mg} : 200 \text{ mL} :: 200 \text{ mg} : x \text{ mL}$
$400x = 40,000$
$x = \dfrac{40,000}{400}$
$x = 100 \text{ mL/h}$

$$\frac{200\ \text{mg}}{\underset{2}{\cancel{400}}\ \text{mg}} \times \overset{1}{\cancel{200}} \text{ mL} =$$

$$\frac{200}{2} = 100 \text{ mL/h}$$

13.

$$\frac{1000\ \text{mL}}{\underset{6}{\cancel{60}}\ \text{min}} \times \overset{1}{\cancel{10}} \text{ gtt/mL} = \frac{1000}{6}$$

$$= 166.6 \text{ rounded to } 167 \text{ gtt/min}$$

14.

$$\frac{500\ \text{mL}}{4\ \text{h}} = 125 \text{ mL/h}$$

ANSWERS

Proportion	Formula

15.

$$\frac{25 \text{ mL}}{\underset{1}{\cancel{15}} \text{ min}} \times \overset{1}{\cancel{15}} \text{ gtt/mL} = 25 \text{ gtt/min}$$

16. 20 mg : 100 mL :: 0.5 mg : x mL
$20x = 50$
$x = \dfrac{50}{20}$
$x = 2.5$ or 3 mL/h

$$\frac{0.5 \text{ mg}}{\underset{1}{\cancel{20}} \text{ mg}} \times \overset{5}{\cancel{100}} \text{ mL} =$$
$$\frac{0.5}{1} \times 5 = 2.5 \text{ or } 3 \text{ mL/h}$$

17.

$$\frac{25 \text{ mL}}{\underset{3}{\cancel{15}} \text{ min}} \times \overset{4}{\cancel{20}} \text{ gtt/mL} = \frac{100}{3}$$
$$= 33.3 \text{ rounded to } 33 \text{ gtt/min}$$

18. 2 g : 100 mL :: 1 g : x mL
$2x = 100$
$x = \dfrac{100}{2}$
$x = 50$ mL/h

$$\frac{1 \text{ g}}{\underset{1}{\cancel{2}} \text{ g}} \times \overset{50}{\cancel{100}} \text{ mL} =$$
$$\frac{50}{1} = 50 \text{ mL/h}$$

19.

$$\frac{250 \text{ mL}}{\underset{12}{\cancel{240}} \text{ min}} \times \overset{1}{\cancel{20}} \text{ gtt/mL} = \frac{250}{12}$$
$$= 20.8 \text{ rounded to } 21 \text{ gtt/min}$$

20.

$$\frac{100 \text{ mL}}{0.25 \text{ h}} = 400 \text{ mL/h}$$

21. 40 mEq : 200 mL :: 10 mEq : x mL
$40x = 2000$
$x = \dfrac{2000}{40}$
$x = 50$ mL/h

$$\frac{10 \text{ mEq}}{\underset{1}{\cancel{40}} \text{ mEq}} \times \overset{5}{\cancel{200}} \text{ mL} =$$
$$\frac{10}{1} \times 5 = 50 \text{ mL/h}$$

22.

$$\frac{1350 \text{ mL}}{10 \text{ h}} = 135 \text{ mL/h}$$

23. 2 g : 50 mL :: 1 g : x mL
$2x = 50$
$x = \dfrac{50}{2}$
$x = 25$ mL/h

$$\frac{1 \text{ g}}{\underset{1}{\cancel{2}} \text{ g}} \times \overset{25}{\cancel{50}} \text{ mL} =$$
$$\frac{25}{1} = 25 \text{ mL/h}$$

24.

$$\frac{200 \text{ mL}}{1 \text{ h}} = 200 \text{ mL/h}$$

25.

$$\frac{100 \text{ mL}}{\underset{3}{\cancel{30}} \text{ min}} \times \overset{2}{\cancel{20}} \text{ gtt/mL} = \frac{200}{3}$$
$$= 66.6 \text{ rounded to } 67 \text{ gtt/min}$$

26.

$$\frac{50 \text{ mL}}{0.5 \text{ h}} = 100 \text{ mL/h}$$

Proportion	Formula
27.	$\dfrac{200 \text{ mL}}{\underset{3}{\cancel{60}} \text{ min}} \times \overset{1}{\cancel{20}} \text{ gtt/mL} = \dfrac{200}{3}$ $= 66.66$ rounded to 67 gtt/min
28.	$\dfrac{500 \text{ mL}}{8 \text{ h}} = 62.5$ or 63 mL/h
29. 200 mg : 250 mL :: 5 mg : x mL $200x = 1250$ $x = \dfrac{1250}{200}$ $x = 6.3$ or 6 mL/h	$\dfrac{5 \text{ mg}}{\underset{4}{\cancel{200}} \text{ mg}} \times \overset{5}{\cancel{250}} \text{ mL} = 6.3$ or 6 mL/h
30.	$\dfrac{50 \text{ mL}}{\underset{1}{\cancel{30}} \text{ min}} \times \overset{2}{\cancel{60}} \text{ gtt/mL} = 100$ gtt/min
31.	$\dfrac{250 \text{ mL}}{2 \text{ h}} = 125$ mL/h
32.	$\dfrac{1000 \text{ mL}}{10 \text{ h}} = 100$ mL/h
33.	$\dfrac{9600 \text{ mL}}{8 \text{ h}} = 1200$ mL/h
34.	$\dfrac{100 \text{ mL}}{3 \text{ h}} = 33.3$ or 33 mL/h
35. 100 mg : 100 mL :: 20 mg : x mL $100x = 2000$ $x = \dfrac{2000}{100}$ $x = 20$ mL/h	$\dfrac{20 \text{ mg}}{\underset{1}{\cancel{100}} \text{ mg}} \times \overset{1}{\cancel{100}} \text{ mL} = 20$ mL/h
36.	$\dfrac{100 \text{ mL}}{0.25 \text{ h}} = 400$ mL/h
37.	$\dfrac{300 \text{ mL}}{2 \text{ h}} = 150$ mL/h

CHAPTER 15 Proportion/Formula Method—Posttest 1, pp. 443–446

Proportion	Formula
1.	$\dfrac{500 \text{ mL}}{2 \text{ h}} = 250$ mL/h
2.	$\dfrac{500 \text{ mL}}{4 \text{ h}} = 125$ mL/h
3.	$\dfrac{120 \text{ mL}}{\underset{5}{\cancel{60}} \text{ min}} \times \overset{1}{\cancel{12}} \text{ gtt/mL} = \dfrac{120}{5} = 24$ gtt/min

ANSWERS

Proportion	**Formula**

4.

$$\frac{\overset{50}{\cancel{500}} \text{ mL}}{\underset{24}{\cancel{240}} \text{ min}} \times 15 \text{ gtt/mL} = \frac{750}{24}$$

$$= 31.2 \text{ rounded to } 31 \text{ gtt/min}$$

5.

$$\frac{1500 \text{ mL}}{8 \text{ h}} = 187.5 \text{ or } 188 \text{ mL/h}$$

6.

$$\frac{250 \text{ mL}}{\underset{15}{\cancel{180}} \text{ min}} \times \overset{1}{\cancel{12}} \text{ gtt/mL} = \frac{250}{15}$$

$$= 16.6 \text{ rounded to } 17 \text{ gtt/min}$$

7.

$$\frac{1000 \text{ mL}}{\underset{48}{\cancel{720}} \text{ min}} \times \overset{1}{\cancel{15}} \text{ gtt/mL} = \frac{1000}{48}$$

$$= 20.8 \text{ rounded to } 21 \text{ gtt/min}$$

8. $2 \text{ g} : 50 \text{ mL} :: 1 \text{ g} : x \text{ mL}$
$2x = 50$
$x = \dfrac{50}{2}$
$x = 25 \text{ mL/h}$

$$\frac{1 \text{ g}}{2 \text{ g}} \times 50 \text{ mL} =$$

$$\frac{50}{2} = 25 \text{ mL/h}$$

9.

$$\frac{150 \text{ mL}}{\underset{1}{\cancel{60}} \text{ min}} \times \overset{1}{\cancel{60}} \text{ gtt/mL} = \frac{150}{1} = 150 \text{ gtt/min}$$

10.

$$\frac{2500 \text{ mL}}{24 \text{ h}} = 104.1 \text{ or } 104 \text{ mL/h}$$

11. $30 \text{ mOsm} : 200 \text{ mL} :: 10 \text{ mOsm} : x \text{ mL}$
$30x = 2000$
$x = \dfrac{2000}{30}$
$x = 66.7 \text{ or } 67 \text{ mL/h}$

$$\frac{\overset{1}{\cancel{10}} \text{ mOsm}}{\underset{3}{\cancel{30}} \text{ mOsm}} \times 200 \text{ mL} =$$

$$\frac{200}{3} = 66.7 \text{ or } 67 \text{ mL/h}$$

12.

$$\frac{25 \text{ mL}}{\underset{1}{\cancel{15}} \text{ min}} \times \overset{4}{\cancel{60}} \text{ gtt/mL} = \frac{25}{1} \times 4 = 100 \text{ gtt/min}$$

13. $100 \text{ mg} : 200 \text{ mL} :: 15 \text{ mg} : x \text{ mL}$
$100x = 3000$
$x = \dfrac{3000}{100}$
$x = 30 \text{ mL/h}$

$$\frac{15 \text{ mg}}{\underset{1}{\cancel{100}} \text{ mg}} \times \overset{2}{\cancel{200}} \text{ mL} =$$

$$\frac{15}{1} \times 2 = 30 \text{ mL/h}$$

14.

$$\frac{200 \text{ mL}}{4 \text{ h}} = 50 \text{ mL/h}$$

15.

$$\frac{100 \text{ mL}}{\underset{1}{\cancel{60}} \text{ min}} \times \overset{1}{\cancel{60}} \text{ gtt/mL} = 100 \text{ gtt/min}$$

CHAPTER 15 Proportion/Formula Method—Posttest 2, pp. 447–450

Proportion	Formula
1.	$\dfrac{200\ mL}{6\ h} = 33.3\ or\ 33\ mL/h$
2.	$\dfrac{250\ mL}{\cancel{60}\ min\ _{6}} \times \overset{1}{\cancel{10}}\ gtt/mL = \dfrac{250}{6}$ $= 41.6\ rounded\ to\ 42\ gtt/min$
3.	$\dfrac{200\ mL}{6\ h} = 33.3\ or\ 33\ mL/h$
4.	$\dfrac{500\ mL}{\cancel{180}\ min\ _{12}} \times \overset{1}{\cancel{15}}\ gtt/mL = \dfrac{500}{12}$ $= 41.6\ rounded\ to\ 42\ gtt/min$
5.	$\dfrac{1000\ mL}{\cancel{360}\ min\ _{36}} \times \overset{1}{\cancel{10}}\ gtt/mL = \dfrac{1000}{36}$ $= 27.7\ rounded\ to\ 28\ gtt/min$
6.	$\dfrac{50\ mL}{0.5\ h} = 100\ mL/h$
7. $100\ mg : 100\ mL :: 8\ mg : x$ $100x = 800$ $x = \dfrac{800}{100}$ $x = 8\ mL/h$	$\dfrac{8\ mg}{\underset{1}{\cancel{100}}\ mg} \times \overset{1}{\cancel{100}}\ mL =$ $\dfrac{8}{1} = 8\ mL/h$
8.	$\dfrac{50\ mL}{\underset{1}{\cancel{15}}\ min} \times \overset{4}{\cancel{60}}\ gtt/mL = \dfrac{200}{1} = 200\ gtt/min$
9.	$\dfrac{50\ mL}{\underset{1}{\cancel{15}}\ min} \times \overset{1}{\cancel{15}}\ gtt/mL = \dfrac{50}{1} - 50\ gtt/min$
10.	$\dfrac{1000\ mL}{6\ h} = 166.7\ or\ 167\ mL/h$
11. $8\ mg : 100\ mL :: 0.4\ mg : x\ mL$ $8x = 40$ $x = \dfrac{40}{8}$ $x = 5\ mL/h$	$\dfrac{0.4\ mg}{\underset{2}{\cancel{8}}\ mg} \times \overset{25}{\cancel{100}}\ mL -$ $\dfrac{10}{2} = 5\ mL/h$
12.	$\dfrac{1200\ mL}{8\ h} = 150\ mL/h$
13.	$\dfrac{25\ mL}{0.25\ h} = 100\ mL/h$

ANSWERS

Proportion	Formula
14.	$$\dfrac{1000 \text{ mL}}{\underset{18}{\cancel{180}} \text{ min}} \times \overset{1}{\cancel{10}} \text{ gtt/mL} = \dfrac{1000}{18}$$ $$= 55.5 \text{ rounded to } 56 \text{ gtt/min}$$
15.	$$\dfrac{500 \text{ mL}}{6 \text{ h}} = 83.3 \text{ or } 83 \text{ mL/h}$$

ANSWERS

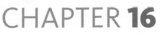

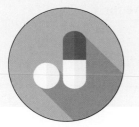

Intravenous Flow Rates for Dosages Measured in Units

LEARNING OBJECTIVES

Upon completion of the materials provided in this chapter, you will be able to perform computations accurately by mastering the following mathematical concepts:

1 Calculating the IV flow rate of medications in units per hour or international units per hour

2 Calculating the units per hour of medications from the IV flow rate

3 Calculating the IV flow rate of medications in units per kilogram per hour (weight-based heparin)

Some intravenous (IV) medications are ordered by units per hour, international units per hour, or units per kilogram per hour. IV heparin and IV insulin are among the medications ordered in this way. Medications ordered in this manner must be delivered with an IV controller or pump for safe administration. Because infusion pumps are set by milliliters per hour (mL/h), the health care provider needs to be familiar with the steps to convert the ordered drug dosage to milliliters per hour.

Calculating Milliliters/Hour from Units/Hour— Dimensional Analysis Method

EXAMPLE 1: A patient has an order for regular insulin IV at a rate of 5 units/h. The concentration is insulin 100 units/100 mL 0.9% NS. At what rate, in milliliters per hour, should the IV pump be programmed?

a. On the left side of the equation, place what you are solving for.

$$x \text{ mL/h} =$$

b. On the right side of the equation, place the available information related to the measurement or abbreviation that was placed on the left side. In this example the measurement we are solving for is *mL/h*. We will deal with the numerator portion of our answer first, the mL. We also know from the problem that 100 units of insulin are diluted in the 100 mL. This information is placed in the equation as a fraction, with the numerator matching.

$$x \frac{\text{mL}}{\text{h}} = \frac{100 \text{ mL}}{100 \text{ units}}$$

c. Next, find the information that matches the measurement used in the denominator of the fraction you created. In this example, *units* is the denominator and our order is for 5 units/h. The equation now looks like

$$x \frac{\text{mL}}{\text{h}} = \frac{100 \text{ mL}}{100 \text{ units}} \times \frac{5 \text{ units}}{1 \text{ h}}$$

d. Then cancel out the like abbreviations on the right side of the equation. If you have set up the problem correctly, the remaining measurements should match the measurements on the left side of the equation. Now solve for x.

$$\frac{x \text{ mL}}{h} = \frac{100 \text{ mL}}{100 \text{ units}} \times \frac{5 \text{ units}}{1 \text{ h}}$$

$$x = \frac{5 \text{ mL}}{100 \text{ h}}$$

$$x = 5 \text{ mL/h}$$

> **❗ ● ALERT**
>
> Medications ordered by units per hour, international units per hour, or units per kilogram per hour must be delivered with an IV controller or pump for safe administration.

Therefore the nurse will program the IV pump for 5 mL/h, and the insulin will be infused at a rate of 5 units/h.

EXAMPLE 2: A patient with a femoral thrombus has an order for heparin IV at 1200 units/h. The concentration is heparin 20,000 units in 250 mL of D_5W. At what rate, in milliliters per hour, should the IV pump be programmed?

a. On the left side of the equation, place what you are solving for.

$$x \text{ mL/h} =$$

b. On the right side of the equation, place the available information related to the measurement or abbreviation that was placed on the left side. In this example the measurement we are solving for is *mL/h*. We will deal with the numerator portion of our answer first, the mL. We know from the problem that there are 20,000 units of heparin in 250 mL. This information is placed in the equation as a fraction, with the numerators matching.

$$\frac{x \text{ mL}}{h} = \frac{250 \text{ mL}}{20,000 \text{ units}}$$

c. Next, find the information that matches the measurement used in the denominator of the fraction you created. In this example, *units* is the denominator. The order is for 1200 units/h. The equation now looks like

$$\frac{x \text{ mL}}{h} = \frac{250 \text{ mL}}{20,000 \text{ units}} \times \frac{1200 \text{ units}}{1 \text{ h}}$$

d. Then cancel out the like abbreviations on the right side of the equation. If you have set up the problem correctly, the remaining measurements should match the measurements on the left side of the equation. Now solve for x.

$$\frac{x \text{ mL}}{h} = \frac{250 \text{ mL}}{20,000 \text{ units}} \times \frac{1200 \text{ units}}{1 \text{ h}}$$

$$x = \frac{250 \text{ mL} \times 1200}{20,000 \text{ h}}$$

$$x = \frac{300,000 \text{ mL}}{20,000 \text{ h}}$$

$$x = 15 \text{ mL/h}$$

Therefore the nurse will program the IV pump for 15 mL/h, and the heparin will be infused at a rate of 1200 units/h.

Calculating Units/Hours from Milliliters/Hour—
Dimensional Analysis Method

EXAMPLE 1: A patient has a continuous insulin infusion at 8 mL/h. The insulin concentration is regular insulin 100 units in 200 mL of 0.9% NS. The nurse needs to calculate how many units per hour of insulin the patient is receiving.

a. On the left side of the equation, place what you are solving for:

$$\frac{x \text{ units}}{h} =$$

b. On the right side of the equation, place the available information related to the measurement that was placed on the left side. In this example, the measurement we are solving for is *units/h*. We will deal with the numerator portion of our answer first, the *units*. We know from the problem that that there are 100 units of regular insulin in 200 mL of 0.9% NS. This information is placed in the equation as a fraction, with the numerators matching.

$$\frac{x \text{ units}}{h} = \frac{100 \text{ units}}{200 \text{ mL}}$$

c. Next, find the information that matches the measurement used in the denominator of the fraction you created. In this example, *mL* is in the denominator, so 8 mL/h is used. The equation now looks like

$$\frac{x \text{ units}}{h} = \frac{100 \text{ units}}{200 \text{ mL}} \times \frac{8 \text{ mL}}{h}$$

d. Then cancel out the like abbreviations on the right side of the equation. If you have set up the problem correctly, the remaining measurements should match the measurements on the left side of the equation. Now solve for *x*.

$$\frac{x \text{ units}}{h} = \frac{100 \text{ units}}{200 \text{ mL}} \times \frac{8 \text{ mL}}{h}$$

$$\frac{x \text{ units}}{h} = \frac{100 \times 8}{200}$$

$$x = 4 \text{ units/h}$$

Therefore the patient is receiving 4 units/h of regular insulin.

EXAMPLE 2: A patient has a continuous heparin infusion at 14 mL/h. The heparin concentration is heparin 25,000 units/250 mL of 0.9% NS. The nurse needs to calculate how many units per hour of heparin the patient is receiving.

a. On the left side of the equation, place what you are solving for:

$$\frac{x \text{ units}}{h} =$$

b. On the right side of the equation, place the available information related to the measurement or abbreviation that was placed on the left side of the equation. In this example, the measurement we are solving for is *units/h*. We will deal with the numerator portion of our answer first, the *units*. We know from the problem that there are 25,000 units of heparin in 250 mL of 0.9% NS. This information is placed in the equation as a fraction, with the numerators matching.

$$\frac{x \text{ units}}{h} = \frac{25,000 \text{ units}}{250 \text{ mL}}$$

c. Next, find the information that matches the measurement used in the denominator of the fraction you created. In this example, *mL* is in the denominator, so 14 mL/h is used. The equation now looks like

$$\frac{x \text{ units}}{h} = \frac{25,000 \text{ units}}{250 \text{ mL}} \times \frac{14 \text{ mL}}{h}$$

d. Then cancel out the like abbreviations on the right side of the equation. If you have set up the problem correctly, the remaining measurements should match the measurements on the left side of the equation. Now solve for *x*.

$$\frac{x \text{ units}}{h} = \frac{25,000 \text{ units}}{250 \text{ mL}} \times \frac{14 \text{ mL}}{h}$$

$$\frac{x \text{ units}}{h} = \frac{25,000 \times 14}{250}$$

$$x = 1400 \text{ units/h}$$

Therefore the patient is receiving heparin at 1400 units/h.

Calculating Weight-Based Heparin—Dimensional Analysis Method

EXAMPLE 1: The order is to start a heparin infusion using the heparin protocol. The patient's weight is 143 lb. Using the weight-based heparin protocol example below, the nurse needs to do two calculations: the heparin bolus and the rate, in milliliters per hour, at which to program the IV pump.

Weight-Based Heparin Protocol (Example)

1. Bolus dose of 70 units/kg, rounded to the nearest 100 units (e.g., 6850 units would be rounded to 6900 units).
2. Begin infusion of heparin at 17 units/kg/h (25,000 units/250 mL = 100 units/mL).
3. Obtain partial thromboplastin time (PTT) every 6 hours, and adjust the infusion using the following scale:

PTT Result	Heparin Dosing
<35	Bolus 70 units/kg and increase drip by 4 units/kg/h
35–54	Bolus 35 units/kg and increase drip by 3 units/kg/h
55–85	Therapeutic—no change
86–100	Decrease drip by 2 units/kg/h
>100	Hold infusion 1 hour; decrease drip by 3 units/kg/h, then restart drip

Bolus. The protocol calls for 70 units/kg, rounded to the nearest hundred.

a. On the left side of the equation, place what you are solving for.

$$x \text{ units} =$$

b. On the right side of the equation, place the available information related to the measurement that was placed on the left side. In this example, the measurement we are solving for is *units*. We will deal with the numerator portion of our answer first, the *units*. We know from the protocol that 70 units/kg is needed; this information is placed in the equation, with the numerators matching.

$$x \text{ units} = \frac{70 \text{ units}}{1 \text{ kg}}$$

c. Next, find the information that matches the measurement used in the denominator of the fraction you created. In this example, *kg* is the denominator. The conversion of 1 kg = 2.2 lb is used as the next fraction. The equation now looks like

$$x \text{ units} = \frac{70 \text{ units}}{\text{kg}} \times \frac{1 \text{ kg}}{2.2 \text{ lb}}$$

d. Next, the *lb* in the denominator must be canceled out. We know from the problem that the patient weighs 143 lb.

$$x \text{ units} = \frac{70 \text{ units}}{1 \text{ kg}} \times \frac{1 \text{ kg}}{2.2 \text{ lb}} \times \frac{143 \text{ lb}}{1}$$

e. Then cancel out the like abbreviations on the right side of the equation. If you have set up the problem correctly, the remaining measurement should match the measurement on the left side of the equation. Now solve for *x*.

$$x \text{ units} = \frac{70 \text{ units}}{\cancel{\text{kg}}} \times \frac{1 \cancel{\text{ kg}}}{2.2 \cancel{\text{ lb}}} \times \frac{143 \cancel{\text{ lb}}}{1}$$

$$x \text{ units} = \frac{70 \times 143}{2.2}$$

$$x \text{ units} = \frac{10{,}010}{2.2}$$

$$x = 4550 \text{ or } 4600 \text{ units IV bolus}$$

IV Infusion. The health care provider needs to calculate how many milliliters are needed to deliver 17 units/kg (protocol states 17 units/kg/h, rounded to the nearest tenth).

a. On the left side of the equation, place what you are solving for.

$$x \frac{\text{mL}}{\text{h}} =$$

b. On the right side of the equation, place the available information related to the measurement or abbreviation that was placed on the left side. In this example the measurement we are solving for is *mL*. We know from the protocol that there are 100 units of heparin in 1 mL. This information is placed in the equation with the numerators matching.

$$x \frac{\text{mL}}{\text{h}} = \frac{1 \text{ mL}}{100 \text{ units}}$$

c. Next, find the information that matches the measurement used in the denominator of the fraction you created. In this example, *units* is the denominator. The order is for 17 units/kg/h. The equation now looks like

$$x \frac{\text{mL}}{\text{h}} = \frac{1 \text{ mL}}{100 \text{ units}} \times \frac{17 \text{ units}}{\text{kg/h}}$$

d. Now, the kg is the denominator that needs to be canceled. The conversion of 1 kg = 2.2 lb is used as the next fraction. Continue this process until all the denominators can be canceled.

$$x \frac{\text{mL}}{\text{h}} = \frac{1 \text{ mL}}{100 \text{ units}} \times \frac{17 \text{ units}}{\text{kg/h}} \times \frac{1 \text{ kg}}{2.2 \text{ lb}} \times \frac{143 \text{ lb}}{1}$$

e. Then cancel out the like abbreviations on the right side of the equation. If you have set up the problem correctly, the remaining measurement should match the measurement on the left side of the equation. Now solve for x.

$$x\ \frac{\text{mL}}{\text{h}} = \frac{1\ \text{mL}}{100\ \cancel{\text{units}}} \times \frac{17\ \cancel{\text{units}}}{\cancel{\text{kg}}/\text{h}} \times \frac{1\ \cancel{\text{kg}}}{2.2\ \cancel{\text{lb}}} \times \frac{143\ \cancel{\text{lb}}}{1}$$

$$x\ \frac{\text{mL}}{\text{h}} = \frac{17 \times 143}{100 \times 2.2}$$

$$x\ \frac{\text{mL}}{\text{h}} = \frac{2431}{220}$$

$$x = 11.1 \text{ or } 11 \text{ mL/h}$$

Therefore the nurse will program the IV pump for 11.1 mL/h, and the heparin will be infused at a rate of 17 units/kg/h.

> **! ALERT**
>
> An IV machine is required for medications that are titrated.

Facilities that administer high-risk medications have IV controllers that allow the health care professional to program medication rates with a decimal. Therefore answers should be **rounded to the nearest tenth decimal place.**

Calculating Milliliters/Hour from Units/Hour— Ratio-Proportion and Formula Methods

EXAMPLE 1: 200 units of regular insulin have been added to 500 mL of 0.9% normal saline (NS). The order states to infuse the regular insulin IV at 10 units/h. The nurse needs to calculate how many milliliters per hour the IV pump should be programmed for.

Using the Ratio-Proportion Method

$$\text{(Formula setup)} \quad 200 \text{ units} : 500 \text{ mL} :: 10 \text{ units} : x \text{ mL}$$

$$200x = 5000$$

$$x = \frac{5000}{200}$$

$$x = 25 \text{ mL}$$

Therefore the nurse will program the IV pump for 25 mL/h to infuse the insulin at 10 units/h.

Using the $\frac{\text{D}}{\text{A}} \times \text{Q}$ Method

$$\text{(Formula setup)} \quad \frac{10 \text{ units}}{200 \text{ units}} \times 500 \text{ mL} = x \text{ mL}$$

$$\text{(Cancel)} \quad \frac{10 \ \cancel{\text{units}}}{\underset{2}{\cancel{200}} \ \cancel{\text{units}}} \times \overset{5}{\cancel{500}} \text{ mL} = x \text{ mL}$$

$$\text{(Calculate)} \quad \frac{50}{2} = 25 \text{ mL}$$

EXAMPLE 2: 25,000 units of heparin have been added to 250 mL of dextrose 5% in water (D_5W). The order is to infuse the heparin drip at 2000 units/h. The health care provider needs to calculate how many milliliters per hour to program the IV pump for.

Using the Ratio-Proportion Method

(Formula setup)   25,000 units : 250 mL :: 2000 units : x mL

$$25,000x = 500,000$$

$$x = \frac{500,\cancel{000}}{25,\cancel{000}}$$

$$x = \frac{500}{25}$$

$$x = 20 \text{ mL}$$

Therefore the nurse will program the IV pump for 20 mL/h to deliver the heparin at 2000 units/h.

Using the $\frac{D}{A} \times Q$ Method

(Formula setup) $\dfrac{2000 \text{ units}}{25,000 \text{ units}} \times 250 \text{ mL} = x \text{ mL}$

(Cancel) $\dfrac{2000 \cancel{\text{ units}}}{\underset{100}{\cancel{25,000} \cancel{\text{ units}}}} \times \overset{1}{\cancel{250}} \text{ mL} = x \text{ mL}$

(Calculate) $\dfrac{2000 \text{ mL}}{100} = 20 \text{ mL}$

Calculating Units/Hour from Milliliter/Hour—Ratio-Proportion and Formula Methods

EXAMPLE 1: A patient has a continuous insulin drip infusing at 8 mL/h. The insulin concentration is regular insulin 100 units in 200 mL of 0.9% NS. The nurse needs to calculate how many units per hour of insulin the patient is receiving.

Using the Ratio-Proportion Method

(Formula setup)   100 units : 200 mL :: x units : 8 mL

$$200x = 800$$

$$x = \frac{800}{200}$$

$$x = 4 \text{ units}$$

Therefore the patient is receiving 4 units/h of regular insulin.

EXAMPLE 2: A patient has a continuous heparin drip infusing at 14 mL/h. The heparin concentration is heparin 25,000 units/250 mL of 0.9% NS. The nurse needs to calculate how many units per hour of heparin the patient is receiving.

Using the Ratio-Proportion Method

$$\text{(Formula setup)} \quad 25{,}000 \text{ units} : 250 \text{ mL} :: x \text{ units} : 14 \text{ mL}$$

$$250x = 350{,}000$$

$$x = \frac{350{,}000}{250}$$

$$x = 1400 \text{ units}$$

Therefore the patient is receiving 1400 units/h of heparin.

> **❗ ALERT**
>
> Weight-based heparin requires 2 calculations: bolus and infusion.

Calculating Weight-Based Heparin—Ratio-Proportion and Formula Methods

Weight-Based Heparin Protocol (Example)

1. Bolus dose of 70 units/kg, rounded to the nearest 100 units (e.g., 6850 units would be rounded to 6900 units).
2. Begin infusion of heparin at 17 units/kg/h (25,000 units/250 mL = 100 units/mL).
3. Obtain partial thromboplastin time (PTT) every 6 hours, and adjust the infusion using the following scale:

PTT Result	Heparin Dosing
<35	Bolus 70 units/kg and increase drip by 4 units/kg/h
35-54	Bolus 35 units/kg and increase drip by 3 units/kg/h
55-85	Therapeutic—no change
86-100	Decrease drip by 2 units/kg/h
>100	Hold infusion 1 hour; decrease drip by 3 units/kg/h, then restart drip

EXAMPLE: The order is to start a heparin infusion using the heparin protocol. The patient's weight is 143 lb. The nurse needs to do two calculations: the heparin bolus and the rate, in milliliters per hour, at which to program the IV pump.

Bolus. The protocol calls for 70 units/kg, rounded to the nearest hundred.

    a. Convert pounds to kilograms.

$$\text{(Formula setup)} \quad 2.2 \text{ lb} : 1 \text{ kg} :: 143 \text{ lb} : x \text{ kg}$$

$$2.2x = 143$$

$$x = \frac{143}{2.2}$$

$$x = 65 \text{ kg}$$

    b. Calculate the units required for the IV bolus.

$$\text{(Formula setup)} \quad 1 \text{ kg} : 70 \text{ units} :: 65 \text{ kg} : x \text{ units}$$

$$x = 70 \times 65$$

$$x = 4550 \text{ or } 4600 \text{ units IV bolus}$$

IV Infusion. The protocol states 17 units/kg/h, rounded to the nearest tenth.

 a. Calculate how many units are needed for a patient weighing 65 kg.

$$\text{(Formula setup)} \quad 1 \text{ kg} : 17 \text{ units/h} :: 65 \text{ kg} : x \text{ units/h}$$

$$x = 17 \times 65$$

$$x = 1105$$

The formula shows that 1105 units/h are required for a 65-kg patient.

 b. Calculate mL/hr for the IV pump.

Using the Ratio-Proportion Method

$$\text{(Formula setup)} \quad 100 \text{ units} : 1 \text{ mL} :: 1105 \text{ units} : x \text{ mL}$$

$$100x = 1105$$

$$x = \frac{1105}{100}$$

$$x = 11.1 \text{ or } 11 \text{ mL/h}$$

Therefore the nurse will set the IV pump for 11.1 mL/h to infuse the heparin at 17 units/kg/h.

Using $\frac{D}{A} \times Q$ Method

$$\text{(Formula setup)} \quad \frac{1105 \text{ units}}{100 \text{ units}} \times 1 \text{ mL} = x \text{ mL}$$

$$\text{(Cancel)} \quad \frac{1105 \text{ units}}{100 \text{ units}} \times 1 \text{ mL} = x \text{ mL}$$

$$\text{(Calculate)} \quad \frac{1105}{100} = 11.1 \text{ or } 11 \text{ mL/h}$$

Complete the following work sheet, which provides for practice of intravenous flow rates for dosages measured in units. Check your answers. If you have difficulties, go back and review the necessary material. An acceptable score as indicated on the posttest signifies that you have successfully completed the chapter. An unacceptable score signifies a need for further study before taking the second posttest.

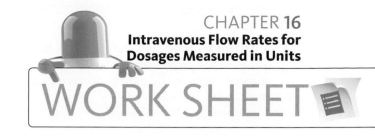

WORK SHEET

DIRECTIONS: The IV fluid order is listed in each problem. Calculate the IV flow rates using the appropriate formula required for the problem.

1. Mr. Sinks has undergone aortic valve repair and has orders for heparin at 1000 units/h. The concentration is heparin 25,000 units in 250 mL of 0.9% NS. How many milliliters per hour should the IV pump be programmed for? _____

2. You have an order for your patient with diabetes to receive regular insulin IV at 12 units/h. The concentration is insulin 100 units in 250 mL of 0.9% NS. How many milliliters per hour should the IV pump be programmed for? _____

3. The insulin order for the patient in problem 2 is reduced to 8 units/h. How many milliliters per hour should the IV pump be programmed for? _____

4. A patient who has undergone mitral valve repair has heparin ordered at 1000 units/h. The concentration is heparin 10,000 units in 500 mL of D_5W. How many milliliters per hour should the IV pump be programmed for? _____

5. Ms. Moreno has a brachial thrombus and has streptokinase ordered at 100,000 international units/h. The concentration is 250,000 international units of streptokinase in 45 mL of 0.9% NS. How many milliliters per hour should the IV pump be programmed for? _____

6. A patient with deep vein thrombosis has a heparin infusion at 15 mL/h. The heparin concentration is 25,000 units in 500 mL of D_5W. How many units per hour is the patient receiving? _____

7. A patient with diabetic ketoacidosis has a continuous insulin drip at 10 mL/h. The insulin comes in a concentration of 100 units of regular insulin in 100 mL of 0.9% NS. How many units per hour is the patient receiving? _____

8. The physician orders heparin per protocol (use protocol on p. 462). The patient's weight is 60 kg.

Bolus:

Infusion:

9. Six hours after the heparin protocol is begun (see question 8), the activated PTT (aPTT) returns at 98 seconds. Using the protocol on p. 462, does the heparin need to be changed? _____

Bolus:

Infusion:

10. The physician orders heparin per protocol (use protocol on p. 462). The patient's weight is 80 kg. Calculate the heparin bolus and infusion.

Bolus:

Infusion:

11. Six hours after the heparin protocol is begun (see question 10), the aPTT returns at 48 seconds. Using the protocol on p. 462, does the heparin need to be changed? _____

Bolus:

Infusion:

ANSWERS ON PP. 474 AND 475–477.

NAME _____

DATE _____

ACCEPTABLE SCORE ___4___

YOUR SCORE _____

POSTTEST 1

DIRECTIONS: The IV fluid order is listed in each problem. Calculate the appropriate rate for each problem.

1. Your patient with diabetes has an order for regular insulin IV at 9 units/h. The concentration is insulin 500 units in 500 mL of 0.9% NS. How many milliliters per hour should the IV pump be programmed for? _____

2. Mrs. Allen has deep vein thrombosis and has an order for heparin at 800 units/h. The concentration is heparin 50,000 units in 500 mL of D$_5$W. How many milliliters per hour should the IV pump be programmed for? _____

3. A patient with a thrombosis has a heparin infusion at 15 mL/h. The heparin concentration is 25,000 units in 250 mL of D$_5$W. How many units per hour is the patient receiving? _____

4. Begin heparin per protocol (use protocol example on p. 462). Patient's weight is 105 kg.

   Bolus:

   Infusion:

ANSWERS ON PP. 474 AND 477.

NAME _____

DATE _____

ACCEPTABLE SCORE ___4___

YOUR SCORE _____

POSTTEST 2

DIRECTIONS: The IV fluid order is listed in each problem. Calculate the rate needed in each problem to deliver the correct dose.

1. A patient with a pulmonary embolus has an order for streptokinase to be infused at 100,000 international units/h. The concentration is streptokinase 750,000 international units in 200 mL of 0.9% NS. How many milliliters per hour should the IV pump be programmed for? _____

2. A patient with diabetic ketoacidosis has a continuous insulin drip at 6 mL/h. The insulin comes in a concentration of 100 units of regular insulin in 200 mL of 0.9% NS. How many units per hour is the patient receiving? _____

3. Your patient has a blood clot in his arm, and the physician has ordered heparin to be infused at 1500 units/h. The concentration is heparin 20,000 units in 200 mL of D_5W. How many milliliters per hour should the IV pump be programmed for? _____

4. Begin heparin per protocol (use protocol example on p. 462). The patient's weight is 75 kg.

   Bolus:

   Infusion:

ANSWERS ON PP. 475 AND 478.

evolve For additional practice problems, refer to the Advanced Calculations section of *Drug Calculations Companion,* Version 5, on Evolve.

ANSWERS

CHAPTER 16 Dimensional Analysis—Work Sheet, pp. 469–470

1. $\dfrac{x \text{ mL}}{h} = \dfrac{250 \text{ mL}}{25,000 \text{ units}} \times \dfrac{1000 \text{ units}}{1 \text{ h}} = 10 \text{ mL/h}$

2. $\dfrac{x \text{ mL}}{h} = \dfrac{250 \text{ mL}}{100 \text{ units}} \times \dfrac{12 \text{ units}}{1 \text{ h}} = 30 \text{ mL/h}$

3. $\dfrac{x \text{ mL}}{h} = \dfrac{250 \text{ mL}}{100 \text{ units}} \times \dfrac{8 \text{ units}}{1 \text{ h}} = 20 \text{ mL/h}$

4. $\dfrac{x \text{ mL}}{h} = \dfrac{500 \text{ mL}}{10,000 \text{ units}} \times \dfrac{1000 \text{ units}}{1 \text{ h}} = 50 \text{ mL/h}$

5. $\dfrac{x \text{ mL}}{h} = \dfrac{45 \text{ mL}}{250,000 \text{ IU}} \times \dfrac{100,000 \text{ IU}}{1 \text{ h}} = 18 \text{ mL/h}$

6. $\dfrac{x \text{ units}}{h} = \dfrac{25,000 \text{ units}}{500 \text{ mL}} \times \dfrac{15 \text{ mL}}{1 \text{ h}} = 750 \text{ units/h}$

7. $\dfrac{x \text{ units}}{h} = \dfrac{100 \text{ units}}{100 \text{ mL}} \times \dfrac{10 \text{ mL}}{1 \text{ h}} = 10 \text{ units/h}$

8. Bolus: $x \text{ units} = \dfrac{70 \text{ units}}{1 \text{ kg}} \times 60 \text{ kg} = 4200 \text{ units}$

   Infusion: $\dfrac{x \text{ mL}}{h} = \dfrac{1 \text{ mL}}{100 \text{ units}} \times \dfrac{17 \text{ units}}{1 \text{ kg/h}} \times \dfrac{60 \text{ kg}}{1} = 10.2 \text{ or } 10 \text{ mL/h}$

9. Yes, the heparin drip needs to be reduced by 2 units/kg/h.
   Bolus: No bolus is needed.

   Infusion: $\dfrac{x \text{ mL}}{h} = \dfrac{1 \text{ mL}}{100 \text{ units}} \times \dfrac{15 \text{ units}}{1 \text{ kg/h}} \times \dfrac{60 \text{ kg}}{1} = 9 \text{ mL/h}$

10. Bolus: $x \text{ units} = \dfrac{70 \text{ units}}{1 \text{ kg}} \times 80 \text{ kg} = 5600 \text{ units}$

    Infusion: $\dfrac{x \text{ mL}}{h} = \dfrac{1 \text{ mL}}{100 \text{ units}} \times \dfrac{17 \text{ units}}{1 \text{ kg/h}} \times \dfrac{80 \text{ kg}}{1} = 13.6 \text{ or } 14 \text{ mL/h}$

11. Yes, provide a bolus of 35 units/kg and increase the heparin drip by 3 units/kg/h.
    Bolus: $x \text{ units} = \dfrac{35 \text{ units}}{1 \text{ kg}} \times 80 \text{ kg} = 2800 \text{ units}$

    Infusion: $\dfrac{x \text{ mL}}{h} = \dfrac{1 \text{ mL}}{100 \text{ units}} \times \dfrac{20 \text{ units}}{1 \text{ kg/h}} \times \dfrac{80 \text{ kg}}{1} = 16 \text{ mL/h}$

CHAPTER 16 Dimensional Analysis—Posttest 1, p. 471

1. $\dfrac{x \text{ mL}}{h} = \dfrac{500 \text{ mL}}{500 \text{ units}} \times \dfrac{9 \text{ units}}{1 \text{ h}} = 9 \text{ mL/h}$

2. $\dfrac{x \text{ mL}}{h} = \dfrac{500 \text{ mL}}{50,000 \text{ units}} \times \dfrac{800 \text{ units}}{1 \text{ h}} = 8 \text{ mL/h}$

3. $\dfrac{x \text{ units}}{h} = \dfrac{25,000 \text{ units}}{250 \text{ mL}} \times \dfrac{15 \text{ mL}}{1 \text{ h}} = 1500 \text{ units/h}$

4. Bolus: $x \text{ units} = \dfrac{70 \text{ units}}{1 \text{ kg}} \times 105 \text{ kg} = 7350 \text{ or } 7400 \text{ units}$

   Infusion: $\dfrac{x \text{ mL}}{h} = \dfrac{1 \text{ mL}}{100 \text{ units}} \times \dfrac{17 \text{ units}}{1 \text{ kg/h}} \times \dfrac{105 \text{ kg}}{1} = 17.9 \text{ or } 18 \text{ mL/h}$

CHAPTER 16 Dimensional Analysis—Posttest 2, p. 473

1. $\dfrac{x \text{ mL}}{\text{h}} = \dfrac{200 \text{ mL}}{750,000 \text{ units}} \times \dfrac{100,000 \text{ units}}{1 \text{ h}} = 26.7 \text{ or } 27 \text{ mL/h}$

2. $\dfrac{x \text{ units}}{\text{h}} = \dfrac{100 \text{ units}}{200 \text{ mL}} \times \dfrac{6 \text{ mL}}{1 \text{ h}} = 3 \text{ units/h}$

3. $\dfrac{x \text{ mL}}{\text{h}} = \dfrac{200 \text{ mL}}{20,000 \text{ units}} \times \dfrac{1500 \text{ units}}{1 \text{ h}} = 15 \text{ mL/h}$

4. Bolus: $x \text{ units} = \dfrac{70 \text{ units}}{1 \text{ kg}} \times \dfrac{75 \text{ kg}}{1} = 5250 \text{ or } 5300 \text{ units}$

   Infusion: $\dfrac{x \text{ mL}}{\text{h}} = \dfrac{1 \text{ mL}}{100 \text{ units}} \times \dfrac{17 \text{ units}}{1 \text{ kg/h}} \times \dfrac{75 \text{ kg}}{1} = 12.8 \text{ or } 13 \text{ mL/h}$

CHAPTER 16 Proportion/Formula Method—Work Sheet, pp. 469–470

Proportion	Formula

1. $25,000 \text{ units} : 250 \text{ mL} :: 1000 \text{ units} : x \text{ mL}$
   $25,000x = 250,000$
   $x = \dfrac{250,000}{25,000}$
   $x = 10 \text{ mL/h}$

   $\dfrac{1000 \text{ units}}{\overset{100}{\cancel{25,000}} \text{ units}} \times \overset{1}{\cancel{250}} \text{ mL} =$
   $\dfrac{1000}{100} = 10 \text{ mL/h}$

2. $100 \text{ units} : 250 \text{ mL} :: 12 \text{ units} : x \text{ mL}$
   $100x = 3000$
   $x = \dfrac{3000}{100}$
   $x = 30 \text{ mL/h}$

   $\dfrac{12 \text{ units}}{\underset{2}{\cancel{100}} \text{ units}} \times \overset{5}{\cancel{250}} \text{ mL} =$
   $\dfrac{60}{2} = 30 \text{ mL/h}$

3. $100 \text{ units} : 250 \text{ mL} :: 8 \text{ units} : x \text{ mL}$
   $100x = 2000$
   $x = \dfrac{2000}{100}$
   $x = 20 \text{ mL/h}$

   $\dfrac{8 \text{ units}}{\underset{2}{\cancel{100}} \text{ units}} \times \overset{5}{\cancel{250}} \text{ mL} =$
   $\dfrac{40}{2} = 20 \text{ mL/h}$

4. $10,000 \text{ units} : 500 \text{ mL} :: 1000 \text{ units} : x \text{ mL}$
   $10,000x - 500,000$
   $x = \dfrac{500,000}{10,000}$
   $x = 50 \text{ mL/h}$

   $\dfrac{1000 \text{ units}}{\underset{20}{\cancel{10,000}} \text{ units}} \times \overset{1}{\cancel{500}} \text{ mL} =$
   $\dfrac{1000}{20} = 50 \text{ mL/h}$

5. $250,000 \text{ IU} : 45 \text{ mL} :: 100,000 \text{ IU} : x \text{ mL}$
   $250,000x = 4,500,000$
   $x = \dfrac{4,500,000}{250,000}$
   $x = 18 \text{ mL/h}$

   $\dfrac{\overset{10}{\cancel{100,000}} \text{ IU}}{\underset{25}{\cancel{250,000}} \text{ IU}} \times 45 \text{ mL} =$
   $\dfrac{450}{25} = 18 \text{ mL/h}$

6. $25,000 \text{ units} : 500 \text{ mL} :: x \text{ units} : 15 \text{ mL}$
   $500x = 375,000$
   $x = \dfrac{375,000}{500}$
   $x = 750 \text{ units/h}$

ANSWERS

Proportion	Formula

7. 100 units : 100 mL :: x units : 10 mL
   $100x = 1000$
   $$x = \frac{1000}{100}$$
   $x = 10$ units/h

8. Bolus: 1 kg : 70 units :: 60 kg : x units
   $x = 4200$ units IV bolus

   Infusion: *Step 1*
   1 kg : 17 units/h :: 60 kg : x units/h
   $x = 17(60) = 1020$ units/h

   Step 2
   100 units : 1 mL :: 1020 units : x mL $\dfrac{1020 \text{ units}}{100 \text{ units}} \times 1 \text{ mL} = 10.2$ or 10 mL/h
   $100x = 1020$
   $$x = \frac{1020}{100}$$
   $x = 10.2$ or 10 mL/h

9. Yes, the heparin drip needs to be reduced by
   2 units/kg/h.
   Bolus: No bolus is needed.
   Infusion: *Step 1* (17 units/kg/h − 2 units/kg/h =
   15 units/kg/h)
   1 kg : 15 units/h :: 60 kg : x units/h
   $x = 900$ units/h

   Step 2
   100 units : 1 mL :: 900 units : x mL $\dfrac{900 \text{ units}}{100 \text{ units}} \times 1 \text{ mL} = 9$ mL/h
   $100x = 900$
   $$x = \frac{900}{100}$$
   $x = 9$ mL/h

10. Bolus: 1 kg : 70 units :: 80 kg : x units
    $x = 5600$ units IV bolus

    Infusion: *Step 1*
    1 kg : 17 units/h :: 80 kg : x units/h
    $x = 1360$ units/h

    Step 2
    100 units : 1 mL :: 1360 units : x mL $\dfrac{1360 \text{ units}}{100 \text{ units}} \times 1 \text{ mL} = 13.6$ or 14 mL/h
    $100x = 1360$
    $$x = \frac{1360}{100}$$
    $x = 13.6$ or 14 mL/h

ANSWERS

Proportion	Formula

11. Yes, provide a bolus of 35 units/kg and increase the heparin drip by 3 units/kg/h.

    Bolus: 1 kg : 35 units :: 80 kg : x units
                 x = 2800 units IV bolus

    Infusion: *Step 1*
              1 kg : 20 units/h :: 80 kg : x units/h
              x = 20(80) = 1600 units/h

              Step 2
              100 units : 1 mL :: 1600 units : x mL
              100x = 1600

$$x = \frac{1600}{100}$$

              x = 16 mL/h

CHAPTER 16 Proportion/Formula Method—Posttest 1, p. 471

Proportion	Formula

1. 500 units : 500 mL :: 9 units : x mL
   500x = 4500

$$x = \frac{4500}{500}$$

   x = 9 mL/h

$$\frac{\overset{9 \text{ units}}{\cancel{500} \text{ units}}}{1} \times \overset{1}{\cancel{500}} \text{ mL} =$$

$$\frac{9}{1} = 9 \text{ mL/h}$$

2. 50,000 units : 500 mL :: 800 units : x mL
   50,000x = 400,000

$$x = \frac{400,000}{50,000}$$

   x = 8 mL/h

$$\frac{800 \text{ units}}{\underset{100}{\cancel{50,000}} \text{ units}} \times \overset{1}{\cancel{500}} \text{ mL} =$$

$$\frac{800}{100} = 8 \text{ mL/h}$$

3. 25,000 units : 250 mL :: x units : 15 mL
   250x = 375,000

$$x = \frac{375,000}{250}$$

   x = 1500 units/h

4. Bolus: 1 kg : 70 units :: 105 kg : x units
              x = 7350 or 7400 units IV bolus

   Infusion: *Step 1*
            1 kg : 17 units/h :: 105 kg : x units/h
            x = 1785 units/h

            Step 2
            100 units : 1 mL :: 1785 units : x mL
            100x = 1785

$$x = \frac{1785}{100}$$

            x = 17.9 or 18 mL/h

$$\frac{1785 \text{ units}}{100 \text{ units}} \times 1 \text{ mL} = 17.9 \text{ or } 18 \text{ mL/h}$$

ANSWERS

CHAPTER 16 Proportion/Formula Method—Posttest 2, p. 473

Proportion	**Formula**

1. $750{,}000 \text{ IU} : 200 \text{ mL} :: 100{,}000 \text{ IU} : x \text{ mL}$

$750{,}000x = 20{,}000{,}000$

$x = \dfrac{20{,}000{,}000}{750{,}000}$

$x = 26.7 \text{ or } 27 \text{ mL/h}$

$\dfrac{\overset{10}{\cancel{100{,}000}} \text{ IU}}{\underset{75}{\cancel{750{,}000}} \text{ IU}} \times 200 \text{ mL} =$

$\dfrac{2000}{75} = 26.7 \text{ or } 27 \text{ mL/h}$

2. $100 \text{ units} : 200 \text{ mL} :: x \text{ units} : 6 \text{ mL}$

$200x = 600$

$x = \dfrac{600}{200}$

$x = 3 \text{ units/h}$

3. $20{,}000 \text{ units} : 200 \text{ mL} :: 1500 \text{ units} : x \text{ mL}$

$20{,}000x = 300{,}000$

$x = \dfrac{300{,}000}{20{,}000}$

$x = 15 \text{ mL/h}$

$\dfrac{1500 \text{ units}}{\underset{100}{\cancel{20{,}000}} \text{ units}} \times \overset{1}{\cancel{200}} \text{ mL} =$

$\dfrac{1500}{100} = 15 \text{ mL/h}$

4. Bolus: $1 \text{ kg} : 70 \text{ units} :: 75 \text{ kg} : x \text{ units}$

$x = 5250 \text{ or } 5300 \text{ units IV bolus}$

Infusion: *Step 1*

$1 \text{ kg} : 17 \text{ units/h} :: 75 \text{ kg} : x \text{ units/h}$

$x = 1275 \text{ units/h}$

Step 2

$100 \text{ units} : 1 \text{ mL} :: 1275 \text{ units} : x \text{ mL}$

$100x = 1275$

$x = \dfrac{1275}{100}$

$x = 12.8 \text{ or } 13 \text{ mL/h}$

$\dfrac{1275 \text{ units}}{100 \text{ units}} \times 1 \text{ mL} = 12.8 \text{ or } 13 \text{ mL/h}$

ANSWERS

CHAPTER 17

Critical Care Intravenous Flow Rates

LEARNING OBJECTIVES

Upon completion of the materials provided in this chapter, you will be able to perform computations accurately by mastering the following mathematical concepts:

1 Calculating the IV flow rate of medications in milligrams per minute

2 Calculating the IV flow rate of medications in micrograms per minute

3 Calculating the IV flow rate of medications in micrograms per kilogram per minute

4 Calculating the milligrams per minute of medications from the IV flow rate

5 Calculating the micrograms per minute of medications from the IV flow rate

6 Calculating the micrograms per kilogram per minute of medications from the IV flow rate

Critically ill patients in a hospital often receive special medications that are very potent and therefore need to be monitored closely. Some of these medications, such as regular insulin or heparin, may be ordered as a set amount of the drug measured in units to be infused over a given period. Other drugs used in the critical care setting may be ordered to be infused by amount of drug per kilogram of body weight per minute. These are called **titrations**. They are based on the manufacturer's provided recommended dosage and the patient's body weight measured in kilograms. In most health care institutions, these situations will occur in the emergency department, an intensive care unit, or a step-down unit. It is extremely important to accurately monitor the flow of these medications; therefore an intravenous (IV) machine is required. Because of the nature of these drugs, route of administration, and state of the patient, the importance of accuracy in calculating the drug dosage and IV flow rates cannot be overemphasized. It is truly a matter of life and death.

The following sections focus on medications that are ordered by micrograms per kilogram per minute (mcg/kg/min), micrograms per minute (mcg/min), and milligrams per minute (mg/min). All the following medications *must* be delivered with an IV controller or pump for safe administration. Because infusion pumps are set by milliliters per hour (mL/h), the health care provider needs to be familiar with the steps to convert the ordered drug dosage to milliliters per hour.

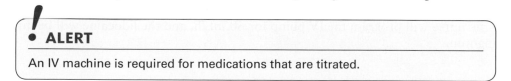

> **! ALERT**
>
> An IV machine is required for medications that are titrated.

Facilities that administer medications with a hemodynamic effect usually have IV controllers that allow the health care professional to program medication rates with a decimal. Therefore answers should be **rounded to the nearest tenth decimal place.**

Calculating Milliliters/Hour from Milligrams/Minute— Dimensional Analysis Method

EXAMPLE: Lidocaine 1 g has been added to 500 mL of D$_5$W. The order states to infuse the lidocaine at 2 mg/min. The nurse needs to calculate the rate, in milliliters per hour, at which the IV pump should be set (rounded to the nearest tenth).

a. On the left side of the equation, place what you are solving for.

$$\frac{x \text{ mL}}{\text{h}} =$$

b. On the right side of the equation, place the available information related to the measurement or abbreviation that was placed on the left side. In this example the measurement we are solving for is *mL/h*. We will deal with the numerator portion of our answer first, the *mL*. We know from the problem that there is 1 g of lidocaine in 500 mL of D$_5$W. This information becomes the first fraction of our equation. This information is placed in the equation as a fraction with the numerators matching.

$$\frac{x \text{ mL}}{\text{h}} = \frac{500 \text{ mL}}{1 \text{ g}}$$

c. Next, find the information that matches the measurement used in the denominator of the fraction you created. In this example, *g* is the denominator. The conversion of 1 g = 1000 mg is used. The equation now looks like

$$\frac{x \text{ mL}}{\text{h}} = \frac{500 \text{ mL}}{1 \text{ g}} \times \frac{1 \text{ g}}{1000 \text{ mg}}$$

d. Now, the *mg* is the denominator that needs to be canceled. The order for 2 mg/min is used as the next fraction. Continue this process until all the denominators except *hour* can be canceled.

$$\frac{x \text{ mL}}{\text{h}} = \frac{500 \text{ mL}}{1 \text{ g}} \times \frac{1 \text{ g}}{1000 \text{ mg}} \times \frac{2 \text{ mg}}{1 \text{ min}} \times \frac{60 \text{ min}}{1 \text{ h}}$$

e. Then cancel out the like abbreviations on the right side of the equation. If you have set up the problem correctly, the remaining measurement should match the measurement on the left side of the equation. Now solve for *x*.

$$\frac{x \text{ mL}}{\text{h}} = \frac{500 \text{ mL}}{1 \cancel{\text{ g}}} \times \frac{1 \cancel{\text{ g}}}{1000 \cancel{\text{ mg}}} \times \frac{2 \cancel{\text{ mg}}}{1 \cancel{\text{ min}}} \times \frac{60 \cancel{\text{ min}}}{1 \text{ h}}$$

$$\frac{x \text{ mL}}{\text{h}} = \frac{500 \times 2 \times 60}{1000}$$

$$\frac{x \text{ mL}}{\text{h}} = \frac{60,000}{1000}$$

$$x = 60 \text{ mL/h}$$

Therefore the nurse will program the IV pump for 60 mL/h, and the lidocaine will be infused at a rate of 2 mg/min.

Calculating Milliliters/Hour from Micrograms/Minute—Dimensional Analysis Method

EXAMPLE: The order is to infuse nitroglycerin at 5 mcg/min; 50 mg of nitroglycerin has been added to 500 mL of 0.9% NS. The nurse needs to calculate the rate, in milliliters per hour, at which to set the IV pump.

a. On the left side of the equation, place what you are solving for.

$$\frac{x\ \text{mL}}{\text{h}} =$$

b. On the right side of the equation, place the available information related to the measurement or abbreviation that was placed on the left side. In this example, the measurement we are solving for is *mL/h*. We will deal with the numerator portion of our answer first, the *mL*. We know from the problem that there are 50 mg of nitroglycerin in 500 mL of 0.9% NS. This information is placed in the equation as a fraction with the numerators matching.

$$\frac{x\ \text{mL}}{\text{h}} = \frac{500\ \text{mL}}{50\ \text{mg}}$$

c. Next, find the information that matches the measurement used in the denominator of the fraction you created. In this example, *mg* is the denominator. The conversion of 1 mg = 1000 mcg is used. The equation now looks like

$$\frac{x\ \text{mL}}{\text{h}} = \frac{500\ \text{mL}}{50\ \text{mg}} \times \frac{1\ \text{mg}}{1000\ \text{mcg}}$$

d. Now, *mcg* is the denominator that needs to be canceled. The order for 5 mcg/min is used as the next fraction. Continue this process until all the denominators except *hour* can be canceled.

$$\frac{x\ \text{mL}}{\text{h}} = \frac{500\ \text{mL}}{50\ \text{mg}} \times \frac{1\ \text{mg}}{1000\ \text{mcg}} \times \frac{5\ \text{mcg}}{1\ \text{min}} \times \frac{60\ \text{min}}{1\ \text{h}}$$

e. Then cancel out the like abbreviations on the right side of the equation. If you have set up the problem correctly, the remaining measurements should match the measurement on the left side of the equation. Now solve for *x*.

$$\frac{x\ \text{mL}}{\text{h}} = \frac{500\ \text{mL}}{50\ \cancel{\text{mg}}} \times \frac{1\ \cancel{\text{mg}}}{1000\ \cancel{\text{mcg}}} \times \frac{5\ \cancel{\text{mcg}}}{1\ \cancel{\text{min}}} \times \frac{60\ \cancel{\text{min}}}{1\ \text{h}}$$

$$\frac{x\ \text{mL}}{\text{h}} = \frac{500 \times 5 \times 60}{50 \times 1000}$$

$$\frac{x\ \text{mL}}{\text{h}} = \frac{150,000}{50,000}$$

$$x = 3\ \text{mL/h}$$

Therefore the nurse will program the IV pump for 3 mL/h, and the nitroglycerin will be infused at a rate of 5 mcg/min.

Calculating Milliliters/Hour from Micrograms/Kilogram/Minute—Dimensional Analysis Method

EXAMPLE: The order is to begin a dopamine infusion at 3 mcg/kg/min; 800 mg of dopamine is added to 250 mL of 0.9% NS. The patient's weight is 70 kg. The nurse needs to calculate the rate, in milliliters per hour, at which to set the IV pump.

a. On the left side of the equation, place what you are solving for.

$$\frac{x \text{ mL}}{h} =$$

b. On the right side of the equation, place the available information related to the measurement or abbreviation that was placed on the left side. In this example the measurement we are solving for is *mL/h*. We will deal with the numerator portion of our answer first: the *mL*. We know from the problem that there are 800 mg of dopamine in 250 mL of 0.9% NS. This information becomes the first fraction of our equation. This information is placed in the equation as a fraction with the numerators matching.

$$\frac{x \text{ mL}}{h} = \frac{250 \text{ mL}}{800 \text{ mg}}$$

c. Next, find the information that matches the measurement used in the denominator of the fraction you created. In this example, *mg* is the denominator. The conversion of 1 mg = 1000 mcg is used. The equation now looks like

$$\frac{x \text{ mL}}{h} = \frac{250 \text{ mL}}{800 \text{ mg}} \times \frac{1 \text{ mg}}{1000 \text{ mcg}}$$

d. Now, the mcg is the denominator that needs to be canceled. The order for 3 mcg/kg/min is used as the next fraction. Continue this process until all the denominators except *hour* can be canceled.

$$\frac{x \text{ mL}}{h} = \frac{250 \text{ mL}}{800 \text{ mg}} \times \frac{1 \text{ mg}}{1000 \text{ mcg}} \times \frac{3 \text{ mcg}}{\text{kg/min}} \times \frac{60 \text{ min}}{1 \text{ h}} \times \frac{70 \text{ kg}}{1}$$

e. Then cancel out the like abbreviations on the right side of the equation. If you have set up the problem correctly, the remaining measurements should match the measurements on the left side of the equation. Now solve for *x*.

$$\frac{x \text{ mL}}{h} = \frac{250 \text{ mL}}{800 \text{ mg}} \times \frac{1 \text{ mg}}{1000 \text{ mcg}} \times \frac{3 \text{ mcg}}{\text{kg min}} \times \frac{60 \text{ min}}{1 \text{ h}} \times \frac{70 \text{ kg}}{1}$$

$$\frac{x \text{ mL}}{h} = \frac{250 \times 3 \times 60 \times 70}{800 \times 1000}$$

$$\frac{x \text{ mL}}{h} = \frac{3,150,000}{800,000}$$

$$x = 3.9 \text{ or } 4 \text{ mL/h}$$

Therefore the nurse will program the IV pump for 3.9 mL/h, and the dopamine will be infused at a rate of 3 mcg/kg/min.

Calculations for critical care medications do not stop with taking an order and calculating milliliters per hour. A nurse may receive in report, "Mr. Douglas is receiving dopamine at 15 mL/h, which is 10 mcg/kg/min." Because the nurse administering the medication during the upcoming shift is the final link in safety, this nurse needs to be able to take the milliliters per hour and calculate the exact dose of dopamine the patient is receiving. This situation also can be applied to medications that are ordered in milligrams per minute and micrograms per minute.

Calculating Milligrams/Minute from Milliliters/Hour— Dimensional Analysis Method

EXAMPLE: A patient is receiving lidocaine at 60 mL/h. The concentration of lidocaine is 1 g/500 mL of D$_5$W. The nurse needs to calculate the milligrams per minute the patient is receiving.

a. On the left side of the equation, place what you are solving for:

$$\frac{x \text{ mg}}{\text{min}} =$$

b. On the right side of the equation, place the available information related to the measurement or abbreviation that was placed on the left side. In this example the measurement we are solving for is *mg/min*. We will deal with the numerator portion of our answer first, the *mg*. Milligrams are not in the problem, but grams are, so the first fraction created for the equation will be the conversion between milligrams and grams. This information is placed in the equation as a fraction with the numerators matching.

$$\frac{x \text{ mg}}{\text{min}} = \frac{1000 \text{ mg}}{1 \text{ g}}$$

c. Next, find the information that matches the measurement used in the denominator of the fraction you created. In this example, g is in the denominator, so 1 g of lidocaine in 500 mL D$_5$W is used. Continue this process until all of the denominators except *minute* can be canceled.

$$\frac{x \text{ mg}}{\text{min}} = \frac{1000 \text{ mg}}{1 \text{ g}} \times \frac{1 \text{ g}}{500 \text{ mL}} \times \frac{60 \text{ mL}}{1 \text{ h}} \times \frac{1 \text{ h}}{60 \text{ min}}$$

d. Then cancel out the abbreviations on the right side of the equation. If you have set up the problem correctly, the remaining measurements should match the measurement on the left side of the equation. Now solve for *x*.

$$\frac{x \text{ mg}}{\text{min}} = \frac{1000 \text{ mg}}{1 \text{ \cancel{g}}} \times \frac{1 \text{ \cancel{g}}}{500 \text{ \cancel{mL}}} \times \frac{60 \text{ \cancel{mL}}}{1 \text{ \cancel{h}}} \times \frac{1 \text{ \cancel{h}}}{60 \text{ min}}$$

$$\frac{x \text{ mg}}{\text{min}} = \frac{1000 \times 60}{500 \times 60}$$

$$x = 2 \text{ mg/min}$$

Therefore when the lidocaine is infusing at 60 mL/h, the patient is receiving a lidocaine dose of 2 mg/min.

Calculating Micrograms/Minute from Milliliters/Hour—Dimensional Analysis Method

EXAMPLE: A patient is receiving nitroglycerin at 3 mL/h. The concentration of nitroglycerin is 50 mg in 500 mL of 0.9% NS. The nurse needs to calculate the micrograms per minute the patient is receiving.

a. On the left side of the equation, place what you are solving for:

$$\frac{x \text{ mcg}}{\text{min}} =$$

b. On the right side of the equation, place the available information related to the measurement or abbreviation that was placed on the left side. In this example the measurement we are solving for is *mcg/min*. We will deal with the numerator portion of our answer first, the *mcg*. Micrograms are not in the problem, but milligrams are, so the first fraction will be the conversion between micrograms and milligrams. This information is placed in the equation as a fraction, with the numerators matching.

$$\frac{x \text{ mcg}}{\min} = \frac{1000 \text{ mcg}}{1 \text{ mg}}$$

c. Next, find the information that matches the measurement used in the denominator of the fraction you created. In this example, *mg* is in the denominator, so 50 mg of nitroglycerin in 500 mL 0.9% NS is used. Continue this process until all of the denominators except for *minute* can be canceled.

$$\frac{x \text{ mcg}}{\min} = \frac{1000 \text{ mcg}}{1 \text{ mg}} \times \frac{50 \text{ mg}}{500 \text{ mL}} \times \frac{3 \text{ mL}}{1 \text{ h}} \times \frac{1 \text{ h}}{60 \text{ min}}$$

d. Then cancel out the abbreviations on the right side of the equation. If you have set up the problem correctly, the remaining measurements should match the measurement on the left side of the equation. Now solve for *x*.

$$\frac{x \text{ mcg}}{\min} = \frac{1000 \text{ mcg}}{1 \text{ mg}} \times \frac{50 \text{ mg}}{500 \text{ mL}} \times \frac{3 \text{ mL}}{1 \text{ h}} \times \frac{1 \text{ h}}{60 \text{ min}}$$

$$\frac{x \text{ mcg}}{\min} = \frac{1000 \times 50 \times 3}{500 \times 60}$$

$$x = 5 \text{ mcg/min}$$

Therefore when the nitroglycerin is infusing at 3 mL/h, the patient is receiving a nitroglycerin dose of 5 mcg/min.

Calculating Micrograms/Kilogram/Minute from Milliliters/Hour—Dimensional Analysis Method

EXAMPLE: A patient is receiving dopamine at 12 mL/h. The concentration of dopamine is 200 mg in 250 mL of 0.9% NS. The nurse needs to calculate the micrograms per kilogram per minute the patient is receiving. The patient's weight is 70 kg.

a. On the left side of the equation, place what you are solving for:

$$\frac{x \text{ mcg}}{\text{kg/min}} =$$

b. On the right side of the equation, place the available information related to the measurement or abbreviation that was placed on the left side. In this example, the measurement we are solving for is *mcg/kg/min*. We will deal with the numerator portion of our answer first, the *mcg*. Micrograms are not in the problem, but milligrams are, so the first fraction will be the conversion between micrograms and milligrams. This information is placed in the equation as a fraction, with the numerators matching.

$$\frac{x \text{ mcg}}{\text{kg/min}} = \frac{1000 \text{ mcg}}{1 \text{ mg}}$$

c. Next, find the information that matches the measurement used in the denominator of the fraction you created. In this example, *mg* is in the denominator, so 200 mg of nitroglycerin in 250 mL 0.9% NS is used. Continue this process until all of the denominators except *minute* can be canceled.

$$\frac{x \text{ mcg}}{\text{kg/min}} = \frac{1000 \text{ mcg}}{1 \text{ mg}} \times \frac{200 \text{ mg}}{250 \text{ mL}} \times \frac{12 \text{ mL}}{1 \text{ h}} \times \frac{1 \text{ h}}{60 \text{ min}} \times \frac{1}{70 \text{ kg}}$$

d. Then cancel out the abbreviations on the right side of the equation. If you have set up the problem correctly, the remaining measurements should match the measurement on the left side of the equation. Now solve for *x*.

$$\frac{x \text{ mcg}}{\text{kg/min}} = \frac{1000 \text{ mcg}}{1 \text{ mg}} \times \frac{200 \text{ mg}}{250 \text{ mL}} \times \frac{12 \text{ mL}}{1 \text{ h}} \times \frac{1 \text{ h}}{60 \text{ min}} \times \frac{1}{70 \text{ kg}}$$

$$\frac{x \text{ mcg}}{\text{kg/min}} = \frac{1000 \times 200 \times 12}{250 \times 60 \times 70}$$

$$x = 2.28 \text{ rounded to } 2.3 \text{ mcg/kg/min}$$

Therefore when the dopamine is infusing at 12 mL/h, the patient is receiving a dopamine dose of 2.3 mcg/kg/min.

Calculating Milliliters/Hour from Milligrams/Minute—Formula Method

EXAMPLE: Lidocaine 1 g has been added to 500 mL of D$_5$W. The order states to infuse the lidocaine at 2 mg/min. The nurse needs to calculate the rate, in milliliters per hour, at which to set the IV pump.

$$\text{The formula: } \frac{\text{Desired mg/min} \times 60 \text{ min/h*}}{\text{Medication concentration (mg/mL)}}$$

*60 min/h is a constant fraction in the formula and represents the equivalency of 60 min = 1 h.

When this formula is used, the answer will always be expressed in milliliters per hour because the pair of values in milligrams will cancel each other, as will the pair of values in minutes.

a. Convert total g in the IV bag to mg.

$$1 \text{ g} = 1000 \text{ mg}$$

b. Calculate mL/h.

(Formula setup) $\dfrac{2 \text{ mg/min} \times 60 \text{ min/h}}{2 \text{ mg/mL}} = x \text{ mL/h}$

(Cancel) $\dfrac{\overset{1}{\cancel{2}} \text{ mg/min} \times 60 \text{ min/h}}{\underset{1}{\cancel{2}} \text{ mg/mL}} = x \text{ mL/h}$

(Calculate) $\dfrac{1 \times 60}{1} = 60 \text{ mL/h}$

Calculating Milliliters/Hour from Micrograms/Minute— Formula Method

EXAMPLE: 50 mg of nitroglycerin has been added to 500 mL of 0.9% NS. The order is to infuse the nitroglycerin at 5 mcg/min. The nurse needs to calculate the rate, in milliliters per hour, at which to set the IV pump.

$$\text{The formula: } \frac{\text{Ordered mcg/min} \times 60 \text{ min/h}}{\text{Medication concentration (mcg/mL)}}$$

When this formula is used, the answer will always be expressed in milliliters per hour because the pair of values in milligrams will cancel each other, as will the pair of values in minutes.

a. Convert total mg in the IV bag to mcg.

$$1 \text{ mg} : 1000 \text{ mcg} :: 50 \text{ mg} : x \text{ mcg}$$

$$x = 50,000 \text{ mcg}$$

b. Calculate the concentration (mcg/mL) by dividing the total mcg by the total amount of fluid in the IV bag.

$$\frac{50,000 \text{ mcg}}{500 \text{ mL}} = 100 \text{ mcg/mL}$$

c. Calculate the mL/h.

$$\text{(Formula setup)} \quad \frac{5 \text{ mcg/min} \times 60 \text{ min/h}}{100 \text{ mcg/mL}} = x \text{ mL/h}$$

$$\text{(Cancel)} \quad \frac{\overset{1}{\cancel{5}} \text{ mcg/\cancel{min}} \times 60 \text{ \cancel{min}/h}}{\underset{20}{\cancel{100}} \text{ \cancel{mcg}/mL}} = x \text{ mL/h}$$

$$\text{(Calculate)} \quad \frac{1 \times 60}{20} = \frac{60}{20} = 3 \text{ mL/h}$$

Calculating Milliliters/Hour from Micrograms/Kilogram/Minute— Formula Method

EXAMPLE: 800 mg of dopamine is added to 250 mL of 0.9% NS. The order is to begin the infusion at 3 mcg/kg/min. The patient's weight is 70 kg. The nurse needs to calculate the rate, in milliliters per hour, at which to set the IV pump.

The formula for calculating the mL/h is:

$$\frac{\text{Ordered mcg/kg/min} \times \text{Patient's weight in kg} \times 60 \text{ min/h}}{\text{Medication concentration (mcg/mL)}}$$

When this formula is used, the result will always be expressed in milliliters per hour because the pair of values in micrograms cancel each other, as do the pair of values in kilograms and the pair of values in minutes.

a. Before the medication concentration can be determined, the total mg in the IV bag must be converted to mcg.

$$1 \text{ mg} : 1000 \text{ mcg} :: 800 \text{ mg} : x \text{ mcg}$$

$$x = 800,000 \text{ mcg}$$

b. Determine the concentration (mcg/mL) by dividing the total mcg in the IV bag by the total amount of fluid in the IV bag.

$$\frac{800,000 \text{ mcg}}{250 \text{ mL}} = \frac{3200 \text{ mcg}}{1 \text{ mL}} = 3200 \text{ mcg/mL}$$

c. Calculate mL/h.

(Formula setup) $\quad \dfrac{3 \text{ mcg/kg/min} \times 70 \text{ kg} \times 60 \text{ min/h}}{3200 \text{ mcg/mL}} = x \text{ mL/h}$

(Cancel) $\quad \dfrac{3 \text{ mcg/kg/min} \times 70 \text{ kg} \times 60 \text{ min/h}}{3200 \text{ mcg/mL}} = x \text{ mL/h}$

(Calculate) $\quad \dfrac{3 \times 70 \times 60}{3200} = \dfrac{12,600}{3200} = 3.93 \text{ or } 3.9 \text{ mL/h}$

Calculations for critical care medications do not stop with taking an order and calculating milliliters per hour. A nurse may receive in report, "Mr. Douglas is receiving dopamine at 15 mL/h, which is 10 mcg/kg/min." Because the nurse administering the medication during the upcoming shift is the final link in safety, this nurse needs to be able to take the milliliters per hour and calculate the exact dose of dopamine the patient is receiving. This situation can also be applied to medications that are ordered in milligrams per minute and micrograms per minute.

Calculating Milligrams/Minute from Milliliters/Hour—Formula Method

EXAMPLE: A patient is receiving lidocaine at 60 mL/h. The concentration of lidocaine is 1 g in 500 mL of D_5W. The nurse needs to calculate the milligrams per minute the patient is receiving.

The formula: $\dfrac{\text{Concentration (mg/mL)} \times \text{Rate (mL/h)}}{60 \text{ min/h}}$

When this formula is used, the answer will always be expressed in milligrams per minute because the pair of values in milliliters cancel each other, as do the pair of values in hours.

a. Convert total g in the IV bag to mg.

$$1 \text{ g} = 1000 \text{ mg}$$

b. Calculate the concentration (mg/mL).

$$\frac{1000 \text{ mg}}{500 \text{ mL}} = 2 \text{ mg/mL}$$

c. Calculate the mg/min.

(Formula setup) $\quad \dfrac{2 \text{ mg/mL} \times 60 \text{ mL/h}}{60 \text{ min/h}}$

(Cancel) $\quad \dfrac{2 \text{ mg/mL} \times \overset{1}{\cancel{60}} \text{ mL/h}}{\underset{1}{\cancel{60}} \text{ min/h}}$

(Calculate) $\quad 2 \text{ mg/min}$

Calculating Micrograms/Minute from Milliliters/Hour— Formula Method

EXAMPLE: A patient is receiving nitroglycerin at 3 mL/h. The concentration of nitroglycerin is 50 mg in 500 mL of 0.9% NS. The nurse needs to calculate the micrograms per minute the patient is receiving.

$$\text{The formula:} \quad \frac{\text{Concentration (mcg/mL)} \times \text{Rate (mL/h)}}{60 \text{ min/h}}$$

When this formula is used, the answer will always be expressed in micrograms per minute because the pair of values in milliliters cancel each other, as do the pair of values in hours.

a. Convert total mg in the IV bag to mcg.

(Formula setup)   1 mg : 1000 mcg :: 50 mg : x mcg

$$x = 1000 \times 50$$
$$x = 50,000 \text{ mcg}$$

b. Calculate the concentration (mcg/mL).

$$\frac{50,000 \text{ mcg}}{500 \text{ mL}} = 100 \text{ mcg/mL}$$

c. Calculate the mcg/min.

(Formula setup) $\dfrac{100 \text{ mcg/mL} \times 3 \text{ mL/h}}{60 \text{ min/h}}$

(Cancel) $\dfrac{100 \text{ mcg/mL} \times \overset{1}{\cancel{3}} \text{ mL/h}}{\underset{20}{\cancel{60}} \text{ min/h}}$

(Calculate) $\dfrac{100}{20} = 5 \text{ mcg/min}$

Calculating Micrograms/Kilogram/Minute from Milliliters/Hour— Formula Method

EXAMPLE: A patient is receiving dopamine at 12 mL/h. The concentration of dopamine is 200 mg in 250 mL of 0.9% NS. The nurse needs to calculate the micrograms per kilogram per minute the patient is receiving. The patient's weight is 70 kg.

$$\text{The formula:} \quad \frac{\text{Concentration (mcg/mL)} \times \text{Rate (mL/h)}}{60 \text{ min/h} \times \text{Weight (kg)}}$$

When this formula is used, the answer will always be expressed in micrograms per kilogram per minute because the pair of values in milliliters cancel each other, as do the pair of values in hours.

a. Convert total mg in the IV bag to mcg.

(Formula setup)   1 mg : 1000 mcg :: 200 mg : x mcg

$$x = 1000 \times 200$$
$$x = 200,000 \text{ mcg}$$

b. Calculate the concentration (mcg/mL).

$$\frac{200,000 \text{ mcg}}{250 \text{ mL}} = 800 \text{ mcg/mL}$$

c. Calculate the mcg/kg/min.

(Formula setup) $$\frac{800 \text{ mcg/mL} \times 12 \text{ mL/h}}{60 \text{ min/h} \times 70 \text{ kg}}$$

(Cancel) $$\frac{800 \text{ mcg/mL} \times \overset{1}{\cancel{12}} \text{ mL/h}}{\underset{5}{\cancel{60}} \text{ min/h} \times 70 \text{ kg}}$$

(Calculate) $$\frac{800}{5 \times 70} = \frac{800}{350} = 2.28 \text{ rounded to } 2.3 \text{ mcg/kg/min}$$

Some IV pumps have the capability of calculating the IV rate required for a specific drug. The nurse can select a drug from the IV pump "library," enter the desired dose, the concentration of the medication, and the patient's weight in kilograms. After all the information is entered, the IV pump will display the mL/h needed for the IV rate (Figure 17-1). Nurses should use this feature as a check of their own dosage calculation answer, not as the only means of dosage calculation.

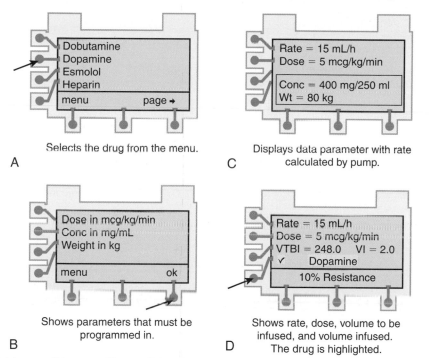

A Selects the drug from the menu.

C Displays data parameter with rate calculated by pump.

B Shows parameters that must be programmed in.

D Shows rate, dose, volume to be infused, and volume infused. The drug is highlighted.

FIGURE 17-1 Using an IV pump library. (Modified from *Volumetric Infusion Manual,* Alaris Medical Systems, San Diego, CA.)

Complete the following work sheet, which provides for practice in the calculation of critical care IV flow rates. Check your answers. If you have difficulties, go back and review the necessary material. An acceptable score as indicated on the posttest signifies that you have successfully completed the chapter. An unacceptable score signifies a need for further study before taking the second posttest.

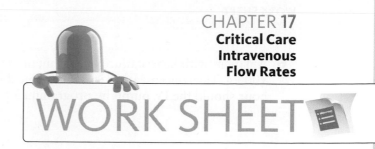

WORK SHEET

DIRECTIONS: The IV fluid order is listed in each problem. Calculate the IV flow rates using the appropriate formula required for the problem.

1. The physician orders dobutamine at 12 mcg/kg/min for Mrs. White, who weighs 75 kg. The concentration is dobutamine 1 g in 250 mL of D_5W. How many milliliters per hour should the IV pump be programmed for? _____

2. Mr. Baxter is having chest pain and has an order for nitroglycerin at 10 mcg/min. The concentration is nitroglycerin 100 mg in 500 mL of D_5W. How many milliliters per hour should the IV pump be programmed for? _____

3. The physician orders dopamine at 5 mcg/kg/min. The concentration is dopamine 2 g in 250 mL of 0.9% NS. The patient's weight is 80 kg. How many milliliters per hour should the IV pump be programmed for? _____

4. The physician has ordered amiodarone at 0.5 mg/min. The concentration is amiodarone 900 mg in 500 mL of D_5W. How many milliliters per hour should the IV pump be programmed for? _____

5. Your patient with malignant hypertension is ordered to have nitroprusside at 3 mcg/kg/min. The concentration is nitroprusside 50 mg in 250 mL of D_5W. The patient's weight is 70 kg. How many milliliters per hour should the IV pump be programmed for? _____

6. A patient with heart failure has dobutamine ordered at 10 mcg/kg/min. The patient weighs 100 kg. The concentration is dobutamine 2 g in 500 mL of D₅W. How many milliliters per hour should the IV pump be programmed for? _____

7. Mr. Nast has propofol ordered at 30 mcg/kg/min. The propofol concentration is 15 mg/mL. The patient's weight is 75 kg. How many milliliters per hour should the IV pump be programmed for? _____

8. A patient with a ventricular dysrhythmia has procainamide ordered at 4 mg/min. The concentration is procainamide 2 g in 250 mL of D₅W. How many milliliters per hour should the IV pump be programmed for? _____

9. Mrs. Waters, who has been resuscitated, has Levophed ordered at 10 mcg/min. The concentration is Levophed 2 mg in 250 mL of 0.9% NS. How many milliliters per hour should the IV pump be programmed for? _____

10. A patient with a dysrhythmia has an order for amiodarone 0.75 mg/min. The concentration is amiodarone 900 mg in 500 mL D₅W. How many milliliters per hour should the IV pump be programmed for? _____

11. A patient with hypotension has a vasopressor ordered at 15 mcg/min. The concentration is vasopressor 4 mg in 250 mL of D₅W. How many milliliters per hour should the IV pump be programmed for? _____

12. Mrs. Roberts has lidocaine ordered at 2 mg/min. The concentration is lidocaine 2 g in 250 mL of D$_5$W. How many milliliters per hour should the IV pump be programmed for? _____

13. The physician orders dopamine at 10 mcg/kg/min. The concentration is dopamine 2 g in 250 mL of 0.9% NS. The patient's weight is 90 kg. How many milliliters per hour should the IV pump be programmed for? _____

14. Mr. Diaz is admitted to your ICU with dopamine infusing at 13.5 mL/h. His weight is 75 kg. The dopamine concentration is 1 g in 250 mL of D$_5$W. At what rate, in micrograms per kilogram per minute, is the dopamine infusing? _____

15. A patient with heart failure has nitroglycerin infusing at 3 mL/h. The nitroglycerin concentration is 100 mg in 500 mL of D$_5$W. At what rate, in micrograms per minute, is the nitroglycerin infusing? _____

16. A patient with supraventricular tachycardia has amiodarone infusing at 17 mL/h. The amiodarone concentration is 900 mg in 500 mL of D$_5$W. At what rate, in milligrams per minute, is the amiodarone infusing? _____

17. Ms. Hart requires mechanical ventilation and is agitated. Propofol is infusing at 9 mL/h. The patient's weight is 75 kg. The propofol concentration is 15 mg/mL. At what rate, in micrograms per kilogram per minute, is the propofol infusing? _____

18. Mr. Simon is admitted with angina. Nitroglycerin is infusing at 5 mL/h. The nitroglycerin concentration is 50 mg in 250 mL of D_5W. How many micrograms per minute is the patient receiving? _____

19. A patient with uncontrolled atrial fibrillation is receiving amiodarone at 20 mL/h. The amiodarone concentration is 900 mg in 500 mL of D_5W. How many milligrams per minute is the patient receiving? _____

20. Mr. McCormick is receiving dopamine at 15 mL/h by IV pump. The patient weighs 80 kg. The dopamine concentration is 2 g in 500 mL of D_5W. Calculate the micrograms per kilogram per minute. _____

21. A patient is receiving nitroglycerin at 10 mL/h by IV pump. The nitroglycerin concentration is 100 mg in 250 mL of D_5W. Calculate the micrograms per minute. _____

22. A patient is receiving amiodarone at 15 mL/h by IV pump. The amiodarone concentration is 900 mg in 250 mL of D_5W. Calculate the milligrams per minute. _____

23. Ms. Nesbitt is receiving lidocaine at 15 mL/h by IV pump. The lidocaine concentration is 1 g in 500 mL of 0.9% NS. Calculate the milligrams per minute. _____

24. Mr. Vargas has supraventricular tachycardia and has a maintenance infusion of Brevibloc 100 mcg/kg/min ordered. The Brevibloc concentration is 10 mg/mL. The patient's weight is 80 kg. At what rate, in milliliters per hour, should the IV pump be set?

ANSWERS ON PP. 499–500 AND 501–502.

NAME _____

DATE _____

ACCEPTABLE SCORE ___9___

YOUR SCORE _____

POSTTEST 1

DIRECTIONS: The IV fluid order is listed in each problem. Calculate the appropriate rate for each problem.

1. Your patient with hypertension has orders for Nipride at 5 mcg/kg/min. The concentration is Nipride 100 mg in 250 mL of D$_5$W. The patient weighs 62 kg. How many milliliters per hour should the IV pump be programmed for? _____

2. Mr. Marshall, who is admitted with pulmonary edema, has dobutamine ordered at 5 mcg/kg/min. The concentration is dobutamine 1 g in 250 mL of 0.9% NS. The patient's weight is 50 kg. How many milliliters per hour should the IV pump be programmed for? _____

3. A patient with an acute myocardial infarction has IV nitroglycerin ordered at 20 mcg/min. The concentration is nitroglycerin 50 mg in 250 mL of D$_5$W. How many milliliters per hour should the IV pump be programmed for? _____

4. A patient with a ventricular dysrhythmia has lidocaine ordered at 3 mg/min. The concentration is lidocaine 2 g in 500 mL of D$_5$W. How many milliliters per hour should the IV pump be programmed for? _____

5. Mrs. Morales has been resuscitated and now has Levophed ordered at 5 mcg/min. The concentration is Levophed 1 mg in 250 mL of 0.9% NS. How many milliliters per hour should the IV pump be programmed for? _____

6. An intubated patient has propofol ordered at 25 mcg/kg/min. The concentration of propofol is 10 mg/mL. The patient's weight is 50 kg. How many milliliters per hour should the IV pump be programmed for? _____

7. Mrs. Green, who has atrial fibrillation, has amiodarone ordered at 0.5 mg/min. The concentration is amiodarone 900 mg in 250 mL of D_5W. How many milliliters per hour should the IV pump be programmed for?

8. A patient with a blood pressure of 240/120 mm Hg is receiving nitroprusside at 63 mL/h. The patient's weight is 70 kg. The nitroprusside concentration is 50 mg in 250 mL of D_5W. How many micrograms per kilogram per minute of nitroprusside is infusing? _____

9. Mr. Messer is receiving vasopressin at 15 mL/h. The vasopressin concentration is 4 mg in 250 mL. How many micrograms per minute of vasopressin is the patient receiving? _____

10. A patient has hypotension after cardiac arrest. Dopamine is infusing at 15 mL/h. The patient's weight is 80 kg. The dopamine concentration is 2 g in 500 mL of D_5W. How many micrograms per kilogram per minute is the patient receiving? _____

ANSWERS ON PP. 500 AND 502.

NAME _____

DATE _____

ACCEPTABLE SCORE ___9___

YOUR SCORE _____

POSTTEST 2

DIRECTIONS: The IV fluid order is listed in each problem. Calculate the rate needed in each problem to deliver the correct dose.

1. A patient with hypotension has dopamine ordered at 3 mcg/kg/min. The patient weighs 85 kg. The concentration is dopamine 2 g in 500 mL of D_5W. How many milliliters per hour should the IV pump be programmed for? _____

2. Ms. Farmer, who has tachycardia, has an order for Brevibloc to be started at 50 mcg/kg/min. The concentration is Brevibloc 5 g in 500 mL of D_5W. The patient weighs 80 kg. How many milliliters per hour should the IV pump be programmed for? _____

3. A patient with a ventricular dysrhythmia has an order for amiodarone at 0.5 mg/min. The concentration is amiodarone 900 mg in 250 mL of D_5W. How many milliliters per hour should the IV pump be programmed for? _____

4. Mr. Wu has an order for a vasopressor at 10 mcg/min. The concentration is vasopressor 4 mg in 500 mL of D_5W. How many milliliters per hour should the IV pump be programmed for? _____

5. Mrs. Davis has an order for dobutamine at 7 mcg/kg/min. The concentration is dobutamine 1 g in 200 mL of 0.9% NS. The patient's weight is 55 kg. How many milliliters per hour should the IV pump be programmed for? _____

6. A patient in shock has an order for Isuprel to be infused at 2 mcg/min. The concentration is Isuprel 1 mg in 500 mL of D$_5$W. How many milliliters per hour should the IV pump be programmed for? _____

7. Ms. Shepard's blood pressure is 60/30 mm Hg. Levophed is infusing at 75 mL/h. The Levophed concentration is 2 mg in 250 mL of 0.9% NS. How many micrograms per minute of Levophed is infusing? _____

8. A patient with ventricular tachycardia is receiving procainamide at 30 mL/h. The procainamide concentration is 2 g in 250 mL of D$_5$W. How many milligrams per minute of procainamide is infusing? _____

9. A hypotensive patient is receiving dopamine at 3 mL/h. The patient's weight is 80 kg. The dopamine concentration is 2 g in 250 mL of 0.9% NS. How many micrograms per kilogram per minute of dopamine is infusing? _____

10. Mr. Flores is receiving nitroprusside at 50 mL/h by IV pump. The patient's weight is 60 kg. The nitroprusside concentration is 50 mg in 250 mL of D$_5$W. Calculate the micrograms per kilogram per minute.

ANSWERS ON PP. 500–501 AND 502.

evolve   For additional practice problems, refer to the Advanced Calculations section of *Drug Calculations Companion,* Version 5, on Evolve.

ANSWERS

CHAPTER 17 Dimensional Analysis—Work Sheet, pp. 491–494

1. $$\frac{x \text{ mL}}{h} = \frac{250 \text{ mL}}{1 \text{ g}} \times \frac{1 \text{ g}}{1,000,000 \text{ mcg}} \times \frac{12 \text{ mcg}}{\text{kg/min}} \times \frac{75 \text{ kg}}{1} \times \frac{60 \text{ min}}{1 \text{ h}} = 13.5 \text{ or } 14 \text{ mL/h}$$

2. $$\frac{x \text{ mL}}{h} = \frac{500 \text{ mL}}{100 \text{ mg}} \times \frac{1 \text{ mg}}{1000 \text{ mcg}} \times \frac{10 \text{ mcg}}{1 \text{ min}} \times \frac{60 \text{ min}}{1 \text{ h}} = 3 \text{ mL/h}$$

3. $$\frac{x \text{ mL}}{h} = \frac{250 \text{ mL}}{2 \text{ mg}} \times \frac{1 \text{ g}}{1,000,000 \text{ mcg}} \times \frac{5 \text{ mcg}}{\text{kg/min}} \times \frac{80 \text{ kg}}{1} \times \frac{60 \text{ min}}{1 \text{ h}} = 3 \text{ mL/h}$$

4. $$\frac{x \text{ mL}}{h} = \frac{500 \text{ mL}}{900 \text{ mg}} \times \frac{0.5 \text{ mg}}{1 \text{ min}} \times \frac{60 \text{ min}}{1 \text{ h}} = 16.7 \text{ or } 17 \text{ mL/h}$$

5. $$\frac{x \text{ mL}}{h} = \frac{250 \text{ mL}}{50 \text{ mg}} \times \frac{1 \text{ mg}}{1000 \text{ mcg}} \times \frac{3 \text{ mcg}}{\text{kg/min}} \times \frac{70 \text{ kg}}{1} \times \frac{60 \text{ min}}{1 \text{ h}} = 63 \text{ mL/h}$$

6. $$\frac{x \text{ mL}}{h} = \frac{500 \text{ mL}}{2 \text{ g}} \times \frac{1 \text{ g}}{1,000,000 \text{ mcg}} \times \frac{10 \text{ mcg}}{\text{kg/min}} \times \frac{100 \text{ kg}}{1} \times \frac{60 \text{ min}}{1 \text{ h}} = 15 \text{ mL/h}$$

7. $$\frac{x \text{ mL}}{h} = \frac{1 \text{ mL}}{15 \text{ mg}} \times \frac{1 \text{ mg}}{1000 \text{ mcg}} \times \frac{30 \text{ mcg}}{\text{kg/min}} \times \frac{75 \text{ kg}}{1} \times \frac{60 \text{ min}}{1 \text{ h}} = 9 \text{ mL/h}$$

8. $$\frac{x \text{ mL}}{h} = \frac{250 \text{ mL}}{2 \text{ g}} \times \frac{1 \text{ g}}{1000 \text{ mg}} \times \frac{4 \text{ mg}}{1 \text{ min}} \times \frac{60 \text{ min}}{1 \text{ h}} = 30 \text{ mL/h}$$

9. $$\frac{x \text{ mL}}{h} = \frac{250 \text{ mL}}{2 \text{ mg}} \times \frac{1 \text{ mg}}{1000 \text{ mcg}} \times \frac{10 \text{ mcg}}{1 \text{ min}} \times \frac{60 \text{ min}}{1 \text{ h}} = 75 \text{ mL/h}$$

10. $$\frac{x \text{ mL}}{h} = \frac{500 \text{ mL}}{900 \text{ mg}} \times \frac{0.75 \text{ mg}}{1 \text{ min}} \times \frac{60 \text{ min}}{1 \text{ h}} = 25 \text{ mL/h}$$

11. $$\frac{x \text{ mL}}{h} = \frac{250 \text{ mL}}{4 \text{ mg}} \times \frac{1 \text{ mg}}{1000 \text{ mcg}} \times \frac{15 \text{ mcg}}{1 \text{ min}} \times \frac{60 \text{ min}}{1 \text{ h}} = 56.3 \text{ or } 56 \text{ mL/h}$$

12. $$\frac{x \text{ mL}}{h} = \frac{250 \text{ mL}}{2 \text{ g}} \times \frac{1 \text{ g}}{1000 \text{ mg}} \times \frac{2 \text{ mg}}{1 \text{ min}} \times \frac{60 \text{ min}}{1 \text{ h}} = 15 \text{ mL/h}$$

13. $$\frac{x \text{ mL}}{h} = \frac{250 \text{ mL}}{2 \text{ g}} \times \frac{1 \text{ g}}{1,000,000 \text{ mcg}} \times \frac{10 \text{ mcg}}{\text{kg/min}} \times \frac{90 \text{ kg}}{1} \times \frac{60 \text{ min}}{1 \text{ h}} = 6.8 \text{ or } 7 \text{ mL/h}$$

14. $$\frac{x \text{ mcg}}{\text{kg/min}} = \frac{1,000,000 \text{ mcg}}{1 \text{ g}} \times \frac{1 \text{ g}}{250 \text{ mL}} \times \frac{13.5 \text{ mL}}{1 \text{ h}} \times \frac{1 \text{ h}}{60 \text{ min}} \times \frac{1}{75 \text{ kg}} = 12 \text{ mcg/kg/min}$$

15. $$\frac{x \text{ mcg}}{\text{min}} = \frac{1000 \text{ mcg}}{1 \text{ mg}} \times \frac{100 \text{ mg}}{500 \text{ mL}} \times \frac{3 \text{ mL}}{1 \text{ h}} \times \frac{1 \text{ h}}{60 \text{ min}} = 10 \text{ mcg/min}$$

16. $$\frac{x \text{ mg}}{\text{min}} = \frac{900 \text{ mg}}{500 \text{ mL}} \times \frac{17 \text{ mL}}{1 \text{ h}} \times \frac{1 \text{ h}}{60 \text{ min}} = 0.51 \text{ rounded to } 0.5 \text{ mg/min}$$

17. $$\frac{x \text{ mcg}}{\text{kg/min}} = \frac{1000 \text{ mcg}}{1 \text{ mg}} \times \frac{15 \text{ mg}}{1 \text{ mL}} \times \frac{9 \text{ mL}}{1 \text{ h}} \times \frac{1 \text{ h}}{60 \text{ min}} \times \frac{1}{75 \text{ kg}} = 30 \text{ mcg/kg/min}$$

18. $$\frac{x \text{ mcg}}{\text{min}} = \frac{1000 \text{ mcg}}{1 \text{ mg}} \times \frac{50 \text{ mg}}{250 \text{ mL}} \times \frac{5 \text{ mL}}{1 \text{ h}} \times \frac{1 \text{ h}}{60 \text{ min}} = 16.66 \text{ rounded to } 16.7 \text{ mcg/min}$$

19. $$\frac{x \text{ mg}}{\text{min}} = \frac{900 \text{ mg}}{500 \text{ mL}} \times \frac{20 \text{ mL}}{1 \text{ h}} \times \frac{1 \text{ h}}{60 \text{ min}} = 0.6 \text{ mg/min}$$

ANSWERS

20. $$\frac{x \text{ mcg}}{\text{kg/min}} = \frac{1{,}000{,}000 \text{ mcg}}{1 \text{ g}} \times \frac{2 \text{ g}}{500 \text{ mL}} \times \frac{15 \text{ mL}}{1 \text{ h}} \times \frac{1 \text{ h}}{60 \text{ min}} \times \frac{1}{80 \text{ kg}} = 12.5 \text{ mcg/kg/min}$$

21. $$\frac{x \text{ mcg}}{\text{min}} = \frac{1000 \text{ mcg}}{1 \text{ mg}} \times \frac{100 \text{ mg}}{250 \text{ mL}} \times \frac{10 \text{ mL}}{1 \text{ h}} \times \frac{1 \text{ h}}{60 \text{ min}} = 66.66 \text{ rounded to } 66.7 \text{ mcg/min}$$

22. $$\frac{x \text{ mg}}{\text{min}} = \frac{900 \text{ mg}}{250 \text{ mL}} \times \frac{15 \text{ mL}}{1 \text{ h}} \times \frac{1 \text{ h}}{60 \text{ min}} = 0.9 \text{ mg/min}$$

23. $$\frac{x \text{ mg}}{\text{min}} = \frac{1000 \text{ mg}}{1 \text{ g}} \times \frac{1 \text{ g}}{500 \text{ mL}} \times \frac{15 \text{ mL}}{1 \text{ h}} \times \frac{1 \text{ h}}{60 \text{ min}} = 0.5 \text{ mg/min}$$

24. $$\frac{x \text{ mL}}{\text{h}} = \frac{1 \text{ mL}}{10 \text{ mg}} \times \frac{1 \text{ mg}}{1000 \text{ mcg}} \times \frac{100 \text{ mcg}}{\text{kg/min}} \times \frac{80 \text{ kg}}{1} \times \frac{60 \text{ min}}{1 \text{ h}} = 48 \text{ mL/h}$$

CHAPTER 17 Dimensional Analysis—Posttest 1, pp. 495–496

1. $$\frac{x \text{ mL}}{\text{h}} = \frac{250 \text{ mL}}{100 \text{ mg}} \times \frac{1 \text{ mg}}{1000 \text{ mcg}} \times \frac{5 \text{ mcg}}{\text{kg/min}} \times \frac{62 \text{ kg}}{1} \times \frac{60 \text{ min}}{1 \text{ h}} = 46.5 \text{ or } 47 \text{ mL/h}$$

2. $$\frac{x \text{ mL}}{\text{h}} = \frac{250 \text{ mL}}{1 \text{ g}} \times \frac{1 \text{ g}}{1{,}000{,}000 \text{ mcg}} \times \frac{5 \text{ mcg}}{\text{kg/min}} \times \frac{50 \text{ kg}}{1} \times \frac{60 \text{ min}}{1 \text{ h}} = 3.8 \text{ or } 4 \text{ mL/h}$$

3. $$\frac{x \text{ mL}}{\text{h}} = \frac{250 \text{ mL}}{50 \text{ mg}} \times \frac{1 \text{ mg}}{1000 \text{ mcg}} \times \frac{20 \text{ mcg}}{1 \text{ min}} \times \frac{60 \text{ min}}{1 \text{ h}} = 6 \text{ mL/h}$$

4. $$\frac{x \text{ mL}}{\text{h}} = \frac{500 \text{ mL}}{2 \text{ g}} \times \frac{1 \text{ g}}{1000 \text{ mg}} \times \frac{3 \text{ mg}}{1 \text{ min}} \times \frac{60 \text{ min}}{1 \text{ h}} = 45 \text{ mL/h}$$

5. $$\frac{x \text{ mL}}{\text{h}} = \frac{250 \text{ mL}}{1 \text{ mg}} \times \frac{1 \text{ mg}}{1000 \text{ mcg}} \times \frac{5 \text{ mcg}}{1 \text{ min}} \times \frac{60 \text{ min}}{1 \text{ h}} = 75 \text{ mL/h}$$

6. $$\frac{x \text{ mL}}{\text{h}} = \frac{1 \text{ mL}}{10 \text{ mg}} \times \frac{1 \text{ mg}}{1000 \text{ mcg}} \times \frac{25 \text{ mcg}}{\text{kg/min}} \times \frac{50 \text{ kg}}{1} \times \frac{60 \text{ min}}{1 \text{ h}} = 7.5 \text{ or } 8 \text{ mL/h}$$

7. $$\frac{x \text{ mL}}{\text{h}} = \frac{250 \text{ mL}}{900 \text{ mg}} \times \frac{0.5 \text{ mg}}{1 \text{ min}} \times \frac{60 \text{ min}}{1 \text{ h}} = 8.3 \text{ or } 8 \text{ mL/h}$$

8. $$\frac{x \text{ mcg}}{\text{kg/min}} = \frac{1000 \text{ mcg}}{1 \text{ mg}} \times \frac{50 \text{ mg}}{250 \text{ mL}} \times \frac{63 \text{ mL}}{1 \text{ h}} \times \frac{1 \text{ h}}{60 \text{ min}} \times \frac{1}{70 \text{ kg}} = 3 \text{ mcg/kg/min}$$

9. $$\frac{x \text{ mcg}}{\text{min}} = \frac{1000 \text{ mcg}}{1 \text{ mg}} \times \frac{4 \text{ mg}}{250 \text{ mL}} \times \frac{15 \text{ mL}}{1 \text{ h}} \times \frac{1 \text{ h}}{60 \text{ min}} = 4 \text{ mcg/min}$$

10. $$\frac{x \text{ mcg}}{\text{kg/min}} = \frac{1{,}000{,}000 \text{ mcg}}{1 \text{ g}} \times \frac{2 \text{ g}}{500 \text{ mL}} \times \frac{15 \text{ mL}}{1 \text{ h}} \times \frac{1 \text{ h}}{60 \text{ min}} \times \frac{1}{80 \text{ kg}} = 12.5 \text{ mcg/kg/min}$$

CHAPTER 17 Dimensional Analysis—Posttest 2, pp. 497–498

1. $$\frac{x \text{ mL}}{\text{h}} = \frac{500 \text{ mL}}{2 \text{ g}} \times \frac{1 \text{ g}}{1{,}000{,}000 \text{ mcg}} \times \frac{3 \text{ mcg}}{\text{kg/min}} \times \frac{85 \text{ kg}}{1} \times \frac{60 \text{ min}}{1 \text{ h}} = 3.8 \text{ or } 4 \text{ mL/h}$$

2. $$\frac{x \text{ mL}}{\text{h}} = \frac{500 \text{ mL}}{5 \text{ g}} \times \frac{1 \text{ g}}{1{,}000{,}000 \text{ mcg}} \times \frac{50 \text{ mcg}}{\text{kg/min}} \times \frac{80 \text{ kg}}{1} \times \frac{60 \text{ min}}{1 \text{ h}} = 24 \text{ mL/h}$$

3. $$\frac{x \text{ mL}}{\text{h}} = \frac{250 \text{ mL}}{900 \text{ mg}} \times \frac{0.5 \text{ mg}}{1 \text{ min}} \times \frac{60 \text{ min}}{1 \text{ h}} = 8.3 \text{ or } 8 \text{ mL/h}$$

4. $\dfrac{x \text{ mL}}{h} = \dfrac{500 \text{ mL}}{4 \text{ mg}} \times \dfrac{1 \text{ mg}}{1000 \text{ mcg}} \times \dfrac{10 \text{ mcg}}{1 \text{ min}} \times \dfrac{60 \text{ min}}{1 \text{ h}} = 75 \text{ mL/h}$

5. $\dfrac{x \text{ mL}}{h} = \dfrac{200 \text{ mL}}{1 \text{ g}} \times \dfrac{1 \text{ g}}{1,000,000 \text{ mcg}} \times \dfrac{7 \text{ mcg}}{\text{kg/min}} \times \dfrac{55 \text{ kg}}{1} \times \dfrac{60 \text{ min}}{1 \text{ h}} = 4.6 \text{ or } 5 \text{ mL/h}$

6. $\dfrac{x \text{ mL}}{h} = \dfrac{500 \text{ mL}}{1 \text{ mg}} \times \dfrac{1 \text{ mg}}{1000 \text{ mcg}} \times \dfrac{2 \text{ mcg}}{1 \text{ min}} \times \dfrac{60 \text{ min}}{1 \text{ h}} = 60 \text{ mL/h}$

7. $\dfrac{x \text{ mcg}}{\min} = \dfrac{1000 \text{ mcg}}{1 \text{ mg}} \times \dfrac{2 \text{ mg}}{250 \text{ mL}} \times \dfrac{75 \text{ mL}}{1 \text{ h}} \times \dfrac{1 \text{ h}}{60 \text{ min}} = 10 \text{ mcg/min}$

8. $\dfrac{x \text{ mg}}{\min} = \dfrac{1000 \text{ mg}}{1 \text{ g}} \times \dfrac{2 \text{ g}}{250 \text{ mL}} \times \dfrac{30 \text{ mL}}{1 \text{ h}} \times \dfrac{1 \text{ h}}{60 \text{ min}} = 4 \text{ mg/min}$

9. $\dfrac{x \text{ mcg}}{\text{kg/min}} = \dfrac{1,000,000 \text{ mcg}}{1 \text{ g}} \times \dfrac{2 \text{ g}}{250 \text{ mL}} \times \dfrac{3 \text{ mL}}{1 \text{ h}} \times \dfrac{1 \text{ h}}{60 \text{ min}} \times \dfrac{1}{80 \text{ kg}} = 5 \text{ mcg/kg/min}$

10. $\dfrac{x \text{ mcg}}{\text{kg/min}} = \dfrac{1000 \text{ mcg}}{1 \text{ mg}} \times \dfrac{50 \text{ mg}}{250 \text{ mL}} \times \dfrac{50 \text{ mL}}{1 \text{ h}} \times \dfrac{1 \text{ h}}{60 \text{ min}} \times \dfrac{1}{60 \text{ kg}} = 2.77 \text{ rounded to } 2.8 \text{ mcg/kg/min}$

CHAPTER 17 Formula Method—Work Sheet, pp. 491–494

1. $\dfrac{12 \text{ mcg} \times 75 \text{ kg} \times 60 \text{ min/h}}{4000 \text{ mcg/mL}} = \dfrac{54,000}{4000}$
   $= 13.5 \text{ or } 14 \text{ mL/h}$

2. $\dfrac{10 \text{ mcg/min} \times 60 \text{ min/h}}{200 \text{ mcg/mL}} = \dfrac{600}{200} = 3 \text{ mL/h}$

3. $\dfrac{5 \text{ mcg} \times 80 \text{ kg} \times 60 \text{ min/h}}{8000 \text{ mcg/mL}} = \dfrac{24,000}{8000}$
   $= 3 \text{ mL/h}$

4. $\dfrac{0.5 \text{ mg/min} \times 60 \text{ min/h}}{1.8 \text{ mg/mL}} = \dfrac{30}{1.8}$
   $= 16.7 \text{ or } 17 \text{ mL/h}$

5. $\dfrac{3 \text{ mcg} \times 70 \text{ kg} \times 60 \text{ min/h}}{200 \text{ mcg/mL}} = \dfrac{12,600}{200}$
   $= 63 \text{ mL/h}$

6. $\dfrac{10 \text{ mcg} \times 100 \text{ kg} \times 60 \text{ min/h}}{4000 \text{ mcg/mL}} = \dfrac{60,000}{4000}$
   $= 15 \text{ mL/h}$

7. $\dfrac{30 \text{ mcg} \times 75 \text{ kg} \times 60 \text{ min/h}}{15,000 \text{ mcg/mL}} = \dfrac{135,000}{15,000}$
   $= 9 \text{ mL/h}$

8. $\dfrac{4 \text{ mg/min} \times 60 \text{ min/h}}{8 \text{ mg/mL}} = \dfrac{240}{8} = 30 \text{ mL/h}$

9. $\dfrac{10 \text{ mcg/min} \times 60 \text{ min/h}}{8 \text{ mcg/mL}} = \dfrac{600}{8} = 75 \text{ mL/h}$

10. $\dfrac{0.75 \text{ mg/min} \times 60 \text{ min/h}}{1.8 \text{ mg/mL}} = \dfrac{45}{1.8} = 25 \text{ mL/h}$

11. $\dfrac{15 \text{ mcg/min} \times 60 \text{ min/h}}{16 \text{ mcg/mL}} = \dfrac{900}{16}$
    $= 56.3 \text{ or } 56 \text{ mL/h}$

12. $\dfrac{2 \text{ mg/min} \times 60 \text{ min/h}}{8 \text{ mg/mL}} = \dfrac{120}{8} = 15 \text{ mL/h}$

13. $\dfrac{10 \text{ mcg} \times 90 \text{ kg} \times 60 \text{ min/h}}{8000 \text{ mcg/mL}} = \dfrac{54,000}{8000}$
    $= 6.8 \text{ or } 7 \text{ mL/h}$

14. $\dfrac{4000 \text{ mcg/mL} \times 13.5 \text{ mL/h}}{60 \text{ min/h} \times 75 \text{ kg}} = \dfrac{54,000}{4500}$
    $= 12 \text{ mcg/kg/min}$

15. $\dfrac{200 \text{ mcg/mL} \times 3 \text{ mL/h}}{60 \text{ min/h}} = \dfrac{600}{60} = 10 \text{ mcg/min}$

16. $\dfrac{1.8 \text{ mg/mL} \times 17 \text{ mL/h}}{60 \text{ min/h}} = \dfrac{30.6}{60}$
    $= 0.51 \text{ rounded to } 0.5 \text{ mg/min}$

17. $\dfrac{15,000 \text{ mcg/mL} \times 9 \text{ mL/h}}{60 \text{ min/h} \times 75 \text{ kg}} = \dfrac{135,000}{4500}$
    $= 30 \text{ mcg/kg/min}$

18. $\dfrac{200 \text{ mcg/mL} \times 5 \text{ mL/h}}{60 \text{ min/h}} = \dfrac{1000}{60}$
    $= 16.66 \text{ rounded to } 16.7 \text{ mcg/min}$

19. $\dfrac{1.8 \text{ mg/mL} \times 20 \text{ mL/h}}{60 \text{ min/h}} = \dfrac{36}{60} = 0.6 \text{ mg/min}$

20. $\dfrac{4000 \text{ mcg/mL} \times 15 \text{ mL/h}}{60 \text{ min/h} \times 80 \text{ kg}} = \dfrac{60,000}{4800}$
    $= 12.5 \text{ mcg/kg/min}$

ANSWERS

21. $\dfrac{400 \text{ mcg/mL} \times 10 \text{ mL/h}}{60 \text{ min/h}} = \dfrac{4000}{60}$
$= 66.66 \text{ rounded to } 66.7 \text{ mcg/min}$

22. $\dfrac{3.6 \text{ mg/mL} \times 15 \text{ mL/h}}{60 \text{ min/h}} = \dfrac{54}{60} = 0.9 \text{ mg/min}$

23. $\dfrac{2 \text{ mg/mL} \times 15 \text{ mL/h}}{60 \text{ min/h}} = \dfrac{30}{60} = 0.5 \text{ mg/min}$

24. $\dfrac{100 \text{ mcg} \times 80 \text{ kg} \times 60 \text{ min/h}}{10,000 \text{ mcg/mL}} = \dfrac{480,000}{10,000}$
$= 48 \text{ mL/h}$

CHAPTER 17 Formula Method—Posttest 1, pp. 495–496

1. $\dfrac{5 \text{ mcg} \times 62 \text{ kg} \times 60 \text{ min/h}}{400 \text{ mcg/mL}} = \dfrac{18,600}{400}$
$= 46.5 \text{ or } 47 \text{ mL/h}$

2. $\dfrac{5 \text{ mcg} \times 50 \text{ kg} \times 60 \text{ min/h}}{4000 \text{ mcg/mL}} = \dfrac{15,000}{4000}$
$= 3.8 \text{ or } 4 \text{ mL/h}$

3. $\dfrac{20 \text{ mcg} \times 60 \text{ min/h}}{200 \text{ mcg/mL}} = \dfrac{1200}{200} = 6 \text{ mL/h}$

4. $\dfrac{3 \text{ mg} \times 60 \text{ min/h}}{4 \text{ mg/mL}} = \dfrac{180}{4} = 45 \text{ mL/h}$

5. $\dfrac{5 \text{ mcg} \times 60 \text{ min/h}}{4 \text{ mcg/mL}} = \dfrac{300}{4} = 75 \text{ mL/h}$

6. $\dfrac{25 \text{ mcg} \times 50 \text{ kg} \times 60 \text{ min/h}}{10,000 \text{ mcg/mL}} = \dfrac{75,000}{10,000}$
$= 7.5 \text{ or } 8 \text{ mL/h}$

7. $\dfrac{0.5 \text{ mg} \times 60 \text{ min/h}}{3.6 \text{ mg/mL}} = \dfrac{30}{3.6} = 8.3 \text{ or } 8 \text{ mL/h}$

8. $\dfrac{200 \text{ mcg/mL} \times 63 \text{ mL/h}}{60 \text{ min/h} \times 70 \text{ kg}} = \dfrac{12,600}{4200}$
$= 3 \text{ mcg/kg/min}$

9. $\dfrac{16 \text{ mcg/mL} \times 15 \text{ mL/h}}{60 \text{ min/h}} = \dfrac{240}{60} = 4 \text{ mcg/min}$

10. $\dfrac{4000 \text{ mcg/mL} \times 15 \text{ mL/h}}{60 \text{ min/h} \times 80 \text{ kg}} = \dfrac{60,000}{4800}$
$= 12.5 \text{ mcg/kg/min}$

CHAPTER 17 Formula Method—Posttest 2, pp. 497–498

1. $\dfrac{3 \text{ mcg} \times 85 \text{ kg} \times 60 \text{ min/h}}{4000 \text{ mcg/mL}} = \dfrac{15,300}{4000}$
$= 3.8 \text{ or } 4 \text{ mL/h}$

2. $\dfrac{50 \text{ mcg} \times 80 \text{ kg} \times 60 \text{ min/h}}{10,000 \text{ mcg/mL}} = \dfrac{240,000}{10,000}$
$= 24 \text{ mL/h}$

3. $\dfrac{0.5 \text{ mg} \times 60 \text{ min/h}}{3.6 \text{ mg/mL}} = \dfrac{30}{3.6} = 8.3 \text{ or } 8 \text{ mL/h}$

4. $\dfrac{10 \text{ mcg} \times 60 \text{ min/h}}{8 \text{ mcg/mL}} = \dfrac{600}{8} = 75 \text{ mL/h}$

5. $\dfrac{7 \text{ mcg} \times 55 \text{ kg} \times 60 \text{ min/h}}{5000 \text{ mcg/mL}} = \dfrac{23,100}{5000}$
$= 4.6 \text{ or } 5 \text{ mL/h}$

6. $\dfrac{2 \text{ mcg} \times 60 \text{ min/h}}{2 \text{ mcg/mL}} = \dfrac{120}{2} = 60 \text{ mL/h}$

7. $\dfrac{8 \text{ mcg/mL} \times 75 \text{ mL/h}}{60 \text{ min/h}} = \dfrac{600}{60} = 10 \text{ mcg/min}$

8. $\dfrac{8 \text{ mg/mL} \times 30 \text{ mL/h}}{60 \text{ min/h}} = \dfrac{240}{60} = 4 \text{ mg/min}$

9. $\dfrac{8000 \text{ mcg/mL} \times 3 \text{ mL/h}}{60 \text{ min/h} \times 80 \text{ kg}} = \dfrac{24,000}{4800}$
$= 5 \text{ mcg/kg/min}$

10. $\dfrac{200 \text{ mcg/mL} \times 50 \text{ mL/h}}{60 \text{ min/h} \times 60 \text{ kg}} = \dfrac{10,000}{3600}$
$= 2.77 \text{ rounded to } 2.8 \text{ mcg/kg/min}$

ANSWERS

Pediatric Dosages

LEARNING OBJECTIVES

Upon completion of the materials provided in this chapter, you will be able to perform computations accurately by mastering the following mathematical concepts:

1 Converting the weight of a child from pounds to kilograms
2 Converting the neonate and infant weight from grams to kilograms
3 Performing pediatric dosage calculations
4 Calculating the single or individual dose of medications
5 Determining whether the prescribed dose is safe and therapeutic
6 Calculating a safe and therapeutic 24-hour dosage range
7 Calculating the single-dose range from a 24-hour dosage range
8 Determining whether the actual dosage (in milligrams per kilograms per 24 hours) is safe to administer
9 Calculating pediatric IV solutions
10 Administering IV medications to pediatric patients
11 Calculating the daily fluid requirements for infants and young children
12 Calculating the body surface area (BSA) for medication administration

Children are more sensitive than adults to medications because of their weight, height, physical condition, immature systems, and metabolism. Nurses who administer medications to infants and children must be vigilant in determining whether the patient is receiving the correct medication. The correct dose is one of the six rights of drug administration: right patient, medication, route, time, dose, and documentation.

The physician or provider will prescribe the medication to be delivered. However, the nurse is responsible for detecting any errors in calculation of dosage, as well as for preparing the medication and administering the drug. The nurse needs to be aware that pediatric dosages are often less than 1 mL; therefore a tuberculin syringe is used for accurate dosing.

Pediatric medications are calculated using the infant or child's kilogram weight. The dosages have been established by the drug companies. Safe and therapeutic (S&T) dosages are readily available from a reliable source such as *The Harriet Lane Handbook*.

> **! ALERT**
>
> Never exceed the adult dose or maximum dose recommended.

In general, pediatric dosages are rounded to the nearest tenth. For infants and young children, doses may be rounded to the nearest hundredth. The child who weighs more than 50 kg **may** receive adult dosages. If the calculated dose is greater than the recommended adult dose, DO NOT administer the medication. A child should not receive higher doses than those recommended for the adult, ever. Many drugs have a "do not exceed" or "max" dose in 24 hours listed; this must always be considered.

Additionally, the physician or pharmacist may use the child's body surface area (BSA) to calculate a dosage of medication to administer. The BSA calculation may be used when an established dosage has not been determined by the drug company, as with some anticancer or specialized drugs.

KILOGRAM CONVERSIONS

Converting Pounds to Kilograms

The conversion: 2.2 lb = 1 kg

The weight of infants and young children must be converted from pounds to kilograms to accurately calculate medication doses and daily fluid requirements. S&T drug dosages have been established using kilogram weights.

Round the kilogram weight to the nearest tenth.

EXAMPLE 1: An infant weighs 24 lb. Convert the infant's weight to kilograms.

Dimensional Analysis

$$x \text{ kg} = \frac{1 \text{ kg}}{2.2 \text{ lb}} \times \frac{24 \text{ lb}}{1}$$

$$x \text{ kg} = \frac{24}{2.2}$$

$$x = 10.9 \text{ kg}$$

Proportion

2.2 lb : 1 kg :: 24 lb : x kg

2.2 : 1 :: 24 : x

2.2x = 24

$$x = \frac{24}{2.2}$$

$$x = 10.9 \text{ kg}$$

Formula Setup

$$\frac{2.2 \text{ lb}}{1 \text{ kg}} = \frac{24 \text{ lb}}{x \text{ kg}}$$

2.2x = 24

x = 10.9 kg

EXAMPLE 2: A child weighs 47 lb. Convert the child's weight to kilograms.

Dimensional Analysis

$$x \text{ kg} = \frac{1 \text{ kg}}{2.2 \text{ lb}} \times \frac{47 \text{ lb}}{1}$$

$$x \text{ kg} = \frac{47}{2.2}$$

$$x = 21.36 \text{ or } 21.4 \text{ kg}$$

Proportion

2.2 lb : 1 kg :: 47 lb : x kg

2.2 : 1 :: 47 : x

2.2x = 47

$$x = \frac{47}{2.2}$$

$$x = 21.36 \text{ or } 21.4 \text{ kg}$$

Formula Setup

$$\frac{2.2 \text{ lb}}{1 \text{ kg}} = \frac{47 \text{ lb}}{x \text{ kg}}$$

2.2x = 47

x = 21.4 kg

Converting Grams to Kilograms

The conversion: 1000 g = 1 kg

Newborn (neonate) and some infant weights are measured in grams. Converting grams to kilograms is done as shown below or by simply dividing the number of grams by 1000.

EXAMPLE 1: A neonate weighs 2300 g. Convert to kilograms.

Dimensional Analysis

$$x \text{ kg} = \frac{1 \text{ kg}}{1000 \text{ g}} \times \frac{2300 \text{ g}}{1}$$

$$x \text{ kg} = \frac{2300}{1000}$$

$$x = 2.3 \text{ kg}$$

Proportion

1000 g : 1 kg :: 2300 g : x kg

1000 : 1 :: 2300 : x

1000x = 2300

$$x = 2.3 \text{ kg}$$

EXAMPLE 2: A newborn weighs 4630 g at birth. Convert to kilograms.

Dimensional Analysis

$$x \text{ kg} = \frac{1 \text{ kg}}{1000 \text{ g}} \times \frac{4630 \text{ g}}{1}$$

$$x \text{ kg} = \frac{4630}{1000}$$

$$x = 4.63 \text{ or } 4.6 \text{ kg}$$

Proportion

1000 g : 1 kg :: 4630 g : x kg

1000 : 1 :: 4630 : x

$1000x = 4630$

$x = 4.63$ or 4.6 kg

Practice Problems. Convert pounds and grams to kilograms.

1. 27 lb _____ kg
2. 38 lb _____ kg
3. 52 lb _____ kg
4. 5220 g _____ kg
5. 3202 g _____ kg
6. 72 lb _____ kg
7. 16 lb _____ kg
8. 92 lb _____ kg

Answers

1. 12.3 kg
2. 17.3 kg
3. 23.6 kg
4. 5.2 kg
5. 3.2 kg
6. 32.7 kg
7. 7.3 kg
8. 41.8 kg

PEDIATRIC DOSAGE CALCULATIONS

In pediatric dosage calculations, you can use the dimensional analysis, proportion, or $\frac{D}{A} \times Q$ method.

EXAMPLE 1: The physician orders Benadryl 12.5 mg po q 4–6 h prn for itching. The nurse has available Benadryl 25 mg/5 mL. How many milliliters would be needed to administer 12.5 mg? Show math.

Dimensional Analysis

$$x \text{ mL} = \frac{5 \text{ mL}}{25 \text{ mg}} \times \frac{12.5 \text{ mg}}{1}$$

$$x \text{ mL} = \frac{5 \times 12.5}{25}$$

$$x = 2.5 \text{ mL}$$

Proportion

25 mg : 5 mL :: 12.5 mg : x mL

$x = 2.5$ mL

$\frac{D}{A} \times Q$

$$\frac{12.5 \text{ mg}}{25 \text{ mg}} \times 5 \text{ mL} = x$$

$$x = 2.5 \text{ mL}$$

EXAMPLE 2: The physician orders morphine 15 mg by intravenous (IV) piggyback (IVPB) now. You have available morphine 10 mg/mL. How much would you give? Show math.

Dimensional Analysis

$$x \text{ mL} = \frac{1 \text{ mL}}{10 \text{ mg}} \times \frac{15 \text{ mg}}{1}$$

$$x \text{ mL} = \frac{15}{10}$$

$$x = 1.5 \text{ mL}$$

Proportion

10 mg : 1 mL :: 15 mg : x mL

$x = 1.5$ mL

$\frac{D}{A} \times Q$

$$\frac{15 \text{ mg}}{10 \text{ mg}} \times 1 \text{ mL} = x$$

$$x = 1.5 \text{ mL}$$

CALCULATING THE SINGLE OR INDIVIDUAL DOSE (MILLIGRAMS/DOSE)

Medications such as acetaminophen and ibuprofen are administered as a single dose. This means that each time the infant or child receives the medication, it is calculated in a single or individual dose based on the kilogram weight.

Most of the medications prescribed in this manner are prn medications, which are given as needed for relief of symptoms such as pain, nausea, and fever. Again, the manufacturer of the drug has established an S&T dosage or range. The nurse is responsible for administering the single dose that is S&T. Therefore it is helpful for the nurse to know how the ordered dose is derived.

To **determine the correct single dose** for the child, you must **calculate the correct dose. A systematic approach is helpful in determining the S&T dose range:**

- Change the child's weight in pounds to kilograms.
- Find the recommended dosage in a reliable source.
- Multiply the kilogram weight by the recommended dose(s).
- The answer is the individual or single dose *(mg/dose)* of medication to be given each time the child receives the medication.

EXAMPLE 1: A child weighs 22 lb. The child needs acetaminophen for pain and fever.

a. Weight   22 lb = 10 kg

b. Recommended   10 to 15 mg/kg/dose q 4–6 h

c. Calculation

(Minimum Recommended Dose)

Dimensional Analysis

$$\frac{x \text{ mg}}{\text{dose}} = \frac{10 \text{ mg}}{\text{kg/dose}} \times \frac{1 \text{ kg}}{2.2 \text{ lb}} \times \frac{22 \text{ lb}}{1}$$

$$\frac{x \text{ mg}}{\text{dose}} = \frac{10 \times 22}{2.2}$$

$$x = 100 \text{ mg/dose}$$

Proportion

$$10 \text{ mg} : 1 \text{ kg} :: x \text{ mg} : 10 \text{ kg}$$

$$x = 10 \times 10$$

$$x = 100 \text{ mg/dose}$$

(Maximum Recommended Dose)

Dimensional Analysis

$$\frac{x \text{ mg}}{\text{dose}} = \frac{15 \text{ mg}}{\text{kg/dose}} \times \frac{1 \text{ kg}}{2.2 \text{ lb}} \times \frac{22 \text{ lb}}{1}$$

$$\frac{x \text{ mg}}{\text{dose}} = \frac{15 \times 22}{2.2}$$

$$x = 150 \text{ mg/dose}$$

Proportion

$$15 \text{ mg} : 1 \text{ kg} :: x \text{ mg} : 10 \text{ kg}$$

$$x = 15 \times 10$$

$$x = 150 \text{ mg/dose}$$

The child may receive 100 to 150 mg each time he or she is given acetaminophen. This is the single or individual dose. The dose is both safe and therapeutic for this child.

- A dose smaller than 100 mg is considered **safe but may not be therapeutic for the child's weight.**
- Doses larger than 150 mg are considered too much for the child's weight and may **exceed the therapeutic range.** There are exceptions—some dosages may be higher. Check *The Hariett Lane Handbook* or other pediatric dosing manuals.

EXAMPLE 2: Calculate an S&T dose range of ibuprofen for a child who weighs 36 lb. Ibuprofen is available as 100 mg/5 mL. How many milliliters would you need to administer for the ordered dose to be S&T?

a. Weight   36 lb = 16.4 kg

b. Recommended   5 to 10 mg/kg/dose q 6–8 h

c. Calculations

(Minimum Recommended Dose)

Dimensional Analysis

$$\frac{x \text{ mg}}{\text{dose}} = \frac{5 \text{ mg}}{\text{kg/dose}} \times \frac{1 \text{ kg}}{2.2 \text{ lb}} \times \frac{36 \text{ lb}}{1}$$

$$\frac{x \text{ mg}}{\text{dose}} = \frac{5 \times 36}{2.2}$$

$$x = 81.8 \text{ mg}$$

Proportion

5 mg : 1 kg :: x mg : 16.4 kg

$$x = 5 \times 16.4$$

$$x = 82 \text{ mg/dose}$$

(Maximum Recommended Dose)

Dimensional Analysis

$$\frac{x \text{ mg}}{\text{dose}} = \frac{10 \text{ mg}}{\text{kg/dose}} \times \frac{1 \text{ kg}}{2.2 \text{ lb}} \times \frac{36 \text{ lb}}{1}$$

$$\frac{x \text{ mg}}{\text{dose}} = \frac{10 \times 36}{2.2}$$

$$x = 163.6 \text{ mg/dose}$$

Proportion

10 mg : 1 kg :: x mg : 16.4 kg

$$x = 10 \times 16.4$$

$$x = 164 \text{ mg/dose}$$

The S&T single dose range for this child is 81.8 to 163.6 mg when using the dimensional analysis method and 82 to 164 mg when using the proportion method.

d. Now perform dosage calculations for the single-dose range using the 100 mg/5 mL strength:

(Minimum Recommended Dose)

Dimensional Analysis

$$x \text{ mL} =$$

$$x \text{ mL} = \frac{5 \text{ mL}}{100 \text{ mg}}$$

$$x \text{ mL} = \frac{5 \text{ mL}}{100 \text{ mg}} \times \frac{81.8 \text{ mg}}{1}$$

$$x = \frac{5 \times 81.8}{100} = 4.09 \text{ mL}$$

Proportion

100 mg : 5 mL :: 82 mg : x mL

$$100x = 5 \times 82$$

$$x = \frac{410}{100}$$

$$x = 4.1 \text{ mL}$$

(Maximum Recommended Dose)

Dimensional Analysis

$x \text{ mL} =$

$$x \text{ mL} = \frac{5 \text{ mL}}{100 \text{ mg}}$$

$$x \text{ mL} = \frac{5 \text{ mL}}{100 \text{ mg}} \times \frac{163.6 \text{ mg}}{1}$$

$$x = \frac{5 \times 163.6}{100} = 8.18 \text{ mL}$$

Proportion

$100 \text{ mg} : 5 \text{ mL} :: 164 \text{ mg} : x \text{ mL}$

$100x = 5 \times 164$

$$x = \frac{820}{100}$$

$x = 8.2 \text{ mL}$

! ● ALERT
_____

Acetaminophen:
Never give more than 5 doses in 24 hours to the infant or young child.
Never exceed 4000 mg/day (4 grams) for the older child and adult.
Teach parents or caregivers.

DETERMINE WHETHER THE PRESCRIBED DOSE IS SAFE AND THERAPEUTIC (MILLIGRAMS/KILOGRAM/DOSE)

This method will **determine whether the child is receiving an S&T dosage** of the drug that is prescribed by the physician. The nurse must determine whether the ordered dose is within the recommended range.

Even though the physician has prescribed the medication to be given, it is the nurse's responsibility to determine whether the dose is S&T to administer to the child. This is done by **dividing the ordered dosage by the child's weight in kilograms (mg/kg/dose)**. A systematic approach is needed.

- Obtain the child's weight in kilograms.
- Obtain the ordered dosage.
- Divide the ordered dose by the child's weight.
- The answer is the mg/kg/dose (for each dose administered).
- Check your drug book to determine whether the ordered dose is S&T (in the recommended dosage range).

EXAMPLE: The doctor has ordered 210 mg of acetaminophen q 4–6 h for pain and fever for a postoperative child. The child weighs 39 lb. The recommended dose range for acetaminophen is 10 to 15 mg/kg/dose q 4–6 h. Acetaminophen is supplied as 160 mg/5 mL.

Is the ordered dose S&T to administer? If the dose ordered is S&T to administer, how many milliliters will be needed?

a. Weight   39 lb = 17.7 kg

b. Ordered   210 mg q 4–6 h

c. Calculation

Dimensional Analysis

$$\frac{x \text{ mg}}{\text{kg/dose}} = \frac{210 \text{ mg}}{\text{dose}} \times \frac{2.2 \text{ lb}}{1 \text{ kg}} \times \frac{}{39 \text{ lb}}$$

$$\frac{x \text{ mg}}{\text{kg/dose}} = \frac{210 \text{ mg}}{\text{dose}} \times \frac{2.2 \text{ lb}}{1 \text{ kg}} \times \frac{}{39 \text{ lb}}$$

$$\frac{x \text{ mg}}{\text{kg/dose}} = \frac{210 \times 2.2}{39}$$

$x = 11.84$ or 11.8 mg/kg/dose

Proportion

$$\frac{210 \text{ mg/dose}}{17.7 \text{ kg}} = 11.86 \text{ or } 11.9 \text{ mg/kg/dose}$$

The dose for this child is 11.8 mg/kg/dose when using the dimensional analysis method and 11.9 mg/kg/dose when using the formula method.

d. Recommended   10 to 15 mg/kg/dose

Yes, it is safe to administer the acetaminophen because it is within the S&T dosage range of 10 to 15 mg/kg/dose.

e. Perform dosage calculation using 160 mg/5 mL concentration:

Dimensional Analysis

$$x \text{ mL} = \frac{5 \text{ mL}}{160 \text{ mg}} \times \frac{210 \text{ mg}}{1}$$

$$x \text{ mL} = \frac{5 \times 210}{160} = 6.56 \text{ or } 6.6 \text{ mL}$$

Proportion

160 mg : 5 mL :: 210 mg : x mL

$160x = 5 \times 210$

$$x = \frac{1050}{160}$$

$x = 6.56$ or 6.6 mL

Remember to round all doses to the nearest tenth. Exceptions: Round all narcotics, antiepileptics, and cardiac medications to *nearest hundredth.* Medications that may be rounded to the nearest hundredth include phenobarbital, morphine, dilantin, digoxin, and anticancer drugs.

CALCULATE THE 24-HOUR DOSAGE (RANGES)

Many drugs are calculated based on the recommended 24-hour dose, then divided into single doses to be given every 12, 8, 6, or 4 hours or as recommended by the drug manufacturers. These divided time schedules vary, and the physician, nurse practitioner, or physician's assistant will order the medication based on the recommended schedules.

Antibiotics especially are given this way. Additionally, an antibiotic may be given in dosages or ranges that have been found to be effective for the child's diagnosis. The physician chooses how often the medication is to be delivered. An example of an antibiotic with many dosing choices is ampicillin.

Recommended dosages for ampicillin may be any of the following:

<2 kg	50 to 100 mg/kg/24 h/q 8 h
>2 kg	100 to 200 mg/kg/24 h/q 8 h
Mild to moderate infection	100 to 200 mg/kg/24 h/q 6 h
Severe infection	200 to 400 mg/kg/24 h/q 4–6 h

The physician must determine the dosage to be given to the infant or child. If an infant or child is diagnosed with otitis media (OM), then the physician may choose the dosage of antibiotic in the mild to moderate range. However, if an infant is admitted with a diagnosis of fever of undetermined origin, sepsis, or meningitis, then the physician may decide to prescribe a larger dosage of the antibiotic, as in the severe infection range.

Knowing the diagnosis is helpful in determining whether the infant or child will be receiving S&T dosages of antibiotics. Nurses who administer antibiotics or antiinfectives can learn how to determine the doses needed for the patient. **However, only the physician, advanced practice nurse, or physician's assistant can prescribe and order the infant's or child's medications.**

EXAMPLE 1: An infant is admitted to the hospital to rule out sepsis. The infant weighs 8 lb. Ampicillin is prescribed. Calculate an S&T 24-hour dosage range for this infant with a possible severe infection.

    a. Weight   8 lb = 3.6 kg

    b. Recommended   200 to 400 mg/kg/24 h q 4–6 h

    c. Calculation

    (Minimum Recommended Dose)

Dimensional Analysis

$$\frac{x \text{ mg}}{\text{day}} = \frac{200 \text{ mg}}{\text{kg/day}} \times \frac{1 \text{ kg}}{2.2 \text{ lb}} \times \frac{8 \text{ lb}}{1}$$

$$\frac{x \text{ mg}}{\text{day}} = \frac{200 \text{ mg}}{\cancel{\text{kg}}/\text{day}} \times \frac{1 \cancel{\text{kg}}}{2.2 \cancel{\text{lb}}} \times \frac{8 \cancel{\text{lb}}}{1}$$

$$\frac{x \text{ mg}}{\text{day}} = \frac{200 \times 8}{2.2}$$

$$x = 727.27 \text{ or } 727.3 \text{ mg/24 h}$$

Formula

3.6 kg × 200 mg/kg/24 h =

3.6 $\cancel{\text{kg}}$ × 200 mg/$\cancel{\text{kg}}$/24 h = 720 mg/24 h

    (Maximum Recommended Dose)

Dimensional Analysis

$$\frac{x \text{ mg}}{\text{day}} = \frac{400 \text{ mg}}{\text{kg/day}} \times \frac{1 \text{ kg}}{2.2 \text{ lb}} \times \frac{8 \text{ lb}}{1}$$

$$\frac{x \text{ mg}}{\text{day}} = \frac{400 \text{ mg}}{\cancel{\text{kg}}/\text{day}} \times \frac{1 \cancel{\text{kg}}}{2.2 \cancel{\text{lb}}} \times \frac{8 \cancel{\text{lb}}}{1}$$

$$\frac{x \text{ mg}}{\text{day}} = \frac{400 \times 8}{2.2}$$

$$x = 1454.54 \text{ or } 1454.5 \text{ mg/24 h}$$

Formula

3.6 kg × 400 mg/kg/24 h =

3.6 $\cancel{\text{kg}}$ × 400 mg/$\cancel{\text{kg}}$/24 h = 1440 mg/24 h

    d. 24-hour dosage range

Dimensional Analysis
727.3 to 1454.5 mg/24 h

Formula
720 to 1440 mg/24 h

This means that the infant can receive 727.3 to 1454.5 mg in a 24-hour period when the dimensional analysis method is used or 720 to 1440 mg in a 24-hour period when the formula method is used.

EXAMPLE 2: The child weighs 35 lb and is diagnosed with OM. The physician prescribes amoxicillin. Calculate an S&T 24-hour dosage range for this patient.

    a. Weight   35 lb = 15.9 kg

    b. Recommended   25 to 50 mg/kg/24 h two or three times a day

                               Adult dosage 250 to 500 mg/dose two times a day

c. Calculation

(Minimum Recommended Dose)

Dimensional Analysis

$$\frac{x \text{ mg}}{\text{day}} = \frac{25 \text{ mg}}{\text{kg/day}} \times \frac{1 \text{ kg}}{2.2 \text{ lb}} \times \frac{35 \text{ lb}}{1}$$

$$\frac{x \text{ mg}}{\text{day}} = \frac{25 \text{ mg}}{\text{kg/day}} \times \frac{1 \text{ kg}}{2.2 \text{ lb}} \times \frac{35 \text{ lb}}{1}$$

$$\frac{x \text{ mg}}{\text{day}} = \frac{25 \times 35}{2.2}$$

$x = 397.72$ or 397.7 mg/24 h

Formula

15.9 kg × 25 mg/kg/24 h =

15.9 kg × 25 mg/kg/24 h = 397.5 mg/24 h

(Maximum Recommended Dose)

Dimensional Analysis

$$\frac{x \text{ mg}}{\text{day}} = \frac{50 \text{ mg}}{\text{kg/day}} \times \frac{1 \text{ kg}}{2.2 \text{ lb}} \times \frac{35 \text{ lb}}{1}$$

$$\frac{x \text{ mg}}{\text{day}} = \frac{50 \text{ mg}}{\text{kg/day}} \times \frac{1 \text{ kg}}{2.2 \text{ lb}} \times \frac{35 \text{ lb}}{1}$$

$$\frac{x \text{ mg}}{\text{day}} = \frac{50 \times 35}{2.2}$$

$x = 795.45$ or 795.5 mg/24 h

Formula

15.9 kg × 50 mg/kg/24 h =

15.9 kg × 50 mg/kg/24 h = 795 mg/24 h

d. 24-hour dosage range

Dimensional Analysis
397.7 to 795.5 mg/24 h

Formula
397.5 to 795 mg/24 h

This means that the child can receive 397.7 to 795.5 mg in a 24-hour period when the dimensional analysis method is used or 397.5 to 795 mg in a 24-hour period when the formula method is used.

Remember not to exceed the adult dose or "max" dose. The physician will now decide how often the child will receive the medication. This is called the individual or single dose, based on 24 hours.

CALCULATE THE INDIVIDUAL DOSE OR SINGLE DOSE (MILLIGRAMS/KILOGRAM/24 HOURS DIVIDED)

The physician will now determine how often the antibiotic will be administered as a single or individual dose. First determine the 24-hour dosage range. Then divide the 24-hour dosage into single doses (the number of times per day the medication is to be given).

- This is the individual dose each time the patient receives the medication.
- These times are established by the drug companies (e.g., q 4 h, q 6 h, q 8 h, q 12 h, or every day).
- **As long as the dose does not exceed the maximum dose established in 24 hours and the dose does not exceed the adult dose, then it can be given safely.**
- The physician will decide how often the medication is to be given.

EXAMPLE 1: A child weighs 22 lb. The physician prescribes ampicillin 100 to 200 mg/kg/24 h divided q 6 h. Calculate the individual dose for ampicillin.

a. Weight   22 lb = 10 kg

b. Recommended   100 to 200 mg/kg/24 h divided q 6 h

3. The physician orders Keflex 300 mg po q 8 h for a child who weighs 34 lb. Keflex is supplied in an oral suspension of 125 mg/5 mL. The recommended daily oral dosage for a child is 50 to 100 mg/kg/24 h divided q 8 h. a. Child's weight is 15.5 kg. b. How many milligrams per kilogram per 24 hours is the child receiving? 58.1 c. If the dosage is S&T, how many milliliters will you administer? 12 mL

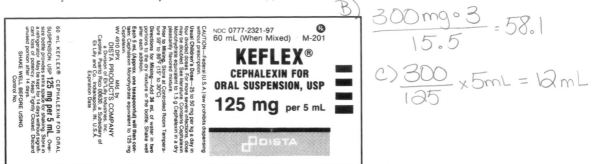

B)
$$\frac{300\,mg \cdot 3}{15.5} = 58.1$$

C) $$\frac{300}{125} \times 5\,mL = 12\,mL$$

4. The physician orders morphine sulfate 4 mg IM STAT for a child weighing 78 lb. Available is morphine sulfate 15 mg/mL. The recommended intramuscular (IM) dosage for a child is 0.1 to 0.2 mg/kg/dose q 2–4 h as needed. a. Child's weight is 35.5 kg. b. What is the safe recommended dosage or range? 3.5-7.1 c. Is the order safe? Prove. yes, 4 in between d. If yes, how many milliliters will you administer? 0.27 mL

B) $$\frac{0.1 \cdot 78}{2.2} = 3.5\,(min)$$

$$\frac{0.2 \cdot 78}{2.2} = 7.1\,(max)$$

C) $$\frac{4}{15} \times 1\,mL = 0.27$$

5. A child has a fever of 101.5° F orally and needs acetaminophen. Calculate an S&T dosage or range of acetaminophen for this child, who weighs 62 lb. Recommended dosage range for acetaminophen is 10 to 15 mg/kg/dose q 4–6 h. It is available as an elixir 160 mg/5 mL.
a. Child's weight is 28.18 kg. b. What is an S&T dosage range for this child? 281.8-422.7
c. How many milliliters are needed for this range? 8.8 - 13.2

B) 281.8-422.7   C) $$\frac{281.8}{160} \times 5 = 8.8\,(min)$$ $$\frac{422.7}{160} \times 5 = 13.2 \,(max)$$

6. The physician orders 1000 mL of 0.9% NS to run over 16 hours. What rate is needed to deliver the ordered fluids? 62.5

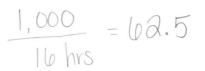

$$\frac{1,000}{16\,hrs} = 62.5$$

7. The physician orders Biaxin 300 mg po twice a day for a child who weighs 92 lb. Available is Biaxin 125 mg/5 mL. The recommended dosage is 15 mg/kg/24 h divided q 12 h.
a. Child's weight is __41.8__ kg. b. What is the S&T dosage for this child? __313.6__
c. Is the order safe? Prove. __yes, does not__ d. If yes, how many milliliters will you administer? __12 mL__ __exceed__

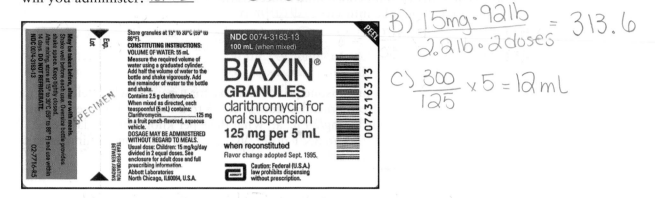

$$B) \frac{15mg \cdot 92lb}{2.2lb \cdot 2\,doses} = 313.6$$

$$C) \frac{300}{125} \times 5 = 12\,mL$$

8. A child is to receive IV fluids at maintenance rate. She weighs 25 lb. a. Child's weight is __11.4__ kg. b. Calculate her 24-hour fluid requirements __1070__ c. How many milliliters per hour are needed to deliver the maintenance fluids? __45 mL/hr__

$$\frac{1000 + 50(11.4) = 1070}{24}$$

9. A patient is to receive vancomycin 650 mg IVPB q 6 h. The patient weighs 96 lb on admission. The recommended dosage is 40 to 60 mg/kg/24 h q 6 h. a. Child's weight is __43.6__ kg. b. How many milligrams per kilogram per 24 hours is the patient receiving? __59.6__ c. Is the written order S&T? Explain. __yes, does not exceed 60__

$$B) \frac{650 \cdot 4}{43.6} = 59.6$$

10. The physician orders Ceclor 300 mg po suspension q 8 h for treatment of otitis media. Recommended oral dosage for infant and child is 20 to 40 mg/kg/24 h q 8 h. Maximum dosage is 2 g/24 h. The patient weighs 95 lb. a. Child's weight is __43.18__ kg. b. How many milligrams per kilogram per 24 hours is the patient receiving? __20.84__ c. Is this an S&T dosage for this patient? Prove. __yes, not above 40__

$$B) \frac{300 \cdot 3}{43.18} = 20.84$$

11. A 10-month-old infant has an order for 100 mL of 0.9% NS to be infused over 6 hours. How many milliliters per hour should the IV pump be programmed for? __16.67__

$$\frac{100}{6hr} = 16.67$$

Handwritten left margin: D) 400 × 2 / 26.4

4. The physician orders Amoxil 400 mg po q 12 h for a child weighing 58 lb. You have Amoxil suspension 250 mg/5 mL. The recommended daily oral dosage for a child is 25 to 50 mg/kg/24 h in divided doses q 12 h. a. Child's weight is *26.4* kg. b. What is the safe 24-hour dosage range for this child? _____ c. What is the single-dose range for this child? _____ d. How many milligrams per kilogram per 24 hours is the patient receiving with this order? *30.3* e. How many milliliters are needed to deliver the ordered dose? *8 mL*

Handwritten (right of Amoxil label):
$$\frac{1 kg}{2.2} \times \frac{58}{1} = 26.4$$
660 – 1320 mg/24 hrs
330 – 660 mg/dose
250/5 = 50 mg/mL
$$\frac{400 mg}{50 mg/mL} = 8 mL$$

AMOXIL® 250mg/5mL

AMOXIL® 250mg/5mL NDC 0029-6009-21

Directions for mixing: Tap bottle until all powder flows freely. Add approximately 1/3 total amount of water for reconstitution (total=59 mL); shake vigorously to wet powder. Add remaining water; again shake vigorously. Each 5 mL (1 teaspoonful) will contain amoxicillin trihydrate equivalent to 250 mg amoxicillin.
Usual Adult Dosage: 250 to 500 mg every 8 hours.
Usual Child Dosage: 20 to 40 mg/kg/day in divided doses every 8 hours, depending on age, weight and infection severity. See accompanying prescribing information.

Keep tightly closed.
Shake well before using.
Refrigeration preferable but not required.
Discard suspension after 14 days.

AMOXIL® AMOXICILLIN FOR ORAL SUSPENSION

80mL (when reconstituted)

SB SmithKline Beecham

NSN 6505-01-153-3442 Net contents: Equivalent to 4.0 grams amoxicillin. Store dry powder at room temperature. Caution: Federal law prohibits dispensing without prescription. SmithKline Beecham Pharmaceuticals Philadelphia, PA 19101

3 0029-6009-21 4

LOT
EXP.
9405783-E

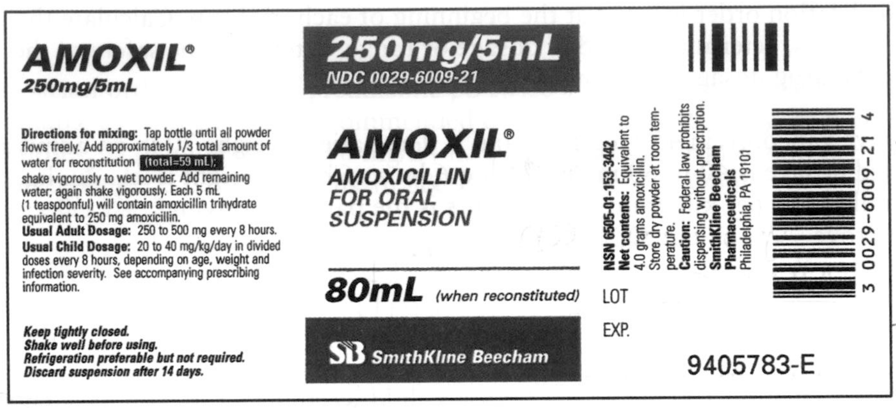

5. The physician orders Keflex 500 mg po q 6 h for a 99-lb school-age child. Available is Keflex 250-mg capsules. The recommended daily oral dosage is 50 to 100 mg/kg/24 h divided q 6 h. Maximum dosage is not to exceed 2 g/24 h. a. Child's weight is *45* kg. b. How many milligrams per kilogram per 24 hours is this child receiving? *44.4* c. Is the order safe? *yes* d. If yes, how many capsules will you administer? *2 caps/dose*

Handwritten (right of Keflex label):
$$\frac{1 kg}{2.2} \times \frac{99 lb}{1} = 45$$
2,250 – 4,500 mg/24 hrs
1,125 – 2,250 mg/dose
$$\frac{2,000 mg}{45 kg} = 44.4 mg/kg/24 hrs$$

CAUTION—Federal (U.S.A.) law prohibits dispensing without prescription.
Keep Tightly Closed
Store at Controlled Room Temperature 59° to 86°F (15° to 30°C)
Manufactured by DISTA PRODUCTS CO. a Division of Eli Lilly Industries, Inc. Carolina, Puerto Rico 00630 a Subsidiary of Eli Lilly and Company Indianapolis, IN, U.S.A.
Expiration Date/Control No.

NDC 0777-0869-02 100 PULVULES® No. 402 Rx
KEFLEX® CEPHALEXIN CAPSULES, USP
250 mg
DISTA

Usual Adult Dose—One PULVULE every 6 hours. For more severe infections, dose may be increased, not to exceed 4 g a day. See literature.
Each PULVULE contains Cephalexin Monohydrate equivalent to 250 mg Cephalexin.
Dispense in a tight container.

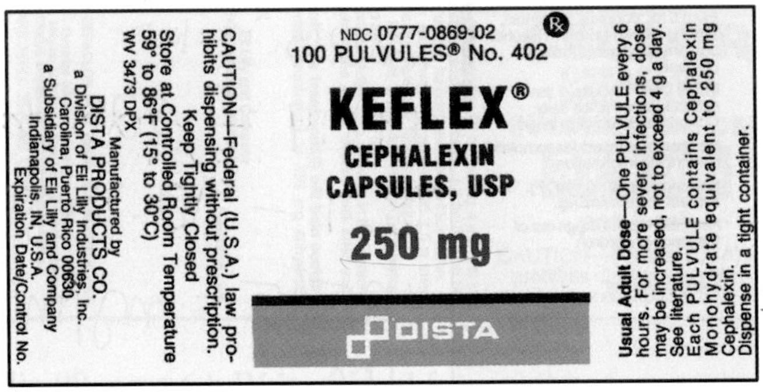

6. The physician orders Omnicef 200 mg po q 12 h for a child weighing 66 lb. Omnicef is available as 125 mg/5 mL. Recommended dosage is 14 mg/kg/24 h divided q 12 h. a. Child's weight is *30* kg. b. How many milligrams per kilogram per 24 hours is the child receiving? *400 mg* c. Is the order safe? *yes* d. If yes, how many milliliters are needed? *8 mL*

Handwritten:
420 mg/24 hrs $\frac{125 mg}{5 mL} = 25 mg/mL$ $\frac{200}{25} = 8 mL/dose$

7. A neonate weighs 2012 g. He is to receive ampicillin 100 to 200 mg/kg/24 h divided q 6 h IV per syringe for otitis media. a. Child's weight is *2.012* kg. b. What 24-hour dosage range is needed? _____ c. What single-dose range is needed? _____

Handwritten:
A) $\frac{2012 g}{1000 kg} = 2.012 kg$ B) 201.2 – 402.4 mg/24 hrs   C) 50.3 – 100.6 mg/dose

8. The physician orders Amoxil 180 mg po q 8 h for a 35-lb child. Available is Amoxil 125 mg/5 mL. Recommended dosage is 25 to 50 mg/kg/24 h divided q 6–8 h. a. Child's weight is 15.9 kg. b. How many milligrams per kilogram per 24 hours is the child receiving? 34 c. Is the order safe? yes d. If yes, how many milliliters are needed? 7.2 mL/Dose

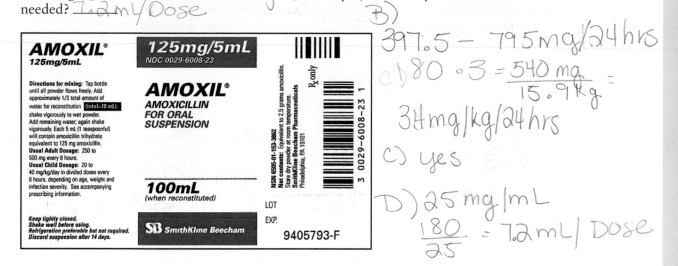

B)
397.5 — 795 mg/24 hrs
C) 180 · 3 = 540 mg / 15.9 kg =
34 mg/kg/24 hrs
C) yes
D) 25 mg/mL
180/25 = 7.2 mL/Dose

9. The physician orders vancomycin 330 mg po q 6 h for a 74-lb child. You have vancomycin 250 mg/5 mL. The recommended daily oral dosage is 40 mg/kg/24 h divided q 6 h. a. Child's weight is 33.6 kg. b. How many milligrams per kilogram per 24 hours is the child receiving? 39.3 c. Is the order safe? yes d. If yes, how many milliliters are needed? 6.6 mL/Dose

B) 330 · 4 = 1,320 mg / 33.6 = 39.3 mg/kg

D) 250/5 = 50
330/50 = 6.6 mL

10. The physician orders morphine sulfate 0.9 mg IV q 4 h for pain. Available is morphine sulfate 0.5 mg/mL. The child weighs 20 lb. The recommended single dose is 0.1 to 0.2 mg/kg q 4 h. a. Child's weight is 9.1 kg. b. What is the safe dose range for this child? ____ c. Is the order safe? yes d. If yes, how many milliliters will you draw up? 1.8 mL

B) 0.91 – 1.82 mg   D) 1.8 mL

C) yes

11. The physician orders an infusion of 200 mL of D₅LR over 3 hours to a 6-year-old child. How many milliliters per hour should the IV pump be programmed for? 66.7

$$\frac{200\,mL}{3\,hrs} = 66.7$$

12. A 60-kg child has an order for vancomycin 500 mg IVPB to be delivered over a 1- to 2-hour period. The vial concentration is 50 mg/mL. The recommended infusion concentration is 5 mg/mL. a. How many milliliters of medication will provide 500 mg of vancomycin? __10__ b. How many milliliters of IV solution need to be added to the medication to equal the recommended concentration? __90__ c. How many drops per minute of vancomycin should be infused? __100__

13. The physician orders Lanoxin 0.013 mg po twice a day for an infant weighing 3036 g. The recommended oral dosage for Lanoxin is 6 to 10 mcg/kg/24 h divided q 12 h. Available is Lanoxin elixir 50 mcg/mL. a. Child's weight is __3.036__ kg. b. What is an S&T 24-hour dosage range for this infant? _____ c. What is a safe single-dose range for this infant? _____ d. Is the order safe? _____ e. If yes, how many milliliters will you give? _____

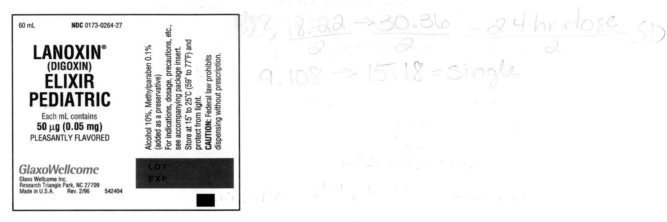

NDC 0173-0264-27 60 mL

LANOXIN®
(DIGOXIN)
ELIXIR PEDIATRIC
Each mL contains
50 µg (0.05 mg)
PLEASANTLY FLAVORED

GlaxoWellcome
Glaxo Wellcome Inc.
Research Triangle Park, NC 27709
Made in U.S.A.   Rev. 2/96   542404

Alcohol 10%, Methylparaben 0.1% (added as a preservative) For indications, dosage, precautions, etc., see accompanying package insert. Store at 15° to 25°C (59° to 77°F) and protect from light. **CAUTION:** Federal law prohibits dispensing without prescription.

LOT EXP

Handwritten: 9.18, 18.22 → 30.36 = 24 hr dose SD, 9.108 → 15.18 = single

14. Calculate the single-dose range of acetaminophen for an infant who weighs 9 lb. Acetaminophen is available as 80 mg/0.8 mL, and the safe dose range is 10 to 15 mg/kg/dose q 6 h. a. Infant's weight is __4.09__ kg. b. What is the single-dose range? _____ c. How many milliliters are needed to deliver the calculated dose range? _____

Handwritten: B) 40.9 → 61.4   C) 0.4 → 0.6

15. Phenobarbital elixir 72 mg po daily is ordered for a child who weighs 37 lb. Phenobarbital is supplied as 20 mg/5 mL. Recommended dosage is 4 to 6 mg/kg/24 h one or two times per day. a. Child's weight is __16.82__ kg. b. What is the 24-hour dosage range needed for this child? _____ c. Is the order safe? __yes__ d. If yes, how many milliliters will you administer? __18mL__

Handwritten: B) 67.27 → 100.9

ANSWERS ON PP. 539–541 AND 546–548.

evolve   For additional practice problems, refer to the Pediatric Calculations section of *Drug Calculations Companion,* Version 5, on Evolve.

ANSWERS

CHAPTER 18 Dimensional Analysis—Work Sheet, pp. 523–526

1. b. $\dfrac{x\ \text{mg}}{\text{day}} = \dfrac{25\ \text{mg}}{\text{kg/day}} \times \dfrac{1\ \text{kg}}{2.2\ \text{lb}} \times \dfrac{50\ \text{lb}}{1} = 568.18$ or 568.2 mg/day (minimum)

   $\dfrac{x\ \text{mg}}{\text{day}} = \dfrac{50\ \text{mg}}{\text{kg/day}} \times \dfrac{1\ \text{kg}}{2.2\ \text{lb}} \times \dfrac{50\ \text{lb}}{1} = 1136.36$ or 1136.4 mg/day (maximum)

   c. Yes, the order is safe to administer.

   d. $x\ \text{cap} = \dfrac{1\ \text{cap}}{250\ \text{mg}} \times \dfrac{250\ \text{mg}}{1} = 1$ capsule

2. b. $\dfrac{x\ \text{mg}}{\text{day}} = \dfrac{0.035\ \text{mg}}{\text{kg/day}} \times \dfrac{1\ \text{kg}}{2.2\ \text{lb}} \times \dfrac{6.5\ \text{lb}}{1} = 0.1$ mg/day (minimum)

   $\dfrac{x\ \text{mg}}{\text{day}} = \dfrac{0.06\ \text{mg}}{\text{kg/day}} \times \dfrac{1\ \text{kg}}{2.2\ \text{lb}} \times \dfrac{6.5\ \text{lb}}{1} = 0.18$ mg/day (maximum)

   c. No, the order is not safe.

   d. Question this order.

3. b. $\dfrac{x\ \text{mg}}{\text{dose}} = \dfrac{5\ \text{mg}}{\text{kg/day}} \times \dfrac{1\ \text{kg}}{2.2\ \text{lb}} \times \dfrac{50\ \text{lb}}{1} \times \dfrac{1\ \text{day}}{4\ \text{doses}} = 28.4$ mg/dose

   c. The order is safe as 25 mg is below 28.4 mg.

   d. $x\ \text{mL} = \dfrac{1\ \text{mL}}{12.5\ \text{mg}} \times \dfrac{25\ \text{mg}}{1} = 2$ mL

4. a. $x\ \text{kg} = \dfrac{1\ \text{kg}}{2.2\ \text{lb}} \times \dfrac{28\ \text{lb}}{1} = 12.7$ kg

   First 10 kg: $x\ \text{mL} = \dfrac{100\ \text{mL}}{\text{kg}} \times \dfrac{10\ \text{kg}}{1} = 1000$ mL/day

   Remaining 2.7 kg: $x\ \text{mL} = \dfrac{50\ \text{mL}}{\text{kg}} \times \dfrac{2.7\ \text{kg}}{1} = 135$ mL/day

   b. $1000 + 135 = 1135$ mL/day

   $\dfrac{x\ \text{mL}}{\text{h}} = \dfrac{1135\ \text{mL}}{24\ \text{h}} = 47.3$ or 47 mL/h

5. b. $\dfrac{x\ \text{mg}}{\text{dose}} = \dfrac{14\ \text{mg}}{\text{kg/day}} \times \dfrac{1\ \text{kg}}{2.2\ \text{lb}} \times \dfrac{22\ \text{lb}}{1} \times \dfrac{1\ \text{day}}{2\ \text{doses}} = 70$ mg/dose

   Yes, 70 mg is ordered.

   c. $x\ \text{mL} = \dfrac{5\ \text{mL}}{125\ \text{mg}} \times \dfrac{70\ \text{mg}}{1} = 2.8$ mL

6. b. $\dfrac{x\ \text{mg}}{\text{day}} = \dfrac{20\ \text{mg}}{\text{kg/day}} \times \dfrac{30.3\ \text{kg}}{1} = 606$ mg/day (minimum)

   $\dfrac{x\ \text{mg}}{\text{day}} = \dfrac{30\ \text{mg}}{\text{kg/day}} \times \dfrac{30.3\ \text{kg}}{1} = 909$ mg/day (maximum)

   c. $\dfrac{x\ \text{mg}}{\text{dose}} = \dfrac{606\ \text{mg}}{\text{day}} \times \dfrac{1\ \text{day}}{2\ \text{doses}} = 303$ mg/dose (minimum)

   $\dfrac{x\ \text{mg}}{\text{dose}} = \dfrac{909\ \text{mg}}{\text{day}} \times \dfrac{1\ \text{day}}{2\ \text{doses}} = 454.5$ mg/dose (maximum)

   d. $x\ \text{mL} = \dfrac{5\ \text{mL}}{250\ \text{mg}} \times \dfrac{300\ \text{mg}}{1} = 6$ mL

7. b. $\dfrac{x \text{ mg}}{\text{day}} = \dfrac{0.5 \text{ mg}}{\text{kg/day}} \times \dfrac{1 \text{ kg}}{2.2 \text{ lb}} \times \dfrac{94 \text{ lb}}{1} = 21.36 \text{ or } 21.4 \text{ mg/day (minimum)}$

$\dfrac{x \text{ mg}}{\text{day}} = \dfrac{2 \text{ mg}}{\text{kg/day}} \times \dfrac{1 \text{ kg}}{2.2 \text{ lb}} \times \dfrac{94 \text{ lb}}{1} = 85.45 \text{ or } 85.5 \text{ mg/day (maximum)}$

c. No, 90 mg exceeds the maximum dose of 85.5 mg.

d. No, call the physician who wrote the order.

8. b. $\dfrac{x \text{ mg}}{\text{day}} = \dfrac{5 \text{ mg}}{\text{kg/day}} \times \dfrac{1 \text{ kg}}{2.2 \text{ lb}} \times \dfrac{40 \text{ lb}}{1} = 90.9 \text{ mg/day (minimum)}$

$\dfrac{x \text{ mg}}{\text{day}} = \dfrac{7 \text{ mg}}{\text{kg/day}} \times \dfrac{1 \text{ kg}}{2.2 \text{ lb}} \times \dfrac{40 \text{ lb}}{1} = 127.27 \text{ or } 127.3 \text{ mg/day (maximum)}$

c. Yes, 60 mg q 12 h = 120 mg/day.

d. $x \text{ tab} = \dfrac{1 \text{ tab}}{30 \text{ mg}} \times \dfrac{60 \text{ mg}}{1} = 2 \text{ chewtabs}$

9. b. $\dfrac{x \text{ mg}}{\text{kg/day}} = \dfrac{750 \text{ mg}}{\text{dose}} \times \dfrac{4 \text{ doses}}{1 \text{ day}} \times \dfrac{2.2 \text{ lb}}{1 \text{ kg}} \times \dfrac{}{68 \text{ lb}} = 97.05 \text{ or } 97.1 \text{ mg/kg/day}$

c. No, it exceeds the recommended range of 40–60 mg/kg/24h.

10. b. $\dfrac{x \text{ mg}}{\text{dose}} = \dfrac{25 \text{ mg}}{\text{kg/day}} \times \dfrac{1 \text{ kg}}{2.2 \text{ lb}} \times \dfrac{42 \text{ lb}}{1} \times \dfrac{1 \text{ day}}{2 \text{ doses}} = 238.63 \text{ mg/dose (minimum)}$

$\dfrac{x \text{ mg}}{\text{dose}} = \dfrac{50 \text{ mg}}{\text{kg/day}} \times \dfrac{1 \text{ kg}}{2.2 \text{ lb}} \times \dfrac{42 \text{ lb}}{1} \times \dfrac{1 \text{ day}}{2 \text{ doses}} = 477.27 \text{ mg/dose (maximum)}$

c. $x \text{ mL} = \dfrac{5 \text{ mL}}{125 \text{ mg}} \times \dfrac{300 \text{ mg}}{1} = 12 \text{ mL}$

11. $\dfrac{x \text{ gtt}}{\text{min}} = \dfrac{60 \text{ gtt}}{1 \text{ mL}} \times \dfrac{100 \text{ mL}}{30 \text{ min}} = 200 \text{ gtt/min}$

12. b. $\dfrac{x \text{ mg}}{\text{dose}} = \dfrac{10 \text{ mg}}{\text{kg/day}} \times \dfrac{1 \text{ kg}}{2.2 \text{ lb}} \times \dfrac{58 \text{ lb}}{1} \times \dfrac{1 \text{ day}}{3 \text{ doses}} = 87.88 \text{ mg/dose (minimum)}$

$\dfrac{x \text{ mg}}{\text{dose}} = \dfrac{20 \text{ mg}}{\text{kg/day}} \times \dfrac{1 \text{ kg}}{2.2 \text{ lb}} \times \dfrac{58 \text{ lb}}{1} \times \dfrac{1 \text{ day}}{3 \text{ doses}} = 175.76 \text{ mg/dose (maximum)}$

c. Yes, the order is safe.

d. $x \text{ mL} = \dfrac{5 \text{ mL}}{100 \text{ mg}} \times \dfrac{150 \text{ mg}}{1} = 7.5 \text{ mL}$

13. a. $x \text{ kg} = \dfrac{1 \text{ kg}}{2.2 \text{ lb}} \times \dfrac{72 \text{ lb}}{1} = 32.7 \text{ kg}$

b. First 20 kg: $x \text{ mL} = \dfrac{1500 \text{ mL}}{\text{day}} = 1500 \text{ mL/day}$

Remaining 12.7 kg: $x \text{ mL} = \dfrac{20 \text{ mL}}{\text{kg}} \times \dfrac{12.7 \text{ kg}}{1} = 254 \text{ mL/day}$

$1500 + 254 = 1754 \text{ mL/24 h}$

c. $\dfrac{x \text{ mL}}{\text{h}} = \dfrac{1754 \text{ mL}}{24 \text{ h}} = 73.1 \text{ or } 73 \text{ mL/h}$

14. b. $\dfrac{x \text{ mg}}{\text{dose}} = \dfrac{5 \text{ mg}}{\text{kg/dose}} \times \dfrac{1 \text{ kg}}{2.2 \text{ lb}} \times \dfrac{52 \text{ lb}}{1} = 118.18 \text{ or } 118.2 \text{ mg/dose (minimum)}$

$\dfrac{x \text{ mg}}{\text{dose}} = \dfrac{10 \text{ mg}}{\text{kg/dose}} \times \dfrac{1 \text{ kg}}{2.2 \text{ lb}} \times \dfrac{52 \text{ lb}}{1} = 236.36 \text{ or } 236.4 \text{ mg/dose (maximum)}$

c. $x \text{ mL} = \dfrac{5 \text{ mL}}{100 \text{ mg}} \times \dfrac{100 \text{ mg}}{1} = 5 \text{ mL}$

ANSWERS

15. b. $\dfrac{x \text{ mg}}{\text{dose}} = \dfrac{25 \text{ mg}}{\text{kg/day}} \times \dfrac{1 \text{ kg}}{2.2 \text{ lb}} \times \dfrac{81 \text{ lb}}{1} \times \dfrac{1 \text{ day}}{4 \text{ doses}} = 230.11 \text{ or } 230.1 \text{ mg/dose (minimum)}$

$\dfrac{x \text{ mg}}{\text{dose}} = \dfrac{50 \text{ mg}}{\text{kg/day}} \times \dfrac{1 \text{ kg}}{2.2 \text{ lb}} \times \dfrac{81 \text{ lb}}{1} \times \dfrac{1 \text{ day}}{4 \text{ doses}} = 460.22 \text{ or } 460.2 \text{ mg/dose (maximum)}$

c. Yes, 350 mg/dose is safe to administer.

d. $x \text{ mL} = \dfrac{5 \text{ mL}}{500 \text{ mg}} \times \dfrac{350 \text{ mg}}{1} = 3.5 \text{ mL}$

16. b. $\dfrac{x \text{ mg}}{\text{dose}} = \dfrac{15 \text{ mg}}{\text{kg/day}} \times \dfrac{1 \text{ kg}}{2.2 \text{ lb}} \times \dfrac{16 \text{ lb}}{1} \times \dfrac{1 \text{ day}}{3 \text{ doses}} = 36.36 \text{ or } 36.4 \text{ mg/dose (minimum)}$

$\dfrac{x \text{ mg}}{\text{dose}} = \dfrac{20 \text{ mg}}{\text{kg/day}} \times \dfrac{1 \text{ kg}}{2.2 \text{ lb}} \times \dfrac{16 \text{ lb}}{1} \times \dfrac{1 \text{ day}}{3 \text{ doses}} = 48.48 \text{ or } 48.5 \text{ mg/dose (maximum)}$

c. No, the order of 60 mg q 8 h exceeds the safe dose range.

d. $\dfrac{x \text{ mg}}{\text{kg/day}} = \dfrac{60 \text{ mg}}{\text{dose}} \times \dfrac{3 \text{ doses}}{\text{day}} \times \dfrac{2.2 \text{ lb}}{1 \text{ kg}} \times \dfrac{1}{16 \text{ lb}} = 24.75 \text{ or } 24.8 \text{ mg/kg/day}$

e. This is not safe; do not administer. Call the physician or pharmacist to check.

17. b. $\dfrac{x \text{ mg}}{\text{day}} = \dfrac{0.5 \text{ mg}}{\text{kg/day}} \times \dfrac{1 \text{ kg}}{2.2 \text{ lb}} \times \dfrac{19 \text{ lb}}{1} = 4.31 \text{ or } 4.3 \text{ mg/day (minimum)}$

$\dfrac{x \text{ mg}}{\text{day}} = \dfrac{2 \text{ mg}}{\text{kg/day}} \times \dfrac{1 \text{ kg}}{2.2 \text{ lb}} \times \dfrac{19 \text{ lb}}{1} = 17.27 \text{ or } 17.3 \text{ mg/day (maximum)}$

c. Yes, it is safe to administer.

d. $x \text{ mL} = \dfrac{5 \text{ mL}}{5 \text{ mg}} \times \dfrac{8 \text{ mg}}{1} = 8 \text{ mL}$

18. b. $\dfrac{x \text{ mg}}{\text{day}} = \dfrac{100 \text{ mg}}{\text{kg/day}} \times \dfrac{1 \text{ kg}}{2.2 \text{ lb}} \times \dfrac{32 \text{ lb}}{1} = 1454.54 \text{ or } 1454.5 \text{ mg/day}$

c. $\dfrac{x \text{ mg}}{\text{day}} = \dfrac{400 \text{ mg}}{\text{dose}} \times \dfrac{3 \text{ doses}}{\text{day}} = 1200 \text{ mg/day}$

Yes, this order is safe.

d. $x \text{ mL} = \dfrac{1 \text{ mL}}{330 \text{ mg}} \times \dfrac{400 \text{ mg}}{1} = 1.2 \text{ mL}$

19. $\dfrac{x \text{ mL}}{\text{h}} = \dfrac{250 \text{ mL}}{3 \text{ h}} = 83.3 \text{ mL/h}$

20. a. $x \text{ mL} = \dfrac{1 \text{ mL}}{10 \text{ mg}} \times \dfrac{40 \text{ mg}}{1} = 4 \text{ mL}$

b. $x \text{ mL} = \dfrac{1 \text{ mL}}{2 \text{ mg}} \times \dfrac{40 \text{ mg}}{1} = 20 \text{ mL}$

20 mL − 4 mL = 16 mL

c. $\dfrac{x \text{ gtt}}{\text{min}} = \dfrac{60 \text{ gtt}}{1 \text{ mL}} \times \dfrac{20 \text{ mL}}{20 \text{ min}} = 60 \text{ gtt/min}$

CHAPTER 18 Dimensional Analysis—Posttest 1, pp. 527–530

1. b. $\dfrac{x \text{ mg}}{\text{dose}} = \dfrac{4 \text{ mg}}{\text{kg/day}} \times \dfrac{1 \text{ kg}}{2.2 \text{ lb}} \times \dfrac{55 \text{ lb}}{1} \times \dfrac{1 \text{ day}}{2 \text{ doses}} = 50 \text{ mg/dose (minimum)}$

$\dfrac{x \text{ mg}}{\text{dose}} = \dfrac{6 \text{ mg}}{\text{kg/day}} \times \dfrac{1 \text{ kg}}{2.2 \text{ lb}} \times \dfrac{55 \text{ lb}}{1} \times \dfrac{1 \text{ day}}{2 \text{ doses}} = 75 \text{ mg/dose (maximum)}$

c. Yes, 60 mg is ordered, and it falls within the 50 to 75 mg/dose range.

d. $x \text{ mL} = \dfrac{5 \text{ mL}}{20 \text{ mg}} \times \dfrac{60 \text{ mg}}{1} = 15 \text{ mL}$

ANSWERS

2. b. $\dfrac{x \text{ mg}}{\text{dose}} = \dfrac{25 \text{ mg}}{\text{kg/day}} \times \dfrac{1 \text{ kg}}{2.2 \text{ lb}} \times \dfrac{44 \text{ lb}}{1} \times \dfrac{1 \text{ day}}{4 \text{ doses}} = 125 \text{ mg/dose (minimum)}$

$\dfrac{x \text{ mg}}{\text{dose}} = \dfrac{50 \text{ mg}}{\text{kg/day}} \times \dfrac{1 \text{ kg}}{2.2 \text{ lb}} \times \dfrac{44 \text{ lb}}{1} \times \dfrac{1 \text{ day}}{4 \text{ doses}} = 250 \text{ mg/dose (maximum)}$

   c. No, 500 mg q 6 h exceeds the recommended dosage for weight.

   d. Question this order.

3. b. $\dfrac{x \text{ mg}}{\text{kg/day}} = \dfrac{300 \text{ mg}}{\text{dose}} \times \dfrac{3 \text{ doses}}{1 \text{ day}} \times \dfrac{2.2 \text{ lb}}{1 \text{ kg}} \times \dfrac{}{34 \text{ lb}} = 58.23 \text{ or } 58.2 \text{ mg/kg/day}$

   c. Dosage is safe and therapeutic; it falls in the recommended range.

$x \text{ mL} = \dfrac{5 \text{ mL}}{125 \text{ mg}} \times \dfrac{300 \text{ mg}}{1} = 12 \text{ mL}$

4. b. $\dfrac{x \text{ mg}}{\text{dose}} = \dfrac{0.1 \text{ mg}}{\text{kg/dose}} \times \dfrac{1 \text{ kg}}{2.2 \text{ lb}} \times \dfrac{78 \text{ lb}}{1} = 3.54 \text{ or } 3.5 \text{ mg/dose (minimum)}$

$\dfrac{x \text{ mg}}{\text{dose}} = \dfrac{0.2 \text{ mg}}{\text{kg/dose}} \times \dfrac{1 \text{ kg}}{2.2 \text{ lb}} \times \dfrac{78 \text{ lb}}{1} = 7.09 \text{ or } 7.1 \text{ mg/dose (maximum)}$

   c. Yes, 4 mg is between 3.54 and 7.09 mg.

   d. $x \text{ mL} = \dfrac{1 \text{ mL}}{15 \text{ mg}} \times \dfrac{4 \text{ mg}}{1} = 0.27 \text{ mL}$

5. b. $\dfrac{x \text{ mg}}{\text{dose}} = \dfrac{10 \text{ mg}}{\text{kg/dose}} \times \dfrac{1 \text{ kg}}{2.2 \text{ lb}} \times \dfrac{62 \text{ lb}}{1} = 281.81 \text{ or } 281.8 \text{ mg/dose (minimum)}$

$\dfrac{x \text{ mg}}{\text{dose}} = \dfrac{15 \text{ mg}}{\text{kg/dose}} \times \dfrac{1 \text{ kg}}{2.2 \text{ lb}} \times \dfrac{62 \text{ lb}}{1} = 422.72 \text{ or } 422.7 \text{ mg/dose (maximum)}$

   c. $x \text{ mL} = \dfrac{5 \text{ mL}}{160 \text{ mg}} \times \dfrac{281.82 \text{ mg}}{1} = 8.8 \text{ mL (minimum)}$

$x \text{ mL} = \dfrac{5 \text{ mL}}{160 \text{ mg}} \times \dfrac{422.73 \text{ mg}}{1} = 13.2 \text{ mL (maximum)}$

6. $\dfrac{x \text{ mL}}{\text{h}} = \dfrac{1000 \text{ mL}}{16 \text{ h}} = 62.5 \text{ mL/h}$

7. b. $\dfrac{x \text{ mg}}{\text{dose}} = \dfrac{15 \text{ mg}}{\text{kg/day}} \times \dfrac{1 \text{ kg}}{2.2 \text{ lb}} \times \dfrac{92 \text{ lb}}{1} \times \dfrac{1 \text{ day}}{2 \text{ doses}} = 313.64 \text{ or } 313.6 \text{ mg/dose}$

   c. Yes, 300 mg does not exceed 313.64 mg, so it is a safe dose.

   d. $x \text{ mL} = \dfrac{5 \text{ mL}}{125 \text{ mg}} \times \dfrac{300 \text{ mg}}{1} = 12 \text{ mL}$

8. a. $x \text{ kg} = \dfrac{1 \text{ kg}}{2.2 \text{ lb}} \times \dfrac{25 \text{ lb}}{1} = 11.4 \text{ kg}$

   b.   First 10 kg: $x \text{ mL} = \dfrac{100 \text{ mL}}{\text{kg}} \times \dfrac{10 \text{ kg}}{1} = 1000 \text{ mL/24 h}$

      Remaining 1.4 kg: $x \text{ mL} = \dfrac{50 \text{ mL}}{\text{kg}} \times \dfrac{1.4 \text{ kg}}{1} = 70 \text{ mL/24 h}$

             $1000 \text{ mL/24 h} + 70 \text{ mL/24 h} = 1070 \text{ mL/24 h}$

   c. $\dfrac{x \text{ mL}}{\text{h}} = \dfrac{1070 \text{ mL}}{24 \text{ h}} = 44.6 \text{ mL/h}$

9. b. $\dfrac{x \text{ mg}}{\text{kg/day}} = \dfrac{650 \text{ mg}}{\text{dose}} \times \dfrac{4 \text{ doses}}{1 \text{ day}} \times \dfrac{2.2 \text{ lb}}{1 \text{ kg}} \times \dfrac{}{96 \text{ lb}} = 59.58 \text{ or } 59.6 \text{ mg/kg/day}$

   c. Yes, it is safe; recommended is 40 to 60 mg/kg/24 h. Child is receiving 59.58 mg/kg/day.

10. b. $\dfrac{x \text{ mg}}{\text{kg/day}} = \dfrac{300 \text{ mg}}{\text{dose}} \times \dfrac{3 \text{ doses}}{1 \text{ day}} \times \dfrac{2.2 \text{ lb}}{1 \text{ kg}} \times \dfrac{}{95 \text{ lb}} = 20.84 \text{ mg/kg/day}$

   c. The child is receiving 20.84 mg/kg/day. Recommended is 20 to 40 mg/kg/day. The ordered dose is both safe and therapeutic.

11. $\dfrac{x \text{ mL}}{\text{h}} = \dfrac{100 \text{ mL}}{6 \text{ h}} = 16.7 \text{ or } 17 \text{ mL/h}$

12. a. $x \text{ mL} = \dfrac{1 \text{ mL}}{250 \text{ mg}} \times \dfrac{400 \text{ mg}}{1} = 1.6 \text{ mL}$

   b. $x \text{ mL} = \dfrac{1 \text{ mL}}{50 \text{ mg}} \times \dfrac{400 \text{ mg}}{1} = 8 \text{ mL}$

     $8 \text{ mL} - 1.6 \text{ mL} = 6.4 \text{ mL}$

   c. $\dfrac{x \text{ gtt}}{\text{min}} = \dfrac{60 \text{ gtt}}{1 \text{ mL}} \times \dfrac{8 \text{ mL}}{30 \text{ min}} = 16 \text{ gtt/min}$

13. a. $\dfrac{x \text{ mg}}{\text{kg/day}} = \dfrac{60 \text{ mg}}{\text{dose}} \times \dfrac{2 \text{ doses}}{1 \text{ day}} \times \dfrac{}{30 \text{ kg}} = 4 \text{ mg/kg/day}$

   b. No, the ordered dosage is more than the recommended 0.5 to 2 mg/kg/24 h. Also, the maximum dose is 80 mg/25 h, and this is exceeded as well.

   c. No, check with the physician.

14. b. $\dfrac{x \text{ mg}}{\text{dose}} = \dfrac{15 \text{ mg}}{\text{kg/day}} \times \dfrac{1 \text{ kg}}{2.2 \text{ lb}} \times \dfrac{89 \text{ lb}}{1} \times \dfrac{1 \text{ day}}{2 \text{ doses}} = 303.4 \text{ mg/dose (minimum)}$

     $\dfrac{x \text{ mg}}{\text{dose}} = \dfrac{20 \text{ mg}}{\text{kg/day}} \times \dfrac{1 \text{ kg}}{2.2 \text{ lb}} \times \dfrac{89 \text{ lb}}{1} \times \dfrac{1 \text{ day}}{2 \text{ doses}} = 404.55 \text{ or } 404.6 \text{ mg/dose (maximum)}$

   c. Yes, 400 mg/dose is within the recommended single-dose range.

   d. $x \text{ mL} = \dfrac{5 \text{ mL}}{375 \text{ mg}} \times \dfrac{400 \text{ mg}}{1} = 5.3 \text{ mL}$

15. b. $\dfrac{x \text{ mg}}{\text{kg/day}} = \dfrac{90 \text{ mg}}{\text{dose}} \times \dfrac{4 \text{ doses}}{1 \text{ day}} \times \dfrac{2.2 \text{ lb}}{1 \text{ kg}} \times \dfrac{}{11 \text{ lb}} = 72 \text{ mg/kg/24 h}$

   c. The order is both safe and therapeutic, between the recommended 50 to 100 mg/kg/24 h.

CHAPTER 18 Dimensional Analysis—Posttest 2, pp. 531–534

1. b. $\dfrac{x \text{ mg}}{\text{kg/day}} = \dfrac{450 \text{ mg}}{\text{dose}} \times \dfrac{4 \text{ doses}}{1 \text{ day}} \times \dfrac{2.2 \text{ lb}}{1 \text{ kg}} \times \dfrac{}{70 \text{ lb}} = 56.57 \text{ mg/kg/24 h}$

   c. Yes, the child is receiving 56.6 mg/kg/24 h, which is between 40 and 60 mg/kg/24 h.

2. b. $\dfrac{x \text{ mg}}{\text{day}} = \dfrac{7 \text{ mg}}{\text{kg/day}} \times \dfrac{1 \text{ kg}}{2.2 \text{ lb}} \times \dfrac{62 \text{ lb}}{1} = 197.27 \text{ mg/day (minimum)}$

     $\dfrac{x \text{ mg}}{\text{day}} = \dfrac{8 \text{ mg}}{\text{kg/day}} \times \dfrac{1 \text{ kg}}{2.2 \text{ lb}} \times \dfrac{62 \text{ lb}}{1} = 225.45 \text{ mg/day (maximum)}$

   c. $\dfrac{x \text{ mg}}{\text{dose}} = \dfrac{197.27 \text{ mg}}{1 \text{ day}} \times \dfrac{1 \text{ day}}{2 \text{ doses}} = 98.64 \text{ or } 98.6 \text{ mg/dose}$

     $\dfrac{x \text{ mg}}{\text{dose}} = \dfrac{225.45 \text{ mg}}{1 \text{ day}} \times \dfrac{1 \text{ day}}{2 \text{ doses}} = 112.73 \text{ or } 112.7 \text{ mg/dose}$

   d. Yes, the ordered dose is both safe and therapeutic because it falls within the recommended 24-hour dosage and single-dose ranges.

   e. $x \text{ mL} = \dfrac{5 \text{ mL}}{125 \text{ mg}} \times \dfrac{100 \text{ mg}}{1} = 4 \text{ mL}$

3. $\dfrac{x \text{ gtt}}{\text{min}} = \dfrac{60 \text{ gtt}}{1 \text{ mL}} \times \dfrac{150 \text{ mL}}{3 \text{ h}} \times \dfrac{1 \text{ h}}{60 \text{ min}} = 50 \text{ gtt/min}$

ANSWERS

4. b. $\dfrac{x\ mg}{day} = \dfrac{25\ mg}{kg/day} \times \dfrac{1\ kg}{2.2\ lb} \times \dfrac{58\ lb}{1} = 659.09$ or 659.1 (minimum)

$\dfrac{x\ mg}{day} = \dfrac{50\ mg}{kg/day} \times \dfrac{1\ kg}{2.2\ lb} \times \dfrac{58\ lb}{1} = 1318.18$ or 1318.2 mg/day (maximum)

c. $\dfrac{x\ mg}{dose} = \dfrac{659.09\ mg}{1\ day} \times \dfrac{1\ day}{2\ doses} = 329.54$ or 329.5 mg/dose

$\dfrac{x\ mg}{dose} = \dfrac{1318.18\ mg}{1\ day} \times \dfrac{1\ day}{2\ doses} = 659.09$ or 659.1 mg/dose

d. $\dfrac{x\ mg}{kg/day} = \dfrac{400\ mg}{dose} \times \dfrac{2\ doses}{1\ day} \times \dfrac{2.2\ lb}{1\ kg} \times \dfrac{}{58\ lb} = 30.3$ mg/kg/24 h

e. $x\ mL = \dfrac{5\ mL}{250\ mg} \times \dfrac{400\ mg}{1} = 8$ mL

5. b. $\dfrac{x\ mg}{kg/day} = \dfrac{500\ mg}{dose} \times \dfrac{4\ doses}{1\ day} \times \dfrac{2.2\ lb}{1\ kg} \times \dfrac{}{99\ lb} = 44.44$ or 44.4 mg/kg/24 h

c. Yes, the recommended dosage is 50 to 100 mg/kg/24 h.

d. $x\ cap = \dfrac{1\ cap}{250\ mg} \times \dfrac{500\ mg}{1} = 2$ capsules

6. b. $\dfrac{x\ mg}{kg/day} = \dfrac{200\ mg}{dose} \times \dfrac{2\ doses}{1\ day} \times \dfrac{2.2\ lb}{1\ kg} \times \dfrac{}{66\ lb} = 13.33$ or 13.3 mg/kg/day

c. Yes, the dose is safe and therapeutic.

d. $x\ mL = \dfrac{5\ mL}{125\ mg} \times \dfrac{200\ mg}{1} = 8$ mL

7. b. $\dfrac{x\ mg}{day} = \dfrac{100\ mg}{kg/day} \times \dfrac{1\ kg}{1000\ g} \times \dfrac{2012\ g}{1} = 201$ mg/day (minimum)

$\dfrac{x\ mg}{day} = \dfrac{200\ mg}{kg/day} \times \dfrac{1\ kg}{1000\ g} \times \dfrac{2012\ g}{1} = 402.4$ mg/day (maximum)

c. $\dfrac{x\ mg}{dose} = \dfrac{201\ mg}{day} \times \dfrac{1\ day}{4\ doses} = 50.25$ or 50.3 mg/dose (minimum)

$\dfrac{x\ mg}{dose} = \dfrac{402.4\ mg}{day} \times \dfrac{1\ day}{4\ doses} = 100.6$ mg/dose (maximum)

8. b. $\dfrac{x\ mg}{kg/day} = \dfrac{180\ mg}{dose} \times \dfrac{3\ doses}{1\ day} \times \dfrac{2.2\ lb}{1\ kg} \times \dfrac{}{35\ lb} = 33.94$ or 33.9 mg/kg/day

c. Yes, the ordered dose is within the safe and therapeutic range.

d. $x\ mL = \dfrac{5\ mL}{125\ mg} \times \dfrac{180\ mg}{1} = 7.2$ mL

9. b. $\dfrac{x\ mg}{kg/day} = \dfrac{330\ mg}{dose} \times \dfrac{4\ doses}{1\ day} \times \dfrac{2.2\ lb}{1\ kg} \times \dfrac{}{74\ lb} = 39.24$ or 39.2 mg/kg/day

c. Yes, the dose ordered is safe to administer.

d. $x\ mL = \dfrac{5\ mL}{250\ mg} \times \dfrac{330\ mg}{1} = 6.6$ mL

10. b. $\dfrac{x\ mg}{dose} = \dfrac{0.1\ mg}{kg/dose} \times \dfrac{1\ kg}{2.2\ lb} \times \dfrac{20\ lb}{1} = 0.91$ mg/dose (minimum)

$\dfrac{x\ mg}{dose} = \dfrac{0.2\ mg}{kg/dose} \times \dfrac{1\ kg}{2.2\ lb} \times \dfrac{20\ lb}{1} = 1.82$ mg/dose (maximum)

c. No, 0.9 mg/dose is not within the safe range to administer. Contact the physician.

d. $x\ mL = \dfrac{1\ mL}{0.5\ mg} \times \dfrac{0.9\ mg}{1} = 1.8$ mL if dose is approved

11. $\dfrac{x\ mL}{h} = \dfrac{200\ mL}{3\ h} = 66.7$ or 67 mL/h

12. a. $x\text{ mL} = \dfrac{1\text{ mL}}{50\text{ mg}} \times \dfrac{500\text{ mg}}{1} = 10\text{ mL}$

b. $x\text{ mL} = \dfrac{1\text{ mL}}{5\text{ mg}} \times \dfrac{500\text{ mg}}{1} = 100\text{ mL} - 10\text{ mL} = 90\text{ mL}$

c. $\dfrac{x\text{ gtt}}{\text{min}} = \dfrac{60\text{ gtt}}{1\text{ mL}} \times \dfrac{100\text{ mL}}{60\text{ min}} = 100\text{ gtt/min}$

13. b. $\dfrac{x\text{ mcg}}{\text{day}} = \dfrac{6\text{ mcg}}{\text{kg/day}} \times \dfrac{1\text{ kg}}{1000\text{ g}} \times \dfrac{3036\text{ g}}{1} = 18.22\text{ mcg/day (minimum)}$

$\dfrac{x\text{ mcg}}{\text{day}} = \dfrac{10\text{ mcg}}{\text{kg/day}} \times \dfrac{1\text{ kg}}{1000\text{ g}} \times \dfrac{3036\text{ g}}{1} = 30.36\text{ mcg/day (maximum)}$

c. $\dfrac{x\text{ mcg}}{\text{dose}} = \dfrac{18.22\text{ mcg}}{\text{day}} \times \dfrac{1\text{ day}}{2\text{ doses}} \times \dfrac{1\text{ mg}}{1000\text{ mcg}} = 0.009\text{ mg/dose (minimum)}$

$\dfrac{x\text{ mcg}}{\text{dose}} = \dfrac{30.36\text{ mcg}}{\text{day}} \times \dfrac{1\text{ day}}{2\text{ doses}} \times \dfrac{1\text{ mg}}{1000\text{ mcg}} = 0.015\text{ mg/dose (maximum)}$

d. Yes, the ordered dose, 0.013 mg, is between 0.009 and 0.015 mg.

e. $x\text{ mL} = \dfrac{1\text{ mL}}{50\text{ mcg}} \times \dfrac{1000\text{ mcg}}{1\text{ mg}} \times \dfrac{0.013\text{ mg}}{1} - 0.26\text{ mL (a drug rounded to the hundredth)}$

14. b. $\dfrac{x\text{ mg}}{\text{dose}} = \dfrac{10\text{ mg}}{\text{kg/dose}} \times \dfrac{1\text{ kg}}{2.2\text{ lb}} \times \dfrac{9\text{ lb}}{1} = 40.9\text{ mg/dose (minimum)}$

$\dfrac{x\text{ mg}}{\text{dose}} = \dfrac{15\text{ mg}}{\text{kg/dose}} \times \dfrac{1\text{ kg}}{2.2\text{ lb}} \times \dfrac{9\text{ lb}}{1} = 61.36\text{ or }61.4\text{ mg/dose (maximum)}$

c. $x\text{ mL} = \dfrac{0.8\text{ mL}}{80\text{ mg}} \times \dfrac{40.9\text{ mg}}{1} = 0.4\text{ mL (minimum)}$

$x\text{ mL} = \dfrac{0.8\text{ mL}}{80\text{ mg}} \times \dfrac{61.36\text{ mg}}{1} = 0.6\text{ mL (maximum)}$

15. b. $\dfrac{x\text{ mg}}{\text{day}} = \dfrac{4\text{ mg}}{\text{kg/day}} \times \dfrac{1\text{ kg}}{2.2\text{ lb}} \times \dfrac{37\text{ lb}}{1} = 67.27\text{ or }67.3\text{ mg/day (minimum)}$

$\dfrac{x\text{ mg}}{\text{day}} = \dfrac{6\text{ mg}}{\text{kg/day}} \times \dfrac{1\text{ kg}}{2.2\text{ lb}} \times \dfrac{37\text{ lb}}{1} = 100.9\text{ mg/day (maximum)}$

Dosage range is 67.27 to 100.9 mg/24 h.

c. Yes, 72 mg/24 h is within the recommended range.

d. $x\text{ mL} = \dfrac{5\text{ mL}}{20\text{ mg}} \times \dfrac{72\text{ mg}}{1} = 18\text{ mL}$

CHAPTER 18 Proportion Method—Work Sheet, pp. 523–526

Proportion Method:

1. a. 2.2 lb : 1 kg :: 50 lb : x kg
   $2.2x = 50$
   $x = \dfrac{50}{2.2}$
   $x = 22.7$ kg

b. 25 mg/24 h : 1 kg :: x mg/24 h : 22.7 kg
   $x = 567.5$ mg/24 h
   50 mg/24 h : 1 kg :: x mg/24 h : 22.7 kg
   $x = 1135$ mg/24 h
   Safe dose range is 567.5 to 1135 mg/24 h.
   250 mg : 1 dose :: x mg : 4 doses
   $x = 1000$ mg/24 h

c. Yes, the order is safe to administer.

d. 250 mg : 1 cap :: 250 mg : x cap
   $250x = 250$
   $x = \dfrac{250}{250}$
   $x = 1$ capsule

Formula Method:

a. 1 kg = 2.2 lb
   $\dfrac{50\text{ lb}}{2.2\text{ kg}} = 22.7$ kg

b. 25 mg/kg/24 h × 22.7 kg = 567.5 mg/24 h

c. 50 mg/kg/24 h × 22.7 kg = 1135 mg/24 h

d. 250 mg × 4 doses/24 h = 1000 mg/24 h

ANSWERS

Proportion Method:

2. a. 2.2 lb : 1 kg :: 6.5 lb : x kg
$2.2x = 6.5$
$x = \dfrac{6.5}{2.2}$
$x = 2.95$ kg or 3 kg
b. 0.035 mg : 1 kg :: x mg : 3 kg
$x = 0.11$ mg/kg/day
0.06 mg : 1 kg :: x mg : 3 kg
$x = 0.18$ mg
The safe range is 0.11 to 0.18 mg/kg/day.
c. No, the order is not safe.
d. Question this order.

3. a. 2.2 lb : 1 kg :: 50 lb : x kg
$2.2x = 50$
$x = \dfrac{50}{2.2}$
$x = 22.7$ kg
b. 5 mg/24 h : 1 kg :: x mg/24 h : 22.7 kg
$x = 113.5$ mg/kg/24 h divided by four doses
c. $\dfrac{113.5 \text{ mg/kg/24 h}}{4 \text{ doses/24 h}} = 28.4$ mg/dose
Safe and therapeutic dose is 28.4 mg/dose, so the 25-mg ordered dose is safe.
d. 12.5 mg : 1 mL :: 25 mg : x mL
$12.5x = 25$
$x = \dfrac{25}{12.5}$
$x = 2$ mL

4. a. 2.2 lb : 1 kg :: 28 lb : x kg
$2.2x = 28$
$x = \dfrac{28}{2.2}$
$x = 12.7$ kg
First 0–10 kg = 100 mL/kg/24 h
10 mL/24 h × 10 kg = 1000 mL/24 h
12.7 kg − 10 kg = 2.7 kg
Remaining 2.7 kg × 50 mL/kg = 135 mL/24 h
1000 + 135 = 1135 mL/24 h
b. $\dfrac{1135 \text{ mL/24 h}}{24 \text{ h}} = 47.3$ or 47 mL/h

5. a. 2.2 lb : 1 kg :: 22 lb : x kg
$2.2x = 22$
$x = \dfrac{22}{2.2}$
$x = 10$ kg

b. 70 mg : 1 dose :: x mg : 2 doses
$x = 140$ mg/24 h
$\dfrac{140 \text{ mg/24 h}}{10 \text{ kg}} = 14$ mg/kg/24 h
Child is receiving the recommended dose.
c. 125 mg : 5 mL :: 70 mg : x mL
$125x = 350$
$x = \dfrac{350}{125}$
$x = 2.8$ mL

6. a. 30.3 kg
b. 20 mg/24 h : 1 kg :: x mg/24 h : 30.3 kg
$x = 606$ mg/24 h
30 mg/24 h : 1 kg :: x mg/24 h : 30.3 kg
$x = 909$ mg/24 h
c. $\dfrac{606 \text{ mg/24 h}}{2 \text{ doses/24 h}} = 303$ mg/dose
$\dfrac{909 \text{ mg/24 h}}{2 \text{ doses/24 h}} = 454.5$ mg/dose
303 to 454.5 mg/dose (single dose)
d. 250 mg : 5 mL :: 300 mg : x mL
$250x = 1500$
$x = \dfrac{1500}{250}$
$x = 6$ mL

7. a. 2.2 lb : 1 kg :: 94 lb : x kg
$2.2x = 94$
$x = \dfrac{94}{2.2}$
$x = 42.7$ kg
b. 42.7 kg × 0.5 mg/kg/24 h = 21.4 mg/24 h
42.7 kg × 2 mg/kg/24 h = 85.4 mg/24 h
NOTE: 80 mg/24 h is the max dose.
c. No, the child would be receiving 90 mg/24 h.
d. No, call the physician who wrote the order.

8. a. 2.2 lb : 1 kg :: 40 lb : x kg
$2.2x = 40$
$x = \dfrac{40}{2.2}$
$x = 18.2$ kg
b. 18.2 kg × 5 mg/kg/24 h = 91 mg/24 h
18.2 kg × 7 mg/kg/24 h = 127.4 mg/24 h
c. Yes, the order is safe to administer.
d. 30 mg : 1 tab :: 60 mg : x tab
$30x = 60$
$x = \dfrac{60}{30}$
$x = 2$ chewtabs

ANSWERS

9. a. 2.2 lb : 1 kg :: 68 lb : x kg
$$2.2x = 68$$
$$x = \frac{68}{2.2}$$
$$x = 30.9 \text{ kg}$$
b. $\dfrac{750 \text{ mg} \times 4 \text{ doses/24 h}}{30.9 \text{ kg}} = \dfrac{3000}{30.9}$
$$= 97.1 \text{ mg/kg/24 h}$$
c. No, it exceeds the recommended 40 to 60 mg/kg/24 h.

10. a. 2.2 lb : 1 kg :: 42 lb : x kg
$$2.2x = 42$$
$$x = \frac{42}{2.2}$$
$$x = 19.1 \text{ kg}$$
b. $\dfrac{19.1 \text{ kg} \times 25 \text{ mg/kg/24 h}}{2 \text{ doses/24 h}} = \dfrac{477.5}{2}$
$$= 238.8 \text{ mg/dose}$$
$\dfrac{19.1 \text{ kg} \times 50 \text{ mg/kg/24 h}}{2 \text{ doses/24 h}} = \dfrac{955}{2}$
$$= 477.5 \text{ mg/dose}$$
Single-dose range is 238.8 to 477.5 mg/dose.
c. 125 mg : 5 mL :: 300 mg : x mL
$$125x = 1500$$
$$x = \frac{1500}{125}$$
$$x = 12 \text{ mL}$$

11. a. $\dfrac{100 \text{ mL}}{30 \text{ min}} \times 60 \text{ gtt/mL} = 200 \text{ gtt/min}$

12. a. 2.2 kg : 1 lb :: 58 lb : x kg
$$2.2x = 58$$
$$x = \frac{58}{2.2}$$
$$x = 26.4 \text{ kg}$$
b. $\dfrac{26.4 \text{ kg} \times 10 \text{ mg/kg/24 h}}{3 \text{ doses/24 h}} = \dfrac{264}{3}$
$$= 88 \text{ mg/dose}$$
$\dfrac{26.4 \text{ kg} \times 20 \text{ mg/kg/24 h}}{3 \text{ doses/24 h}} = \dfrac{528}{3}$
$$= 176 \text{ mg/dose}$$
Single-dose range is 88 to 176 mg/dose.
c. Yes, the dose is safe to administer.
d. 100 mg : 5 mL :: 150 mg : x mL
$$100x = 750$$
$$x = \frac{750}{100}$$
$$x = 7.5 \text{ mL}$$

13. a. 2.2 lb : 1 kg :: 72 lb : x kg
$$2.2x = 72$$
$$x = \frac{72}{2.2}$$
$$x = 32.7 \text{ kg}$$
b. First 20 kg
Next 12.7 kg × 20 mL
$$\begin{array}{r} 1500 \text{ mL/24 h} \\ + 254 \text{ mL/24 h} \\ \hline 1754 \text{ mL/24 h} \end{array}$$
c. $\dfrac{1754 \text{ mL/24 h}}{24 \text{ h}} = 73.1$ or 73 mL/h

14. a. 2.2 lb : 1 kg :: 52 lb : x kg
$$2.2x = 52$$
$$x = \frac{52}{2.2}$$
$$x = 23.6 \text{ kg}$$
b. 23.6 kg × 5 mg/kg/dose = 118 mg/dose
23.6 kg × 10 mg/kg/dose = 236 mg/dose
c. 100 mg : 5 mL :: 100 mg : x mL
$$100x = 500$$
$$x = \frac{500}{100}$$
$$x = 5 \text{ mL}$$

15. a. 2.2 lb : 1 kg :: 81 lb : x kg
$$2.2x = 81$$
$$x = \frac{81}{2.2}$$
$$x = 36.8 \text{ kg}$$
b. $\dfrac{36.8 \text{ kg} \times 25 \text{ mg/kg/24 h}}{4 \text{ doses/24 h}} = \dfrac{920}{4}$
$$= 230 \text{ mg/dose}$$
$\dfrac{36.8 \text{ kg} \times 50 \text{ mg/kg/24 h}}{4 \text{ doses/24 h}} = \dfrac{1840}{4}$
$$= 460 \text{ mg/dose}$$
Single-dose range is 230 to 460 mg/dose.
c. Yes, 350 mg/dose is safe to administer.
d. 500 mg : 5 mL :: 350 mg : x mL
$$500x = 1750$$
$$x = \frac{1750}{500}$$
$$x = 3.5 \text{ mL}$$

16. a. 2.2 lb : 1 kg :: 16 lb : x kg
$$2.2x = 16$$
$$x = \frac{16}{2.2}$$
$$x = 7.3 \text{ kg}$$

ANSWERS

b. $\dfrac{7.3\ \text{kg} \times 15\ \text{mg/kg/24 h}}{3\ \text{doses/24 h}} = \dfrac{109.5}{3}$

$= 36.5\ \text{mg/dose}$

$\dfrac{7.3\ \text{kg} \times 20\ \text{mg/kg/24 h}}{3\ \text{doses/24 h}} = \dfrac{146}{3}$

$= 48.7\ \text{mg/dose}$

c. No, the order of 60 mg q 8 h exceeds the safe range.

d. $\dfrac{60\ \text{mg} \times 3\ \text{doses/24 h}}{7.3\ \text{kg}} = 24.7\ \text{mg/kg/24 h}$

Proof that the ordered dose exceeds the recommended 15 to 20 mg/kg/24 h

e. This is not safe; do not administer. Call the physician or pharmacist to check.

17. a. 2.2 lb : 1 kg :: 19 lb : x kg

$2.2x = 19$

$x = \dfrac{19}{2.2}$

$x = 8.6\ \text{kg}$

b. 8.6 kg × 0.5 mg/kg/24 h = 4.3 mg/24 h
8.6 kg × 2 mg/kg/24 h = 17.2 mg/24 h

c. Yes, it is safe to administer.

d. 5 mg : 5 mL :: 8 mg : x mL

$5x = 40$

$x = \dfrac{40}{5}$

$x = 8\ \text{mL}$

18. a. 2.2 lb : 1 kg :: 32 lb : x kg

$2.2x = 32$

$x = \dfrac{32}{2.2}$

$x = 14.5\ \text{kg}$

b. 14.6 kg × 100 mg/kg/24 h = 1460 mg/24 h
The child may receive up to 1460 mg/24 h.

c. 400 mg : 1 dose :: x mg : 3 doses
$x = 1200\ \text{mg/24 h}$
Yes, this order is safe.

d. 330 mg : 1 mL :: 400 mg : x mL

$330x = 400$

$x = \dfrac{400}{330}$

$x = 1.2\ \text{mL}$

19. $\dfrac{250\ \text{mL}}{3\ \text{h}} = 83.3\ \text{mL/h}$

20. a. 10 mg : 1 mL :: 40 mg : x mL

$10x = 40$

$x = \dfrac{40}{10}$

$x = 4\ \text{mL}$

b. 2 mg : mL :: 40 mg : x mL

$2x = 40$

$x = 40/2 = 20\ \text{mL}$

20 mL − 4 mL = 16 mL

c. $\dfrac{20\ \text{mL}}{20\ \text{min}} \times 60\ \text{gtt/mL} = 60\ \text{gtt/min}$

CHAPTER 18 Proportion Method—Posttest 1, pp. 527–530

1. a. 2.2 lb : 1 kg :: 55 lb : x kg

$2.2x = 55$

$x = \dfrac{55}{2.2}$

$x = 25\ \text{kg}$

b. $\dfrac{25\ \text{kg} \times 4\ \text{mg/kg/24 h}}{2\ \text{doses/24 h}} = \dfrac{100}{2}$

$= 50\ \text{mg/dose}$

$\dfrac{25\ \text{kg} \times 6\ \text{mg/kg/24 h}}{2\ \text{doses/24 h}} = \dfrac{150}{2}$

$= 75\ \text{mg/dose}$

Single-dose range is 50 to 75 mg/dose.

c. Yes, 60 mg is ordered, and it falls within the 50 to 75 mg/dose range.

d. 20 mg : 5 mL :: 60 mg : x mL

$20x = 300$

$x = \dfrac{300}{20}$

$x = 15\ \text{mL}$

2. a. 2.2 lb : 1 kg :: 44 lb : x kg

$2.2x = 44$

$x = \dfrac{44}{2.2}$

$x = 20\ \text{kg}$

b. $\dfrac{20\ \text{kg} \times 25\ \text{mg/kg/24 h}}{4\ \text{doses/24 h}} = \dfrac{500}{4}$

$= 125\ \text{mg/dose}$

$\dfrac{20\ \text{kg} \times 50\ \text{mg/kg/24 h}}{4\ \text{doses/24 h}} = \dfrac{1000}{4}$

$= 250\ \text{mg/dose}$

Single-dose range is 125 to 250 mg/dose.

c. No, 500 mg q 6 h exceeds the recommended dosage for weight.

d. Question this order.

3. a. 2.2 lb : 1 kg :: 34 lb : x kg

$2.2x = 34$

$$x = \frac{34}{2.2}$$

$x = 15.5$

b. $\dfrac{300 \text{ mg} \times 3 \text{ doses/24 h}}{15.5 \text{ kg}} = \dfrac{900}{15.5}$

$= 58.1 \text{ mg/kg/24 h}$

c. Dosage is safe and therapeutic; it falls in the recommended range.

125 mg : 5 mL :: 300 mg : x mL

$125x = 1500$

$$x = \frac{1500}{125}$$

$x = 12 \text{ mL}$

4. a. 2.2 lb : 1 kg :: 78 lb : x kg

$2.2x = 78$

$$x = \frac{78}{2.2}$$

$x = 35.5 \text{ kg}$

b. 35.5 kg × 0.1 mg/kg/dose = 3.55 mg/dose

35.5 kg × 0.2 mg/kg/dose = 7.1 mg/dose

c. Yes, it falls between 3.55 and 7.1 mg/dose.

d. 15 mg : 1 mL :: 4 mg : x mL

$15x = 4$

$$x = \frac{4}{15}$$

$x = 0.27 \text{ mL}$

5. a. 2.2 lb : 1 kg :: 62 lb : x kg

$2.2x = 62$

$$x = \frac{62}{2.2}$$

$x = 28.2 \text{ kg}$

b. 28.2 kg × 10 mg/kg/dose = 282 mg/dose

28.2 kg × 15 mg/kg/dose = 423 mg/dose

Single-dose range is 282 to 423 mg/dose.

c. 160 mg : 5 mL :: 282 mg : x mL

$160x = 1410$

$$x = \frac{1410}{160}$$

$x = 8.8 \text{ mL}$

160 mg : 5 mL :: 423 mg : x mL

$160x = 2115$

$$x = \frac{2115}{160}$$

$x = 13.2 \text{ mL}$

6. $\dfrac{1000 \text{ mL}}{16 \text{ h}} = 62.5$ or 63 mL/h

7. a. 2.2 lb : 1 kg :: 92 lb : x kg

$2.2x = 92 \text{ lb}$

$$x = \frac{92}{2.2}$$

$x = 41.8 \text{ kg}$

b. $\dfrac{41.8 \text{ kg} \times 15 \text{ mg/kg/24 h}}{2 \text{ doses/24 h}} = \dfrac{627}{2}$

$= 313.5 \text{ mg/dose}$

c. Yes, 300 mg is a safe dose to administer; 300 mg does not exceed 313.64 mg.

d. 125 mg : 5 mL :: 300 mg : x mL

$125x = 1500 \text{ mL}$

$$x = \frac{1500}{125}$$

$x = 12 \text{ mL}$

8. a. 2.2 lb : 1 kg :: 25 lb : x kg

$2.2x = 25$

$$x = \frac{25}{2.2}$$

$x = 11.4 \text{ kg}$

b. First 10 kg   1000 mL/24 h

Next 1.4 kg × 50 mL/kg =   + 70 mL/24 h

                         1070 mL/24 h

c. $\dfrac{1070 \text{ mL/24 h}}{24 \text{ h}} = 44.6$ or 45 mL/h

9. a. 2.2 lb : 1 kg :: 96 lb : x kg

$2.2x - 96$

$$x = \frac{96}{2.2}$$

$x = 43.6 \text{ kg}$

b. $\dfrac{650 \text{ mg} \times 4 \text{ doses/24 h}}{43.6 \text{ kg}} = \dfrac{2600}{43.6}$

$- 59.6 \text{ mg/kg/24 h}$

c. Yes, it is safe; recommended is 40 to 60 mg/kg/24 h. Child is receiving 59.6 mg/kg/24 h.

10. a. 2.2 lb : 1 kg :: 95 lb : x kg

$2.2x = 95$

$$x = \frac{95}{2.2}$$

$x = 43.2 \text{ kg}$

b. $\dfrac{300 \text{ mg} \times 3 \text{ doses/24 h}}{43.2 \text{ kg}} = \dfrac{900}{43.2}$

$= 20.8 \text{ mg/kg/24 h}$

c. The child is receiving 20.8 mg/kg/24 h; recommended is 20 to 40 mg/kg/24 h. The ordered dose is both safe and therapeutic.

11. $\dfrac{100 \text{ mL}}{6 \text{ h}} = 16.7$ or 17 mL/h

Copyright © 2016 by Mosby, an imprint of Elsevier Inc.

ANSWERS

12. a. $250 \text{ mg} : 1 \text{ mL} :: 400 \text{ mg} : x \text{ mL}$

$250x = 400$

$x = \dfrac{400}{250}$

$x = 1.6 \text{ mL}$

b. $400 \text{ mg} \times \dfrac{1 \text{ mg}}{50 \text{ mL}} = 8 \text{ mL} \rightarrow$

$8 \text{ mL} - 1.6 \text{ mL} = 6.4 \text{ mL}$

c. $\dfrac{8 \text{ mL}}{30 \text{ min}} \times 60 \text{ gtt/mL} = x \text{ gtt/min}$

$x = \dfrac{480}{30}$

$x = 16 \text{ gtt/min}$

13. a. $\dfrac{60 \text{ mg} \times 2 \text{ doses/24 h}}{30 \text{ kg}} = \dfrac{120}{30}$

$= 4 \text{ mg/kg/24 h}$

b. No, the ordered dosage is more than the recommended 0.5 to 2 mg/kg/24 h. Also, the maximum dose is 80 mg/24 h, and this is exceeded as well.

c. No, check with the physician.

14. a. $2.2 \text{ lb} : 1 \text{ kg} :: 89 \text{ lb} : x \text{ kg}$

$2.2x = 89$

$x = \dfrac{89}{2.2}$

$x = 40.5 \text{ kg}$

b. $\dfrac{40.5 \text{ kg} \times 15 \text{ mg/kg/24 h}}{2 \text{ doses/24 h}} = \dfrac{607.5}{2}$

$= 303.8 \text{ mg/dose}$

$\dfrac{40.5 \text{ kg} \times 20 \text{ mg/kg/24 h}}{2 \text{ doses/24 h}} = \dfrac{810}{2}$

$= 405 \text{ mg/dose}$

Dosage range is 607.5 to 810 mg/24 h. Single-dose range is 303.8 to 405 mg/dose.

c. Yes, 400 mg/dose is within the recommended single-dose range.

d. $375 \text{ mg} : 5 \text{ mL} :: 400 \text{ mg} : x \text{ mL}$

$375x = 2000$

$x = \dfrac{2000}{375}$

$x = 5.3 \text{ mL}$

15. a. $2.2 \text{ lb} : 1 \text{ kg} :: 11 \text{ lb} : x \text{ kg}$

$2.2x = 11$

$x = \dfrac{11}{2.2}$

$x = 5 \text{ kg}$

b. $\dfrac{90 \text{ mg} \times 4 \text{ doses/24 h}}{5 \text{ kg}} = \dfrac{360}{5}$

$= 72 \text{ mg/kg/24 h}$

c. The order is both safe and therapeutic, between the recommended 50 to 100 mg/kg/24 h.

CHAPTER 18 Proportion Method—Posttest 2, pp. 531–534

1. a. $2.2 \text{ lb} : 1 \text{ kg} :: 70 \text{ lb} : x \text{ kg}$

$2.2x = 70$

$x = \dfrac{70}{2.2}$

$x = 31.8 \text{ kg}$

b. $\dfrac{450 \text{ mg} \times 4 \text{ doses/24 h}}{31.8 \text{ kg}} = \dfrac{1800}{31.8}$

$= 56.6 \text{ mg/kg/24 h}$

c. Yes, the child is receiving 56.6 mg/kg/24 h, which is between 40 and 60 mg/kg/24 h.

2. a. $2.2 \text{ lb} : 1 \text{ kg} :: 62 \text{ lb} : x \text{ kg}$

$2.2x = 62$

$x = \dfrac{62}{2.2}$

$x = 28.2 \text{ kg}$

b. $28.2 \text{ kg} \times 7 \text{ mg/kg/24 h} = 197.4 \text{ mg/24 h}$

$28.2 \text{ kg} \times 8 \text{ mg/kg/24 h} = 225.6 \text{ mg/24 h}$

Dosage range is 197.4 to 225.6 mg/24 h.

c. $\dfrac{197.4 \text{ mg/24 h}}{2 \text{ doses/24 h}} = 98.7 \text{ mg/dose}$

$\dfrac{225.6 \text{ mg/24 h}}{2 \text{ doses/24 h}} = 112.8 \text{ mg/dose}$

Single-dose range is 98.7 to 112.8 mg/dose.

d. Yes, the ordered dose is both safe and therapeutic because it falls within the recommended 24-hour dosage and single-dose ranges.

e. $125 \text{ mg} : 5 \text{ mL} :: 100 \text{ mg} : x \text{ mL}$

$125x = 500$

$x = \dfrac{500}{125}$

$x = 4 \text{ mL}$

ANSWERS

3. $\dfrac{150 \text{ mL}}{180 \text{ min}} \times 60 \text{ gtt/mL} = 50 \text{ gtt/min}$

4. a. 2.2 lb : 1 kg :: 58 lb : x kg
   $2.2x = 58$
   $x = \dfrac{58}{2.2}$
   $x = 26.4$ kg

   b. 26.4 kg × 25 mg/kg/24 h = 660 mg/24 h
   26.4 kg × 50 mg/kg/24 h = 1320 mg/24 h
   Dosage range is 660 to 1320 mg/24 h.

   c. $\dfrac{660 \text{ mg/24 h}}{2 \text{ doses/24 h}} = 330$ mg/dose
   $\dfrac{1320 \text{ mg/24 h}}{2 \text{ doses/24 h}} = 660$ mg/dose
   Single-dose range is 330 to 660 mg/dose.

   d. $\dfrac{400 \text{ mg} \times 2 \text{ doses/24 h}}{26.4 \text{ kg}} = \dfrac{800}{26.4}$
   $= 30.3$ mg/kg/24 h

   e. 250 mg : 5 mL :: 400 mg : x mL
   $250x = 2000$
   $x = \dfrac{2000}{250}$
   $x = 8$ mL

5. a. 2.2 lb : 1 kg :: 99 lb : x kg
   $2.2x = 99$
   $x = \dfrac{99}{2.2}$
   $x = 45$ kg

   b. $\dfrac{500 \text{ mg} \times 4 \text{ doses/24 h}}{45 \text{ kg}} = \dfrac{2000}{45}$
   $= 44.4$ mg/kg/24 h

   c. Yes, the recommended daily oral dosage is 50 to 100 mg/kg/24 h.

   d. 250 mg : 1 cap :: 500 mg : x cap
   $250x = 500$
   $x = \dfrac{500}{250}$
   $x = 2$ capsules

6. a. 2.2 lb : 1 kg :: 66 lb : x kg
   $2.2x = 66$ lb
   $x = \dfrac{66}{2.2}$
   $x = 30$ kg

   b. $\dfrac{200 \text{ mg} \times 2 \text{ doses/24 h}}{30 \text{ kg}} = \dfrac{400}{30}$
   $= 13.3$ mg/kg/24 h

   c. Yes, the order is safe to administer.

7. a. 1000 g : 1 kg :: 2012 g : x kg
   $1000x = 2012$
   $x = \dfrac{2012}{1000}$
   $x = 2$ kg

   b. 2 kg × 100 mg/kg/24 h = 200 mg/24 h
   2 kg × 200 mg/kg/24 h = 400 mg/24 h
   Dosage range is 200 to 400 mg/24 h.

   c. $\dfrac{200 \text{ mg/24 h}}{4 \text{ doses/24 h}} = 50$ mg/dose
   $\dfrac{400 \text{ mg/24 h}}{4 \text{ doses/24 h}} = 100$ mg/dose
   Single-dose range is 50 to 100 mg/dose.

d. 125 mg : 5 mL :: 200 mg : x mL
   $125x = 1000$
   $x = \dfrac{1000}{125}$
   $x = 8$ mL

8. a. 2.2 lb : 1 kg :: 35 lb : x kg
   $2.2x = 35$
   $x = \dfrac{35}{2.2}$
   $x = 15.9$ kg

   b. $\dfrac{180 \text{ mg} \times 3 \text{ doses/24 h}}{15.9 \text{ kg}} = \dfrac{540}{15.9}$
   $= 33.96$ mg/kg/24 h

   c. Yes, the ordered dose is within the safe and therapeutic range.

   d. 125 mg : 5 mL :: 180 mg : x mL
   $125x = 900$
   $x = \dfrac{900}{125}$
   $x = 7.2$ mL

9. a. 2.2 lb : 1 kg :: 74 lb : x kg
   $2.2x = 74$
   $x = \dfrac{74}{2.2}$
   $x = 33.6$ kg

   b. $\dfrac{330 \text{ mg} \times 4 \text{ doses/24 h}}{33.6 \text{ kg}} = \dfrac{1320}{33.6}$
   $= 39.29$ mg/kg/24 h

   c. Yes, the dose ordered is safe to administer.

   d. 250 mg : 5 mL :: 330 mg : x mL
   $250x = 1650$
   $x = \dfrac{1650}{250}$
   $x = 6.6$ mL

ANSWERS

10. a. 2.2 lb : 1 kg :: 20 lb : x kg
$2.2x = 20$
$$x = \frac{20}{2.2}$$
$x = 9.1$ kg
  b. 9.1 kg $\times$ 0.1 mg/kg/dose = 0.91 mg/dose
9.1 kg $\times$ 0.2 mg/kg/dose = 1.82 mg/dose
Safe dose range is 0.91 to 1.82 mg/dose
(nearest hundredth with narcotics).
  c. No, 0.9 mg is not within the safe range
to administer. Contact the physician.
  d. 0.5 mg : 1 mL :: 0.9 mg : x mL
$0.5x = 0.9$
$$x = \frac{0.9}{0.5}$$
$x = 1.8$ mL if dose is approved

11. $\dfrac{200 \text{ mL}}{3 \text{ h}} = 66.7$ or 67 mL/h

12. a. 50 mg : 1 mL :: 500 mg : x mL
$50x = 500$
$$x = \frac{500}{50}$$
$x = 10$ mL
  b. 500 mg $\times \dfrac{1 \text{ mL}}{5 \text{ mg}} = 100$ mL $\rightarrow$
100 mL $-$ 10 mL = 90 mL
  c. Drop factor = 60 gtt/mL = microgtt
$\dfrac{100 \text{ mL}}{60 \text{ min}} \times 60$ gtt/min = x gtt/min
$\dfrac{6000}{60} = 100$ gtt/min

13. a. 1000 g : 1 kg :: 3036 g : x kg
$1000x = 3036$
$$x = \frac{3036}{1000}$$
$x = 3.0$ kg or 3 kg
  b. 3 kg $\times$ 6 mcg/kg/24 h = 18 mcg/24 h
3 kg $\times$ 10 mcg/kg/24 h = 30 mcg/24 h
Dosage range is 18 to 30 mcg/24 h.
  c. $\dfrac{18 \text{ mcg/24 h}}{2 \text{ doses/24 h}} = 9$ mcg/dose
$\dfrac{30 \text{ mcg/24 h}}{2 \text{ doses/24 h}} = 15$ mcg/dose
Single dose is 9 to 15 mcg/dose.
9 mcg = 0.009 mg
15 mcg = 0.015 mg

---

  d. Yes, the ordered dose, 0.013 mg, is
between 0.009 mg and 0.015 mg.
  e. 50 mcg = 0.05 mg
0.05 mg : 1 mL :: 0.013 mg : x mL
$0.05x = 0.013$
$$x = \frac{0.013}{0.05}$$
$x = 0.26$ mL (a drug that is
measured to the nearest hundredth)

14. a. 2.2 lb : 1 kg :: 9 lb : x kg
$2.2x = 9$
$$x = \frac{9}{2.2}$$
$x = 4.1$ kg
  b. 4.1 kg $\times$ 10 mg/kg/dose = 41 mg/dose
4.1 kg $\times$ 15 mg/kg/dose = 61.5 mg/dose
Single-dose range is 41 to 61.5 mg/dose.
  c. 80 mg : 0.8 mL :: 41 mg : x mL
$80x = 32.8$
$$x = \frac{32.8}{80}$$
$x = 0.4$ mL
80 mg : 0.8 mL :: 61.5 mg : x mL
$80x = 49.2$
$$x = \frac{49.2}{80}$$
$x = 0.6$ mL
Single-dose range is 0.4 to 0.6 mL/dose.

15. a. 2.2 lb : 1 kg :: 37 lb : x kg
$2.2x = 37$
$$x = \frac{37}{2.2}$$
$x = 16.8$ kg
  b. 16.8 kg $\times$ 4 mg/kg/24 h = 67.2 mg/24 h
16.8 kg $\times$ 6 mg/kg/24 h = 100.8 mg/24 h
Dosage range is 67.2 to 100.8 mg/24 h.
  c. Yes, 72 mg/24 h is within the
recommended dosage range.
  d. 20 mg : 5 mL :: 72 mg : x mL
$20x = 360$
$$x = \frac{360}{20}$$
$x = 18$ mL

Obstetric Dosages

LEARNING OBJECTIVES

Upon completion of the materials in this chapter, you will be able to perform computations accurately by mastering the following mathematical concepts:

1 Calculating the intravenous (IV) rate of oxytocin (Pitocin) ordered in milliunits per minute

2 Calculating the IV rate of magnesium sulfate ordered in milligrams per minute

In obstetric nursing, oxytocin (Pitocin) and magnesium sulfate are commonly used. Oxytocin is used to either augment or induce labor. Magnesium sulfate is used to prevent seizures in mothers diagnosed with preeclampsia and is also used "off label" to control preterm labor contractions. Both these medications can be titrated, which means that the medication can be adjusted up and down based on patient status.

IV ADMINISTRATION OF MEDICATIONS BY MILLIUNITS/MINUTE

EXAMPLE 1: The physician has ordered 1000 mL 5% dextrose in water (D_5W) with 10 units IV oxytocin. Begin at 1 mU/min and then increase by 1 mU/min every 30 minutes until regular contractions occur. Maximum dose is 20 mU/min.

What Is the IV Rate (mL/h) for the Beginning Infusion?

Using the Dimensional Analysis Method

$$\frac{x \text{ mL}}{\text{h}} = \frac{1000 \text{ mL}}{10 \text{ units}} \times \frac{1 \text{ unit}}{1000 \text{ mU}} \times \frac{1 \text{ mU}}{1 \text{ min}} \times \frac{60 \text{ min}}{1 \text{ h}}$$

$$\frac{x \text{ mL}}{\text{h}} = \frac{1000 \times 60}{10 \times 1000}$$

$$x = 6 \text{ mL/h}$$

Using the Ratio-Proportion Method

a. Convert total units in the IV bag to milliunits.

(Formula setup) 1 unit : 1000 mU :: 10 units : x mU

$x = 1000 \times 10 = 10{,}000$ mU

b. Calculate mL/min.

(Formula setup)   10,000 mU : 1000 mL :: 1 mU : x mL

$$10,000x = 1000$$

$$x = \frac{1000}{10,000}$$

$$x = 0.1 \text{ mL/min}$$

c. Calculate mL/h.

(Formula setup)   0.1 mL : 1 min :: x mL : 60 min (h)

$$0.1 : 1 :: x : 60$$

$$x = 6 \text{ mL/h}$$

Using the $\dfrac{D}{A} \times Q$ Method

a. Convert total units in the IV bag to milliunits.

$$10 \text{ units} = 10,000 \text{ mU}$$

b. Calculate mL/min.

(Formula setup) $\dfrac{D}{A} \times Q = \dfrac{1 \text{ mU/min}}{10,000 \text{ mU}} \times 1000 \text{ mL}$

(Cancel) $\dfrac{D}{A} \times Q = \dfrac{1 \text{ mU/min}}{10,000 \text{ mU}} \times 1000 \text{ mL} = 0.1 \text{ mL/min}$

Therefore 0.1 mL/min of oxytocin is infusing.

c. Calculate mL/h.

(Formula setup) $\dfrac{\text{Total mL}}{\text{Total min}} \times \dfrac{60 \text{ min}}{1 \text{ h}}$

$$\dfrac{0.1 \text{ mL}}{1 \text{ min}} \times \dfrac{60 \text{ min}}{1 \text{ h}}$$

(Cancel) $\dfrac{0.1 \text{ mL}}{1 \text{ min}} \times \dfrac{60 \text{ min}}{1 \text{ h}} = 6 \text{ mL/h}$

The infusion pump should be set at 6 mL/h.

What Is the Maximum IV Rate the Oxytocin Infusion May Be Set for?

Using the Dimensional Analysis Method

$$\frac{x \text{ mL}}{h} = \frac{1000 \text{ mL}}{10 \text{ units}} \times \frac{1 \text{ unit}}{1000 \text{ mU}} \times \frac{20 \text{ mU}}{1 \text{ min}} \times \frac{60 \text{ min}}{1 \text{ h}}$$

$$\frac{x \text{ mL}}{h} = \frac{1000 \times 20 \times 60}{10 \times 1000}$$

$$x = 120 \text{ mL/h}$$

Using the Ratio-Proportion Method

a. Convert total units in the IV bag to milliunits.

$$1 \text{ unit} : 1000 \text{ mU} :: 10 \text{ units} : x \text{ mU}$$

$$x = 1000 \times 10 = 10,000 \text{ mU}$$

b. Calculate mL/min.

$$10{,}000 \text{ mU} : 1000 \text{ mL} :: 20 \text{ mU} : x \text{ mL}$$

$$10{,}000x = 1000 \times 20$$

$$x = \frac{1000 \times 20}{10{,}000} = 2 \text{ mL/min}$$

c. Calculate mL/h. $2 \text{ mL} : 1 \text{ min} :: x \text{ mL} : 60 \text{ min (h)}$

$$x = 2 \times 60 = 120 \text{ mL/h}$$

Using the $\dfrac{\text{D}}{\text{A}} \times$ Q Method

a. Convert units to milliunits.

$$10 \text{ units } = 10{,}000 \text{ mU}$$

b. Calculate mL/min.

(Formula setup) $\dfrac{\text{D}}{\text{A}} \times \text{Q} = \dfrac{20 \text{ mU/min}}{10{,}000 \text{ mU}} \times 1000 \text{ mL}$

(Cancel) $\dfrac{\text{D}}{\text{A}} \times \text{Q} = \dfrac{20 \text{ \cancel{mU}/min}}{10{,}000 \text{ \cancel{mU}}} \times 1000 \text{ mL} = 2 \text{ mL/min}$

c. Calculate mL/h.

(Formula setup) $\dfrac{\text{Total mL}}{\text{Total min}} \times \dfrac{60 \text{ min}}{1 \text{ h}}$

$$\dfrac{2 \text{ mL}}{1 \text{ min}} \times \dfrac{60 \text{ min}}{1 \text{ h}}$$

(Cancel) $\dfrac{2 \text{ mL}}{1 \text{ \cancel{min}}} \times \dfrac{60 \text{ \cancel{min}}}{1 \text{ h}} = 120 \text{ mL/h}$

Therefore the maximum IV rate is 120 mL/h.

EXAMPLE 2: The physician has ordered 500 mL D_5W with 10 units IV oxytocin. Begin at 1 mU/min and then increase by 1 mU/min every 30 minutes until active labor begins. Maximum dose is 28 mU/min.

What Is the IV Rate (mL/h) for the Beginning Infusion?
Using the Dimensional Analysis Method

$$\frac{x \text{ mL}}{\text{h}} = \frac{500 \text{ mL}}{10 \text{ units}} \times \frac{1 \text{ unit}}{1000 \text{ mU}} \times \frac{1 \text{ mU}}{1 \text{ min}} \times \frac{60 \text{ min}}{1 \text{ h}}$$

$$\frac{x \text{ mL}}{\text{h}} = \frac{500 \times 60}{10 \times 1000}$$

$$x = 3 \text{ mL/h}$$

Using the Ratio-Proportion Method

a. Convert total units in the IV bag to milliunits.

(Formula setup) $1 \text{ unit} : 1000 \text{ mU} :: 10 \text{ units} : x \text{ mU}$

$$1 : 1000 :: 10 : x$$

$$x = 1000 \times 10$$

$$x = 10{,}000 \text{ mU}$$

b. Calculate mL/min.

(Formula setup)   10,000 mU : 500 mL :: 1 mU : x min

$$10,000x = 500$$

$$x = \frac{500}{10,000}$$

$$x = 0.05 \text{ mL/min}$$

c. Calculate mL/h.

(Formula setup)   0.05 mL : 1 min :: x mL : 60 min/h

$$0.05 : 1 :: x : 60$$

$$x = 3 \text{ mL/h}$$

Using the $\dfrac{D}{A} \times Q$ Method

a. Convert total units in the IV bag to milliunits.

$$10 \text{ units} = 10,000 \text{ mU}$$

b. Calculate mL/min.

(Formula setup) $\dfrac{D}{A} \times Q = \dfrac{1 \text{ mU/min}}{10,000 \text{ mU}} \times 500 \text{ mL}$

(Cancel) $\dfrac{D}{A} \times Q = \dfrac{1 \text{ m\cancel{U}/min}}{10,000 \text{ m\cancel{U}}} \times 500 \text{ mL} = 0.05 \text{ mL/min}$

Therefore 0.05 mL/min of oxytocin is infusing.

c. Calculate mL/h.

(Formula setup) $\dfrac{\text{Total mL}}{\text{Total min}} \times \dfrac{60 \text{ min}}{1 \text{ h}}$

$\dfrac{0.05 \text{ mL}}{1 \text{ min}} \times \dfrac{60 \text{ min}}{1 \text{ h}}$

(Cancel) $\dfrac{0.05 \text{ mL}}{1 \text{ \cancel{min}}} \times \dfrac{60 \text{ \cancel{min}}}{1 \text{ h}} = 3 \text{ mL/h}$

The infusion pump should be set at 3 mL/h.

What Is the Maximum IV Rate the Oxytocin Infusion May Be Set for?

Using the Dimensional Analysis Method

$$\frac{x \text{ mL}}{\text{h}} = \frac{500 \text{ mL}}{10 \text{ units}} \times \frac{1 \text{ unit}}{1000 \text{ mU}} \times \frac{28 \text{ mU}}{1 \text{ min}} \times \frac{60 \text{ min}}{1 \text{ h}}$$

$$\frac{x \text{ mL}}{\text{h}} = \frac{500 \times 28 \times 60}{10 \times 1000}$$

$$x = 84 \text{ mL/h}$$

Using the Ratio-Proportion Method

a. Convert total units in the IV bag to milliunits.

$$1 \text{ unit} : 1000 \text{ mU} :: 10 \text{ units} : x \text{ mU}$$

$$x = 1000 \times 10 = 10,000 \text{ mU}$$

b. Calculate mL/min.

$$10{,}000 \text{ mU} : 500 \text{ mL} :: 28 \text{ mU} : x \text{ mL}$$

$$10{,}000x = 500 \times 28$$

$$x = \frac{500 \times 28}{10{,}000} = 1.4 \text{ mL/min}$$

c. Calculate mL/h.
$$1.4 \text{ mL} : 1 \text{ min} :: x \text{ mL} : 60 \text{ min (h)}$$
$$x = 1.4 \times 60 = 84 \text{ mL/h}$$

Using the $\dfrac{D}{A} \times Q$ Method

a. Convert units to milliunits.

$$10 \text{ units} = 10{,}000 \text{ mU}$$

b. Calculate mL/min.

(Formula setup) $\dfrac{D}{A} \times Q = \dfrac{28 \text{ mU/min}}{10{,}000 \text{ mU}} \times 500 \text{ mL}$

(Cancel) $\dfrac{D}{A} \times Q = \dfrac{28 \cancel{\text{ mU}}\text{/min}}{10{,}000 \cancel{\text{ mU}}} \times 500 \text{ mL} = 1.4 \text{ mL/min}$

Therefore 1.4 mL/min of oxytocin is infusing.

c. Calculate mL/h.

(Formula setup) $\dfrac{\text{Total mL}}{\text{Total min}} \times \dfrac{60 \text{ min}}{1 \text{ h}}$

$\dfrac{1.4 \text{ mL}}{1 \text{ min}} \times \dfrac{60 \text{ min}}{1 \text{ h}}$

(Cancel) $\dfrac{1.4 \text{ mL}}{1 \cancel{\text{ min}}} \times \dfrac{60 \cancel{\text{ min}}}{1 \text{ h}} = 84 \text{ mL/h}$

Therefore the maximum IV rate is 84 mL/h.

IV ADMINISTRATION OF MEDICATIONS BY MILLIGRAMS/MINUTE

EXAMPLE 1: The physician has ordered 1000 mL lactated Ringer's with 20 g magnesium sulfate IV. Bolus with 4 g/30 min and then maintain a continuous infusion at 2 g/h.

What Is the IV Rate (mL/h) for the Bolus Order?
Using the Dimensional Analysis Method

$$\frac{x \text{ mL}}{\text{h}} = \frac{1000 \text{ mL}}{20 \text{ g}} \times \frac{4 \text{ g}}{30 \text{ min}} \times \frac{60 \text{ min}}{1 \text{ h}}$$

$$\frac{x \text{ mL}}{\text{h}} = \frac{1000 \times 4 \times 60}{20 \times 30}$$

$$x = 400 \text{ mL/h}$$

Using the Ratio-Proportion Method

a. Calculate the number of milliliters to infuse 4 g.

$$20 \text{ g} : 1000 \text{ mL} :: 4 \text{ g} : x \text{ mL}$$

$$20 : 1000 :: 4 : x$$

$$20x = 4000$$

$$x = 200 \text{ mL}$$

b. Calculate mL/h.

(Formula setup) $200 \text{ mL} : 30 \text{ min} :: x \text{ mL} : 60 \text{ min/h}$

$$200 : 30 :: x : 60$$

$$12000 = 30x$$

$$x = 400$$

The IV pump should be set at 400 mL/h.

Using the $\dfrac{D}{A} \times Q$ Method

a. Calculate the number of milliliters to infuse 4 g.

(Formula setup) $\dfrac{D}{A} \times Q = \dfrac{4 \text{ g}}{20 \text{ g}} \times 1000 \text{ mL}$

(Cancel) $\dfrac{D}{A} \times Q = \dfrac{4 \cancel{g}}{20 \cancel{g}} \times 1000 \text{ mL} = 200 \text{ mL}$

b. Calculate the bolus rate in mL/h.

(Formula setup) $\dfrac{\text{Total mL}}{\text{Total min}} \times \dfrac{60 \text{ min}}{1 \text{ h}}$

$\dfrac{200 \text{ mL}}{30 \text{ min}} \times \dfrac{60 \text{ min}}{1 \text{ h}}$

(Cancel) $\dfrac{200 \text{ mL}}{30 \cancel{\text{min}}} \times \dfrac{60 \cancel{\text{min}}}{1 \text{ h}} = 400 \text{ mL/h}$

The infusion pump should be set at 400 mL/h.

What Is the IV Rate (mL/h) for the Continuous Infusion?

Using the Dimensional Analysis Method

$$\frac{x \text{ mL}}{\text{h}} = \frac{1000 \text{ mL}}{20 \text{ g}} \times \frac{2 \text{ g}}{1 \text{ h}}$$

$$\frac{x \text{ mL}}{\text{h}} = \frac{1000 \times 2}{20}$$

$$x = 100 \text{ mL/h}$$

Using the Ratio-Proportion Method

Calculate the number of milliliters to infuse 2 g/h.

(Formula setup) $20 \text{ g} : 1000 \text{ mL} :: 2 \text{ g} : x \text{ mL}$

$$20 : 1000 :: 2 : x$$

$$20x = 2000$$

$$x = 100 \text{ mL}$$

The IV pump should be set at 100 mL/h.

Using the $\dfrac{D}{A} \times Q$ Method

Calculate the mL/h to infuse 2 g/h.

(Formula setup) $\dfrac{D}{A} \times Q = \dfrac{2 \text{ g/h}}{20 \text{ g}} \times 1000 \text{ mL}$

(Cancel) $\dfrac{D}{A} \times Q = \dfrac{2 \text{ g/h}}{20 \text{ g}} \times 1000 \text{ mL} = 100 \text{ mL/h}$

The infusion pump should be set at 100 mL/h.

EXAMPLE 2: The physician has ordered 500 mL lactated Ringer's with 10 g magnesium sulfate IV. Bolus with 2 g/20 min and then maintain a continuous infusion at 1 g/h.

What Is the IV Rate (mL/h) for the Bolus Order?

Using the Dimensional Analysis Method

$$\frac{x \text{ mL}}{h} = \frac{500 \text{ mL}}{10 \text{ g}} \times \frac{2 \text{ g}}{20 \text{ min}} \times \frac{60 \text{ min}}{1 \text{ h}}$$

$$\frac{x \text{ mL}}{h} = \frac{500 \times 2 \times 60}{10 \times 20}$$

$$x = 300 \text{ mL/h}$$

Using the Ratio-Proportion Method

a. Calculate the number of milliliters to infuse 2 g.

$$10 \text{ g} : 500 \text{ mL} :: 2 \text{ g} : x \text{ mL}$$

$$10 : 500 :: 2 : x$$

$$10x = 1000$$

$$x = 100 \text{ mL}$$

b. Calculate mL/h.

(Formula setup) $100 \text{ mL} : 20 \text{ min} :: x \text{ mL} : 60 \text{ min (h)}$

$$100 : 20 :: x : 60$$

$$6000 = 20x$$

$$x = 300 \text{ mL/h}$$

The IV pump will be set at 300 mL/h.

Using the $\dfrac{D}{A} \times Q$ Method

a. Calculate the milliliters to infuse 2 g.

(Formula setup) $\dfrac{D}{A} \times Q = \dfrac{2 \text{ g}}{10 \text{ g}} \times 500 \text{ mL}$

(Cancel) $\dfrac{D}{A} \times Q = \dfrac{2 \cancel{g}}{10 \cancel{g}} \times 500 \text{ mL} = 100 \text{ mL}$

b. Calculate the bolus rate in mL/h.

(Formula setup) $\dfrac{\text{Total mL}}{\text{Total min}} \times \dfrac{60 \text{ min}}{1 \text{ h}}$

$\dfrac{100 \text{ mL}}{20 \text{ min}} \times \dfrac{60 \text{ min}}{1 \text{ h}}$

(Cancel) $\dfrac{100 \text{ mL}}{20 \cancel{\text{min}}} \times \dfrac{60 \cancel{\text{min}}}{1 \text{ h}} = 300 \text{ mL/h}$

The IV pump will be set at 300 mL/h.

What Is the IV Rate (mL/h) for the Continuous Infusion?

Using the Dimensional Analysis Method

$$\dfrac{x \text{ mL}}{h} = \dfrac{500 \text{ mL}}{10 \text{ g}} \times \dfrac{1 \text{ g}}{1 \text{ h}}$$

$$\dfrac{x \text{ mL}}{h} = \dfrac{500}{10}$$

$$x = 50 \text{ mL/h}$$

Using the Ratio-Proportion Method

Calculate the number of mL/h to infuse 1 g/h.

$$10 \text{ g} : 500 \text{ mL} :: 1 \text{ g} : x \text{ mL}$$

$$10 : 500 :: 1 : x$$

$$10x = 500$$

$$x = 50$$

The IV pump will be set at 50 mL/h.

Using the $\dfrac{D}{A} \times Q$ Method

Calculate the mL/h to infuse 1 g/h.

(Formula setup) $\dfrac{D}{A} \times Q = \dfrac{1 \text{ g/h}}{10 \text{ g}} \times 500 \text{ mL}$

(Cancel) $\dfrac{D}{A} \times Q = \dfrac{1 \cancel{g}/h}{10 \cancel{g}} \times 500 \text{ mL} = 50 \text{ mL/h}$

The infusion pump should be set at 50 mL/h.

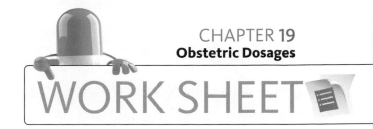

1. The physician has ordered 500 mL D₅W with 10 units IV oxytocin. Begin at 2 mU/min and then increase by 1 mU/min every 30 minutes until regular contractions begin. Maximum dose is 30 mU/min.

    a. What is the IV rate for the beginning infusion? ‾‾‾‾‾‾‾‾

    b. What is the IV rate for the maximum infusion? ‾‾‾‾‾‾‾‾

2. The physician has ordered 500 mL D₅W with 30 units IV oxytocin. Begin at 2 mU/min and then increase by 1 mU/min every 30 minutes until regular contractions begin. Maximum dose is 20 mU/min.

    a. What is the IV rate for the beginning infusion? ‾‾‾‾‾‾‾‾

    b. What is the IV rate for the maximum infusion? ‾‾‾‾‾‾‾‾

3. The physician has ordered 500 mL D₅W with 30 units IV oxytocin. Begin at 1 mU/min and then increase by 1 mU/min every 30 minutes until active labor begins. Maximum dose is 20 mU/min.

    a. What is the IV rate for the beginning infusion? ‾‾‾‾‾‾‾‾

    b. What is the IV rate for the maximum infusion? ‾‾‾‾‾‾‾‾

4. The physician has ordered 1000 mL D₅W with 40 units IV oxytocin. Begin at 2 mU/min and then increase by 1 mU/min every 30 minutes until regular contractions begin. Maximum dose is 20 mU/min.

    a. What is the IV rate for the beginning infusion? ‾‾‾‾‾‾‾‾

    b. What is the IV rate for the maximum infusion? ‾‾‾‾‾‾‾‾

5. The physician has ordered 1000 mL lactated Ringer's with 20 g IV magnesium sulfate. Bolus with 2 g/30 min; then maintain a continuous infusion at 2 g/h.

   a. What is the IV rate for the bolus order? _____

   b. What is the IV rate for the continuous infusion? _____

6. The physician has ordered 1000 mL lactated Ringer's with 40 g IV magnesium sulfate. Bolus with 1 g/20 min; then maintain a continuous infusion at 1 g/h.

   a. What is the IV rate for the bolus order? _____

   b. What is the IV rate for the continuous infusion? _____

7. The physician has ordered 1000 mL lactated Ringer's with 40 g IV magnesium sulfate. Bolus with 6 g/20 min; then maintain a continuous infusion at 4 g/h.

   a. What is the IV rate for the bolus order? _____

   b. What is the IV rate for the continuous infusion? _____

8. The physician has ordered 500 mL lactated Ringer's with 10 g IV magnesium sulfate. Bolus with 4 g/30 min; then maintain a continuous infusion at 2 g/h.

   a. What is the IV rate for the bolus order? _____

   b. What is the IV rate for the continuous infusion? _____

ANSWERS ON PP. 563 AND 564–567.

NAME _____

DATE _____

ACCEPTABLE SCORE ___8___

YOUR SCORE _____

POSTTEST 1

1. The physician orders 500 mL of D_5W with 20 units of IV oxytoxin to begin at 2 mU/min and then increase by 1 mU/min every 20 minutes until regular contractions begin. Maximum dose is 20 mU/min.

   a. What is the IV rate for the beginning infusion? _____

   b. What is the IV rate for the maximum infusion? _____

2. The physician orders 1000 mL of D_5W with 30 units of IV oxytoxin to begin at 2 mU/min and then increase by 1 mU/min every 20 minutes until regular contractions begin. Maximum dose is 30 mU/min.

   a. What is the IV rate for the beginning infusion? _____

   b. What is the IV rate for the maximum infusion? _____

3. The physician orders 500 mL lactated Ringer's with 20 g of magnesium sulfate. Bolus with 2 g/30 minutes; then maintain a continuous infusion at 3 g/h.

   a. What is the IV rate for the bolus order? _____

   b. What is the IV rate for the continuous infusion? _____

4. The physician orders 500 mL lactated Ringer's with 30 g of magnesium sulfate. Bolus with 2 g/20 minutes; then maintain a continuous infusion at 3 g/h.

   a. What is the IV rate for the bolus order? _____

   b. What is the IV rate for the continuous infusion? _____

ANSWERS ON PP. 563–564 AND 567–568.

NAME _____

DATE _____

REQUIRED SCORE __8__

YOUR SCORE _____

CHAPTER 19
Obstetric Dosages

POSTTEST 2

1. The physician orders 1000 mL of D_5W with 10 units of IV oxytoxin to begin at 2 mU/min and then increase by 2 mU/min every 15 minutes until regular contractions begin. Maximum dose is 30 mU/min.

   a. What is the IV rate for the beginning infusion? _____

   b. What is the IV rate for the maximum infusion? _____

2. The physician orders 1000 mL of D_5W with 40 units of IV oxytoxin to begin at 4 mU/min and then increase by 3 mU/min every 20 minutes until regular contractions begin. Maximum dose is 20 mU/min.

   a. What is the IV rate for the beginning infusion? _____

   b. What is the IV rate for the maximum infusion? _____

3. The physician orders 1000 mL lactated Ringer's with 20 g of magnesium sulfate. Bolus with 2 g/30 minutes; then maintain a continuous infusion at 2 g/h.

   a. What is the IV rate for the bolus order? _____

   b. What is the IV rate for the continuous infusion? _____

4. The physician orders 1000 mL lactated Ringer's with 40 g of magnesium sulfate. Bolus with 2 g/15 minutes; then maintain a continuous infusion at 4 g/h.

   a. What is the IV rate for the bolus order? _____

   b. What is the IV rate for the continuous infusion? _____

ANSWERS ON PP. 564 AND 568–570.

ANSWERS

CHAPTER 19 Dimensional Analysis—Work Sheet, pp. 557–558

1. a. $\dfrac{x\ mL}{h} = \dfrac{500\ mL}{10\ units} \times \dfrac{1\ unit}{1000\ mU} \times \dfrac{2\ mU}{1\ min} \times \dfrac{60\ min}{1\ h} = 6\ mL/h$

 b. $\dfrac{x\ mL}{h} = \dfrac{500\ mL}{10\ units} \times \dfrac{1\ unit}{1000\ mU} \times \dfrac{30\ mU}{1\ min} \times \dfrac{60\ min}{1\ h} = 90\ mL/h$

2. a. $\dfrac{x\ mL}{h} = \dfrac{500\ mL}{30\ units} \times \dfrac{1\ unit}{1000\ mU} \times \dfrac{2\ mU}{1\ min} \times \dfrac{60\ min}{1\ h} = 2\ mL/h$

 b. $\dfrac{x\ mL}{h} = \dfrac{500\ mL}{30\ units} \times \dfrac{1\ unit}{1000\ mU} \times \dfrac{20\ mU}{1\ min} \times \dfrac{60\ min}{1\ h} = 20\ mL/h$

3. a. $\dfrac{x\ mL}{h} = \dfrac{500\ mL}{30\ units} \times \dfrac{1\ unit}{1000\ mU} \times \dfrac{1\ mU}{1\ min} \times \dfrac{60\ min}{1\ h} = 1\ mL/h$

 b. $\dfrac{x\ mL}{h} = \dfrac{500\ mL}{30\ units} \times \dfrac{1\ unit}{1000\ mU} \times \dfrac{20\ mU}{1\ min} \times \dfrac{60\ min}{1\ h} = 20\ mL/h$

4. a. $\dfrac{x\ mL}{h} = \dfrac{1000\ mL}{40\ units} \times \dfrac{1\ unit}{1000\ mU} \times \dfrac{2\ mU}{1\ min} \times \dfrac{60\ min}{1\ h} = 3\ mL/h$

 b. $\dfrac{x\ mL}{h} = \dfrac{1000\ mL}{40\ units} \times \dfrac{1\ unit}{1000\ mU} \times \dfrac{20\ mU}{1\ min} \times \dfrac{60\ min}{1\ h} = 30\ mL/h$

5. a. $\dfrac{x\ mL}{h} = \dfrac{1000\ mL}{20\ g} \times \dfrac{2\ g}{30\ min} \times \dfrac{60\ min}{1\ h} = 200\ mL/h$

 b. $\dfrac{x\ mL}{h} = \dfrac{1000\ mL}{20\ g} \times \dfrac{2\ g}{1\ h} = 100\ mL/h$

6. a. $\dfrac{x\ mL}{h} = \dfrac{1000\ mL}{40\ g} \times \dfrac{1\ g}{20\ min} \times \dfrac{60\ min}{1\ h} = 75\ mL/h$

 b. $\dfrac{x\ mL}{h} = \dfrac{1000\ mL}{40\ g} \times \dfrac{1\ g}{1\ h} = 25\ mL/h$

7. a. $\dfrac{x\ mL}{h} = \dfrac{1000\ mL}{40\ g} \times \dfrac{6\ g}{20\ min} \times \dfrac{60\ min}{1\ h} = 450\ mL/h$

 b. $\dfrac{x\ mL}{h} = \dfrac{1000\ mL}{40\ g} \times \dfrac{4\ g}{1\ h} = 100\ mL/h$

8. a. $\dfrac{x\ mL}{h} = \dfrac{500\ mL}{10\ g} \times \dfrac{4\ g}{30\ min} \times \dfrac{60\ min}{1\ h} = 400\ mL/h$

 b. $\dfrac{x\ mL}{h} = \dfrac{500\ mL}{10\ g} \times \dfrac{2\ g}{1\ h} = 100\ mL/h$

CHAPTER 19 Dimensional Analysis—Posttest 1, p. 559

1. a. $\dfrac{x\ mL}{h} = \dfrac{500\ mL}{20\ units} \times \dfrac{1\ unit}{1000\ mU} \times \dfrac{2\ mU}{1\ min} \times \dfrac{60\ min}{1\ h} = 3\ mL/h$

 b. $\dfrac{x\ mL}{h} = \dfrac{500\ mL}{20\ units} \times \dfrac{1\ unit}{1000\ mU} \times \dfrac{20\ mU}{1\ min} \times \dfrac{60\ min}{1\ h} = 30\ mL/h$

2. a. $\dfrac{x\ mL}{h} = \dfrac{1000\ mL}{30\ units} \times \dfrac{1\ unit}{1000\ mU} \times \dfrac{2\ mU}{1\ min} \times \dfrac{60\ min}{1\ h} = 4\ mL/h$

 b. $\dfrac{x\ mL}{h} = \dfrac{1000\ mL}{30\ units} \times \dfrac{1\ unit}{1000\ mU} \times \dfrac{30\ mU}{1\ min} \times \dfrac{60\ min}{1\ h} = 60\ mL/h$

3. a. $\dfrac{x \text{ mL}}{h} = \dfrac{500 \text{ mL}}{20 \text{ g}} \times \dfrac{2 \text{ g}}{30 \text{ min}} \times \dfrac{60 \text{ min}}{1 \text{ h}} = 100 \text{ mL/h}$

  b. $\dfrac{x \text{ mL}}{h} = \dfrac{500 \text{ mL}}{20 \text{ g}} \times \dfrac{3 \text{ g}}{1 \text{ h}} = 75 \text{ mL/h}$

4. a. $\dfrac{x \text{ mL}}{h} = \dfrac{500 \text{ mL}}{30 \text{ g}} \times \dfrac{2 \text{ g}}{20 \text{ min}} \times \dfrac{60 \text{ min}}{1 \text{ h}} = 100 \text{ mL/h}$

  b. $\dfrac{x \text{ mL}}{h} = \dfrac{500 \text{ mL}}{30 \text{ g}} \times \dfrac{3 \text{ g}}{1 \text{ h}} = 50 \text{ mL/h}$

CHAPTER 19 Dimensional Analysis—Posttest 2, p. 561

1. a. $\dfrac{x \text{ mL}}{h} = \dfrac{1000 \text{ mL}}{10 \text{ units}} \times \dfrac{1 \text{ unit}}{1000 \text{ mU}} \times \dfrac{2 \text{ mU}}{1 \text{ min}} \times \dfrac{60 \text{ min}}{1 \text{ h}} = 12 \text{ mL/h}$

  b. $\dfrac{x \text{ mL}}{h} = \dfrac{1000 \text{ mL}}{10 \text{ units}} \times \dfrac{1 \text{ unit}}{1000 \text{ mU}} \times \dfrac{30 \text{ mU}}{1 \text{ min}} \times \dfrac{60 \text{ min}}{1 \text{ h}} = 180 \text{ mL/h}$

2. a. $\dfrac{x \text{ mL}}{h} = \dfrac{1000 \text{ mL}}{40 \text{ units}} \times \dfrac{1 \text{ unit}}{1000 \text{ mU}} \times \dfrac{4 \text{ mU}}{1 \text{ min}} \times \dfrac{60 \text{ min}}{1 \text{ h}} = 6 \text{ mL/h}$

  b. $\dfrac{x \text{ mL}}{h} = \dfrac{1000 \text{ mL}}{40 \text{ units}} \times \dfrac{1 \text{ unit}}{1000 \text{ mU}} \times \dfrac{20 \text{ mU}}{1 \text{ min}} \times \dfrac{60 \text{ min}}{1 \text{ h}} = 30 \text{ mL/h}$

3. a. $\dfrac{x \text{ mL}}{h} = \dfrac{1000 \text{ mL}}{20 \text{ g}} \times \dfrac{2 \text{ g}}{30 \text{ min}} \times \dfrac{60 \text{ min}}{1 \text{ h}} = 200 \text{ mL/h}$

  b. $\dfrac{x \text{ mL}}{h} = \dfrac{1000 \text{ mL}}{20 \text{ g}} \times \dfrac{2 \text{ g}}{1 \text{ h}} = 100 \text{ mL/h}$

4. a. $\dfrac{x \text{ mL}}{h} = \dfrac{1000 \text{ mL}}{40 \text{ g}} \times \dfrac{2 \text{ g}}{15 \text{ min}} \times \dfrac{60 \text{ min}}{1 \text{ h}} = 200 \text{ mL/h}$

  b. $\dfrac{x \text{ mL}}{h} = \dfrac{1000 \text{ mL}}{40 \text{ g}} \times \dfrac{4 \text{ g}}{1 \text{ h}} = 100 \text{ mL/h}$

CHAPTER 19 Ratio-Proportion/Formula Method—Work Sheet, pp. 557–558

Ratio-Proportion	Formula Method

1. a. 1 unit : 1000 mU :: 10 units : x mU
$x = 1000 \times 10 = 10{,}000$ mU
10,000 mU : 500 mL :: 2 mU : x mL/min
$10{,}000x = 500 \times 2$
$x = \dfrac{1000}{10{,}000} = 0.1$ mL/min
0.1 mL : 1 min :: x mL : 60 min
$x = 60 \times 0.1$ mL/h = 6 mL/h

$\dfrac{2 \text{ mU/min}}{10{,}000 \text{ mU}} \times 500 \text{ mL} = 0.1 \text{ mL/min}$

$\dfrac{0.1 \text{ mL}}{1 \text{ min}} \times \dfrac{60 \text{ min}}{1 \text{ h}} = 6 \text{ mL/h}$

  b. 1 unit : 1000 mU :: 10 units : x mU
$x = 1000 \times 10 = 10{,}000$ mU
10,000 mU : 500 mL :: 30 mU : x mL/min
$10{,}000x = 500 \times 30$
$x = \dfrac{15{,}000}{10{,}000}$
$x = 1.5$ mL/min
1.5 mL : 1 min :: x mL : 60 min
$x = 60 \times 1.5 = 90$ mL/h

$\dfrac{30 \text{ mU/min}}{10{,}000 \text{ mU}} \times 500 \text{ mL} = 1.5 \text{ mL/min}$

$\dfrac{1.5 \text{ mL}}{1 \text{ min}} \times \dfrac{60 \text{ min}}{1 \text{ h}} = 90 \text{ mL/h}$

ANSWERS

Ratio-Proportion	Formula Method

2. a. 1 unit : 1000 mU :: 30 units : x mU
$x = 1000 \times 30 = 30{,}000$ mU
30,000 mU : 500 mL :: 2 mU : x mL/min
$30{,}000x = 500 \times 2$
$$x = \frac{1000}{30{,}000} = 0.033 \text{ mL/min}$$
0.033 mL : 1 min :: x mL : 60 min
$x = 60 \times 0.033 = 2$ mL/h

$$\frac{2 \text{ mU/min}}{30{,}000 \text{ mU}} \times 500 \text{ mL} = 0.033 \text{ mL/min}$$
$$\frac{0.033 \text{ mL}}{1 \text{ min}} \times \frac{60 \text{ min}}{1 \text{ h}} = 2 \text{ mL/h}$$

b. 1 unit : 1000 mU :: 30 units : x mU
$x = 1000 \times 30 = 30{,}000$ mU
30,000 mU : 500 mL :: 20 mU : x mL/min
$30{,}000x = 500 \times 20$
$$x = \frac{10{,}000}{30{,}000} = 0.33 \text{ mL/min}$$
0.33 mL : 1 min :: x mL : 60 min
$x = 60 \times 0.33 = 19.8$ or 20 mL/h

$$\frac{20 \text{ mU/min}}{30{,}000 \text{ mU}} \times 500 \text{ mL} = 0.33 \text{ mL/min}$$
$$\frac{0.33 \text{ mL}}{1 \text{ min}} \times \frac{60 \text{ min}}{1 \text{ h}} = 19.8 \text{ or } 20 \text{ mL/h}$$

3. a. 1 unit : 1000 mU :: 30 units : x mU
$x = 1000 \times 30 = 30{,}000$ mU
30,000 mU : 500 mL :: 1 mU : x mL/min
$30{,}000x = 500$
$$x = \frac{500}{30{,}000} = 0.016 \text{ mL/min}$$
0.016 mL : 1 min :: x mL : 60 min
$x = 60 \times 0.016 = 1$ mL/h

$$\frac{1 \text{ mU/min}}{30{,}000 \text{ mU}} \times 500 \text{ mL} = 0.016 \text{ mL/min}$$
$$\frac{0.016 \text{ mL}}{1 \text{ min}} \times \frac{60 \text{ min}}{1 \text{ h}} = 1 \text{ mL/h}$$

b. 1 unit : 1000 mU :: 30 units : x mU
$x = 1000 \times 30 = 30{,}000$ mU
30,000 mU : 500 mL :: 20 mU : x mL/min
$30{,}000x = 500 \times 20$
$$x = \frac{10{,}000}{30{,}000} = 0.33 \text{ mL/min}$$
0.33 mL : 1 min :: x mL : 60 min
$x = 60 \times 0.33 = 19.8$ or 20 mL/h

$$\frac{20 \text{ mU/min}}{30{,}000 \text{ mU}} \times 500 \text{ mL} = 0.33 \text{ mL/min}$$
$$\frac{0.33 \text{ mL}}{1 \text{ min}} \times \frac{60 \text{ min}}{1 \text{ h}} = 19.8 \text{ or } 20 \text{ mL/h}$$

4. a. 1 unit : 1000 mU :: 40 units : x mU
$x = 1000 \times 40 = 40{,}000$ mU
40,000 mU : 1000 mL :: 2 mU : x mL/min
$40{,}000x = 1000 \times 2$
$$x = \frac{2000}{40{,}000} = 0.05 \text{ mL/min}$$
0.05 mL : 1 min :: x mL : 60 min
$x = 60 \times 0.05$ mL/h $= 3$ mL/h

$$\frac{2 \text{ mU/min}}{40{,}000 \text{ mU}} \times 1000 \text{ mL} = 0.05 \text{ mL/min}$$
$$\frac{0.05 \text{ mL}}{1 \text{ min}} \times \frac{60 \text{ min}}{1 \text{ h}} = 3 \text{ mL/h}$$

b. 1 unit : 1000 mU :: 40 units : x mU
$x = 1000 \times 40 = 40{,}000$ mU
40,000 mU : 1000 mL :: 20 mU : x mL/min
$40{,}000x = 1000 \times 20$
$$x = \frac{20{,}000}{40{,}000} = 0.5 \text{ mL/min}$$
0.5 mL : 1 min :: x mL : 60 min
$x = 60 \times 0.5 = 30$ mL/h

$$\frac{20 \text{ mU/min}}{40{,}000 \text{ mU}} \times 1000 \text{ mL} = 0.5 \text{ mL/min}$$
$$\frac{0.5 \text{ mL}}{1 \text{ min}} \times \frac{60 \text{ min}}{1 \text{ h}} = 30 \text{ mL/h}$$

ANSWERS

Ratio-Proportion	**Formula Method**

5. a. $20 \text{ g} : 1000 \text{ mL} :: 2 \text{ g} : x \text{ mL}$
    $20x = 2000$
      $x = 100 \text{ mL}$
    $100 \text{ mL} : 30 \text{ min} :: x \text{ mL} : 60 \text{ min}$
    $30x = 6000$

      $x = \dfrac{6000}{30} = 200 \text{ mL/h}$

$$\frac{100 \text{ mL}}{30 \text{ min}} \times \frac{60 \text{ min}}{1 \text{ h}} = 200 \text{ mL/h}$$

  b. $20 \text{ g} : 1000 \text{ mL} :: 2 \text{ g} : x \text{ mL}$
    $20x = 2000$
      $x = 100 \text{ mL}$
    $100 \text{ mL} : 60 \text{ min} :: x \text{ mL} : 60 \text{ min}$
    $60x = 6000$

      $x = \dfrac{6000}{60} = 100 \text{ mL/h}$

$$\frac{2 \text{ g/h}}{20 \text{ g}} \times 1000 \text{ mL} = 100 \text{ mL/h}$$

6. a. $40 \text{ g} : 1000 \text{ mL} :: 1 \text{ g} : x \text{ mL}$
    $40x = 1000$
      $x = 25 \text{ mL}$
    $25 \text{ mL} : 20 \text{ min} :: x \text{ mL} : 60 \text{ min}$
    $20x = 1500$

      $x = \dfrac{1500}{20} = 75 \text{ mL/h}$

$$\frac{25 \text{ mL}}{20 \text{ min}} \times \frac{60 \text{ min}}{1 \text{ h}} = 75 \text{ mL/h}$$

  b. $40 \text{ g} : 1000 \text{ mL} :: 1 \text{ g} : x \text{ mL}$
    $40x = 1000$
      $x = 25 \text{ mL}$
    $25 \text{ mL} : 60 \text{ min} :: x \text{ mL} : 60 \text{ min}$
    $60x = 1500$

      $x = \dfrac{1500}{60} = 25 \text{ mL/h}$

$$\frac{1 \text{ g/h}}{40 \text{ g}} \times 1000 \text{ mL} = 25 \text{ mL/h}$$

7. a. $40 \text{ g} : 1000 \text{ mL} :: 6 \text{ g} : x \text{ mL}$
    $40x = 6000$
      $x = 150 \text{ mL}$
    $150 \text{ mL} : 20 \text{ min} :: x \text{ mL} : 60 \text{ min}$
    $20x = 9000$

      $x = \dfrac{9000}{20} = 450 \text{ mL/h}$

$$\frac{150 \text{ mL}}{20 \text{ min}} \times \frac{60 \text{ min}}{1 \text{ h}} = 450 \text{ mL/h}$$

  b. $40 \text{ g} : 1000 \text{ mL} :: 4 \text{ g} : x \text{ mL}$
    $40x = 4000$
      $x = 100 \text{ mL}$
    $100 \text{ mL} : 60 \text{ min} :: x \text{ mL} : 60 \text{ min}$
    $60x = 6000$

      $x = \dfrac{6000}{60} = 100 \text{ mL/h}$

$$\frac{4 \text{ g/h}}{40 \text{ g}} \times 1000 \text{ mL} = 100 \text{ mL/h}$$

Ratio-Proportion	**Formula Method**

8. a. $10\text{ g} : 500\text{ mL} :: 4\text{ g} : x\text{ mL}$
$10x = 2000$
$x = 200\text{ mL}$
$200\text{ mL} : 30\text{ min} :: x\text{ mL} : 60\text{ min}$
$30x = 12{,}000$
$x = \dfrac{12{,}000}{30} = 400\text{ mL/h}$

$\dfrac{200\text{ mL}}{30\text{ min}} \times \dfrac{60\text{ min}}{1\text{ h}} = 400\text{ mL/h}$

b. $10\text{ g} : 500\text{ mL} :: 2\text{ g} : x\text{ mL}$
$10x = 1000$
$x = 100\text{ mL}$
$100\text{ mL} : 60\text{ min} :: x\text{ mL} : 60\text{ min}$
$60x = 6000$
$x = \dfrac{6000}{60} = 100\text{ mL/h}$

$\dfrac{2\text{ g/h}}{10\text{ g}} \times 500\text{ mL} = 100\text{ mL/h}$

CHAPTER 19 Ratio-Proportion/Formula Method—Posttest 1, p. 559

Ratio-Proportion	**Formula**

1. a. $1\text{ unit} : 1000\text{ mU} :: 20\text{ units} : x\text{ mU}$
$x = 1000 \times 20 = 20{,}000\text{ mU}$
$20{,}000\text{ mU} : 500\text{ mL} :: 2\text{ mU} : x\text{ mL/min}$
$20{,}000x = 500 \times 2$
$x = \dfrac{1000}{20{,}000} = 0.05\text{ mL/min}$
$0.05\text{ mL} : 1\text{ min} :: x\text{ mL} : 60\text{ min}$
$x = 60 \times 0.05 = 3\text{ mL/h}$

$\dfrac{2\text{ mU/min}}{20{,}000\text{ mU}} \times 500\text{ mL} = 0.05\text{ mL/min}$
$\dfrac{0.05\text{ mL}}{1\text{ min}} \times \dfrac{60\text{ min}}{1\text{ h}} = 3\text{ mL/h}$

b. $1\text{ unit} : 1000\text{ mU} :: 20\text{ units} : x\text{ mU}$
$x = 1000 \times 20 = 20{,}000\text{ mU}$
$20{,}000\text{ mU} : 500\text{ mL} :: 20\text{ mU} : x\text{ mL/min}$
$20{,}000x = 500 \times 20$
$x = \dfrac{10{,}000}{20{,}000} = 0.5\text{ mL/min}$
$0.5\text{ mL} : 1\text{ min} :: x\text{ mL} : 60\text{ min}$
$x = 60 \times 0.5 = 30\text{ mL/h}$

$\dfrac{20\text{ mU/min}}{20{,}000\text{ mU}} \times 500\text{ mL} = 0.05\text{ mL/min}$
$\dfrac{0.5\text{ mL}}{1\text{ min}} \times \dfrac{60\text{ min}}{1\text{ h}} = 30\text{ mL/h}$

2. a. $1\text{ unit} : 1000\text{ mU} :: 30\text{ units} : x\text{ mU}$
$x = 1000 \times 30 = 30{,}000\text{ mU}$
$30{,}000\text{ mU} : 1000\text{ mL} :: 2\text{ mU} : x\text{ mL/min}$
$30{,}000x = 1000 \times 2$
$x = \dfrac{2000}{30{,}000} = 0.066\text{ mL/min}$
$0.066\text{ mL} : 1\text{ min} :: x\text{ mL} : 60\text{ min}$
$x = 60 \times 0.066 = 4\text{ mL/h}$

$\dfrac{2\text{ mU/min}}{30{,}000\text{ mU}} \times 1000\text{ mL} = 0.066\text{ mL/min}$
$\dfrac{0.066\text{ mL}}{1\text{ min}} \times \dfrac{60\text{ min}}{1\text{ h}} = 4\text{ mL/h}$

b. $1\text{ unit} : 1000\text{ mU} :: 30\text{ units} : x\text{ mU}$
$x = 1000 \times 30 = 30{,}000\text{ mU}$
$30{,}000\text{ mU} : 1000\text{ mL} :: 30\text{ mU} : x\text{ mL/min}$
$30{,}000x = 1000 \times 30$
$x = \dfrac{30{,}000}{30{,}000} = 1\text{ mL/min}$
$1\text{ mL} : 1\text{ min} :: x\text{ mL} : 60\text{ min}$
$x = 60 \times 1 = 60\text{ mL/h}$

$\dfrac{30\text{ mU/min}}{30{,}000\text{ mU}} \times 1000\text{ mL} = 1\text{ mL/min}$
$\dfrac{1\text{ mL}}{1\text{ min}} \times \dfrac{60\text{ min}}{1\text{ h}} = 60\text{ mL/h}$

ANSWERS

Ratio-Proportion	Formula
3. a. 20 g : 500 mL :: 2 g : x mL $\quad$ $20x = 1000$ $\quad\quad$ $x = 50$ mL $\quad$ 50 mL : 30 min :: x mL : 60 min $\quad$ $30x = 3000$ $\quad\quad$ $x = \dfrac{3000}{30} = 100$ mL/h	$\dfrac{50 \text{ mL}}{30 \text{ min}} \times \dfrac{60 \text{ min}}{1 \text{ h}} = 100$ mL/h
$\quad$ b. 20 g : 500 mL :: 3 g : x mL $\quad$ $20x = 1500$ $\quad\quad$ $x = 75$ mL $\quad$ 75 mL : 60 min :: x mL : 60 min $\quad$ $60x = 4500$ $\quad\quad$ $x = \dfrac{4500}{60} = 75$ mL/h	$\dfrac{3 \text{ g/h}}{20 \text{ g}} \times 500 \text{ mL} = 75$ mL/h
4. a. 30 g : 500 mL :: 2 g : x mL $\quad$ $30x = 1000$ $\quad\quad$ $x = 33.3$ mL $\quad$ 33.3 mL : 20 min :: x mL : 60 min $\quad$ $20x = 1998$ $\quad\quad$ $x = \dfrac{1998}{20} = 100$ mL/h	$\dfrac{33.3 \text{ mL}}{20 \text{ min}} \times \dfrac{60 \text{ min}}{1 \text{ h}} = 100$ mL/h
$\quad$ b. 30 g : 500 mL :: 3 g : x mL $\quad$ $30x = 1500$ $\quad\quad$ $x = 50$ mL $\quad$ 50 mL : 60 min :: x mL : 60 min $\quad$ $60x = 3000$ $\quad\quad$ $x = \dfrac{3000}{60} = 50$ mL/h	$\dfrac{3 \text{ g/h}}{30 \text{ g}} \times 500 \text{ mL} = 50$ mL/h

CHAPTER 19 Ratio-Proportion/Formula Method—Posttest 2, p. 561

Ratio-Proportion	Formula
1. a. 1 unit : 1000 mU :: 10 units : x mU $\quad$ $x = 1000 \times 10 = 10{,}000$ mU $\quad$ 10,000 mU : 1000 mL :: 2 mU : x mL/min $\quad$ $10{,}000x = 1000 \times 2$ $\quad\quad$ $x = \dfrac{2000}{10{,}000} = 0.2$ mL/min $\quad$ 0.2 mL : 1 min :: x mL : 60 min $\quad$ $x = 60 \times 0.2$ mL/h $= 12$ mL/h	$\dfrac{2 \text{ mU/min}}{10{,}000 \text{ mU}} \times 1000 \text{ mL} = 0.2$ mL/min $\dfrac{0.2 \text{ mL}}{1 \text{ min}} \times \dfrac{60 \text{ min}}{1 \text{ h}} = 12$ mL/h

Ratio-Proportion	Formula

b. 1 unit : 1000 mU :: 10 units : x mU
$x = 1000 \times 10 = 10,000$ mU
10,000 mU : 1000 mL :: 30 mU : x mL/min
$10,000x = 1000 \times 30$
$x = \dfrac{30,000}{10,000} = 3$ mL/min
3 mL : 1 min :: x mL : 60 min
$x = 60 \times 3 = 180$ mL/h

$$\dfrac{30 \text{ mU/min}}{10,000 \text{ mU}} \times 1000 \text{ mL} = 3 \text{ mL/min}$$
$$\dfrac{3 \text{ mL}}{1 \text{ min}} \times \dfrac{60 \text{ min}}{1 \text{ h}} = 180 \text{ mL/h}$$

2. a. 1 unit : 1000 mU :: 40 units : x mU
$x = 1000 \times 40 = 40,000$ mU
40,000 mU : 1000 mL :: 4 mU : x mL/min
$40,000x = 1000 \times 4$
$x = \dfrac{4000}{40,000} = 0.1$ mL/min
0.1 mL : 1 min :: x mL : 60 min
$x = 60 \times 0.1 = 6$ mL/h

$$\dfrac{4 \text{ mU/min}}{40,000 \text{ mU}} \times 1000 \text{ mL} = 0.1 \text{ mL/min}$$
$$\dfrac{0.1 \text{ mL}}{1 \text{ min}} \times \dfrac{60 \text{ min}}{1 \text{ h}} = 6 \text{ mL/h}$$

b. 1 unit : 1000 mU :: 40 units : x mU
$x = 1000 \times 40 = 40,000$ mU
40,000 mU : 1000 mL :: 20 mU : x mL/min
$40,000x = 1000 \times 20$
$x = \dfrac{20,000}{40,000} = 0.5$ mL/min
0.5 mL : 1 min :: x mL : 60 min
$x = 60 \times 0.5 = 30$ mL/h

$$\dfrac{20 \text{ mU/min}}{40,000 \text{ mU}} \times 1000 \text{ mL} = 0.5 \text{ mL/min}$$
$$\dfrac{0.5 \text{ mL}}{1 \text{ min}} \times \dfrac{60 \text{ min}}{1 \text{ h}} = 30 \text{ mL/h}$$

3. a. 20 g : 1000 mL :: 2 g : x mL
$20x = 2000$
$x = 100$ mL
100 mL : 30 min :: x mL : 60 min
$30x = 6000$
$x = \dfrac{6000}{30} = 200$ mL/h

$$\dfrac{100 \text{ mL}}{30 \text{ min}} \times \dfrac{60 \text{ min}}{1 \text{ h}} = 200 \text{ mL/h}$$

b. 20 g : 1000 mL :: 2 g : x mL
$20x = 2000$
$x = 100$ mL
100 mL : 60 min :: x mL : 60 min
$60x = 6000$
$x = \dfrac{6000}{60} = 100$ mL/h

$$\dfrac{2 \text{ g/h}}{20 \text{ g}} \times 1000 \text{ mL} = 100 \text{ mL/h}$$

Ratio-Proportion

Formula

4. a. 40 g : 1000 mL :: 2 g : x mL
$40x = 2000$
$x = 50$ mL
50 mL : 15 min :: x mL : 60 min
$15x = 3000$
$x = \dfrac{3000}{15} = 200$ mL/h

$$\dfrac{50 \text{ mL}}{15 \text{ min}} \times \dfrac{60 \text{ min}}{1 \text{ h}} = 200 \text{ mL/h}$$

   b. 40 g : 1000 mL :: 4 g : x mL
$40x = 4000$
$x = 100$ mL
100 mL : 60 min :: x mL : 60 min
$60x = 6000$
$x = \dfrac{6000}{60} = 100$ mL/h

$$\dfrac{4 \text{ g/h}}{40 \text{ g}} \times 1000 \text{ mL} = 100 \text{ mL/h}$$

NAME _____

DATE _____

ACCEPTABLE SCORE __**95**__

YOUR SCORE _____

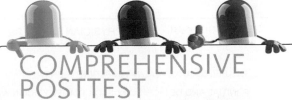

COMPREHENSIVE POSTTEST

DIRECTIONS: This test contains 56 questions with a total of 100 points (pts) possible. Each of the nine separate case sections includes a variety of patient diagnoses. Test items focus on medication dosages, medication calculations, and medication transcription. Use the forms provided, and mark syringes where indicated.

CASE 1 *(20 pts)*

Mr. Jones is transferred to your floor from the intensive care unit (ICU). You receive Mr. Jones and look over his orders. It is 1700 on 2/3/19. Refer to the physician's order sheet and medication profile sheet on p. 572 for the following questions. Show your work where applicable.

1. Mr. Jones complains of pain to his incision. Percocet 5/500 tablets are ordered on the physician's order sheet. Percocet is supplied in single tablets issued from the pharmacy. Give _____ *(1 pt)*

2. What regularly scheduled medications would Mr. Jones receive at 0900 each day? Include the amount of medication. a. _____ b. _____ c. _____ d. _____ *(4 pts)*

3. How much intravenous (IV) fluid will Mr. Jones receive every 8 hours? _____ mL *(1 pt)*

PHYSICIAN'S ORDERS

1. LABEL BEFORE PLACING IN PATIENT'S CHART ▶
2. INITIAL AND DETACH COPY EACH TIME PHYSICIAN WRITES ORDERS
3. TRANSMIT COPY TO PHARMACY
4. ORDERS MUST BE DATED AND TIMED

Mr. Jones

☐ Inpatient   ☐ Outpatient

DATE	TIME	ORDERS	TRANS BY
		Diagnosis: S/P Coronary Art. Bypass Graft Weight: 184.5 lb Height: 5'11"	
		Sensitivities/Drug Allergies: NKDA	
2/3/19	2250	1. Transfer to step-down unit from ICU	
		2. VS q.4. h. × 24 hours then q. 8 hours	
		3. Up in chair 3×day, asst. to walk in hall 2×day	
		4. Intake and output q. 8 hours	
		5. Daily WT.	
		6. TED Hose	
		7. Incentive spirometer q.1 h. while awake	
		8. Diet: 3 g Na^+, low cholesterol	
		9. Percocet 5/500, 2 tablets p.o. q.4 h. p.r.n. pain	
		10. Tylenol 650 mg p.o. q.4 h. p.r.n. pain or Temp. ≥38 C	
		11. MOM 30 mL p.o. q.day p.r.n. constipation	
		12. Mylanta 30 mL p.o. q.4 h. p.r.n. indigestion	
		13. Ambien 10 mg p.o. at bedtime p.r.n. insomnia	
		14. O_2 3 L per nasal cannula	
		15. IVF: D_5 1/2 NS @ $50^{mL}/_{hr}$, maximum 1200 mL IVF/day	
		16. Digoxin 0.25 mg p.o. daily	
		17. E.C. ASA 325 mg p.o. daily	
		18. Cimetidine 300 mg p.o. three times a day	
		19. Lasix 20 mg I.V. q.8 h.	
		20. Slow-K 10 mEq p.o. twice a day	
		21. Labs A_7, CBC, CXR q. a.m.	
		M. Doctor, M.D.	

Do Not Write Orders If No Copies Remain; Begin New Form   Copies
Remaining

MEDICAL RECORDS COPY		**PHYSICIAN'S ORDERS**						**T-5**
B-CLIN. NOTES	E-LAB	G-X-RAY	K-DIAGNOSTIC	M-SURGERY	Q-THERAPY	T-ORDERS	W-NURSING	Y-MISC.

4. Transcribe each as-needed (prn) medication from the physician's orders. Include date, medication, dose, route, interval, and time schedule. *(5 pts)*

	dose	route	interval									
	dose	route	interval									
	dose	route	interval									
	dose	route	interval									
	dose	route	interval									

5. Transcribe each regularly scheduled medication from the physician's order sheet. Include date, medication, dose, route, interval, and time schedule. *(5 pts)*

	dose	route	interval									
	dose	route	interval									
	dose	route	interval									
	dose	route	interval									
	dose	route	interval									

6. Mr. Jones complains of insomnia at 2300. What prn medication is available for him? _____
(1 pt)

7. It is time to give Mr. Jones his Lasix. You have a premixed intravenous piggyback (IVPB) of Lasix 20 mg in 50 mL of normal saline solution (NS). Infusion time is 30 minutes. Drop factor is 60 gtt/mL. How many drops per minute will you administer? _____ *(1 pt)*

8. Mr. Jones complains of constipation. What medication will you give? _____ How much will you administer? _____ *(1 pt)*

9. What regularly scheduled medication would Mr. Jones receive at 0800 each day? Include the amount of medication. Give _____ *(1 pt)*

CASE 2 *(12 pts)*

Mrs. Smith is received by you from the recovery room. You review her orders. It is 1700 on 2/3/19. Refer to the physician's order sheet for the following questions. Show your work where applicable.

PHYSICIAN'S ORDERS

1. LABEL BEFORE PLACING IN PATIENT'S CHART ▶
2. INITIAL AND DETACH COPY EACH TIME PHYSICIAN WRITES ORDERS
3. TRANSMIT COPY TO PHARMACY
4. ORDERS MUST BE DATED AND TIMED

Mrs. Smith

☐ Inpatient   ☐ Outpatient

DATE	TIME	ORDERS	TRANS BY
2/3/19	1650	Diagnosis: S/P Thyroidectomy Weight: 146.0 lb Height: 5'10"	
		Sensitivities/Drug Allergies: PCN	
		STATUS: ASSIGN TO OBSERVATION ☐ ; ADMIT AS INPATIENT ☐	
		1. Transfer to ward from recovery room.	
		2. VS q.1 hour ×2 hours, then q.4 hours	
		3. HOB ↑45 degrees	
		4. Up in chair 3× day, support head and neck	
		5. Intake and output q. 8 hours	
		6. Incentive spirometer q.1 hour while awake	
		7. Diet: Full liquid	
		8. Dilaudid 2 mg I.M. q.4 hours p.r.n. pain	
		9. Phenergan 12.5 mg I.M. q.4 hours p.r.n. nausea	
		10. Tylenol 650 mg p.o. q.4 hours p.r.n. pain or Temp >38°C	
		11. Ambien 5 mg p.o. at bedtime p.r.n. insomnia	
		12. O_2 4 L per nasal cannula	
		13. IVF: NS 75 mL/h	
		14. Synthroid 0.15 mg. p.o. daily	
		15. Tagamet 300 mg. p.o. daily	
		16. Labs: Ca^+ q. 8 hours × 3 days A_7, CBC q. a.m.	
		17. JP drains × 2 to bulb suction, record output q. 8 hours	
		M. Doctor, M.D.	

Do Not Write Orders If No Copies Remain; Begin New Form   Copies Remaining

MEDICAL RECORDS COPY	PHYSICIAN'S ORDERS	T-5

B-CLIN. NOTES	E-LAB	G-X-RAY	K-DIAGNOSTIC	M-SURGERY	Q-THERAPY	T-ORDERS	W-NURSING	Y-MISC.

1. What regularly scheduled medications would Mrs. Smith receive at 0900 each day? Include the amount of each medication. a. _____ b. _____ *(2 pts)*

2. Mrs. Smith complains of nausea. You have Phenergan 25 mg/2 mL available. How many milliliters will you administer? _____ *(1 pt)*

3. How much IV fluid will Mrs. Smith receive per shift? _____ Per day? _____ *(2 pts)*

4. Mrs. Smith complains of insomnia at 2200. Ambien is supplied in 10-mg tablets. Give _____ tablet(s). *(1 pt)*

5. What prn medications are available for complaints of pain? a. _____ b. _____ *(2 pts)*

6. Your patient complains of pain shortly after she is received on the ward from the recovery room. Dilaudid is available 1 mg/1 mL for injection. How many milliliters will you administer? _____ *(1 pt)*

7. Your patient has a fever of 38.6° C. You have Tylenol 325-mg tablets available. How many tablets will you administer? _____ *(1 pt)*

   nscribe all regularly scheduled medications from the physician's orders. Include date, med-
   n, dose, route, interval, and time schedule. *(2 pts)*

CASE 3

(9 pts)

Mrs. Hutsen is received by you after vaginal delivery childbirth without complications. Refer to the physician's order sheet for the following questions. Show your work where applicable.

		PHYSICIAN'S ORDERS			
		1. LABEL BEFORE PLACING IN PATIENT'S CHART ▶		Mrs. Hutsen	
		2. INITIAL AND DETACH COPY EACH TIME PHYSICIAN WRITES ORDERS			
		3. TRANSMIT COPY TO PHARMACY			
		4. ORDERS MUST BE DATED AND TIMED		☐ Inpatient ☐ Outpatient	

DATE	TIME	ORDERS	TRANS BY
4/27/19	0815	Diagnosis: S/P Childbirth Weight: 146.0 lb Height: 5'8"	
		Sensitivities/Drug Allergies: PCN	
		STATUS: ASSIGN TO OBSERVATION [ ]; ADMIT AS INPATIENT [ ]	
		1. Diet: Regular	
		2. Activity: Up ad lib c̄ assistance as needed	
		3. Vital signs: Routine	
		4. Breast care: per protocol manual breast pump if desired.	
		5. Incentive spirometer X10 breaths q.1 h. while awake	
		6. May shower as desired	
		7. If pt. unable to void within 8 h. or fundus boggy, bladder distended, or uterus displaced, may in and out cath.	
		8. Notify M.D. if unable to void 6 h. after catheterization.	
		9. Call physician for temp >38.5° C, urinary output <240 mL/shift.	
		10. DSLR 50mL/h, may D/C I.V. when tolerating p.o. well.	
		11. Ferrous sulfate 0.3 g p.o. twice daily	
		12. Percocet 7.5/500, 1 tablet p.o. q.6 h. p.r.n. pain	
		13. Tucks to peri-area for discomfort p.r.n. at bedside.	
		14. Senokot 1 tablet p.o. daily p.r.n. for constipation	
		15. Ibuprofen 400 mg p.o. q.6 hours p.r.n. mild pain	
		M. Dundar, M.D.	

Do Not Write Orders If No Copies Remain; Begin New Form   **Copies Remaining**

MEDICAL RECORDS COPY			PHYSICIAN'S ORDERS						T-5
B-CLIN. NOTES	E-LAB	G-X-RAY	K-DIAGNOSTIC	M-SURGERY	Q-THERAPY	T-ORDERS	W-NURSING	Y-MISC.	

1. What regularly scheduled medication would your patient receive each day? _____ Include the amount. _____ *(2 pts)*

2. Your patient is tolerating oral intake well. Her IV fluid was stopped 2 hours before the evening shift (1500-2330) ended. How many milliliters did the patient receive on the evening shift? _____ mL. *(1 pt)*

3. Your patient complains of pain and has ibuprofen ordered. Ibuprofen is supplied as 200-mg tablets. How many tablets will you administer? _____ *(1 pt)*

4. Transcribe all prn medications from the physician's orders. Include date, medication, dose, route, interval, and time schedule. *(5 pts)*

	dose	route	interval							
	dose	route	interval							
	dose	route	interval							
	dose	route	interval							
	dose	route	interval							

CASE 4

(15 pts)

J. Todd is received on your floor with a diagnosis of acute lymphocytic leukemia. Refer to the physician's order sheet for the following questions. Show your work where applicable.

	PHYSICIAN'S ORDERS		

PHYSICIAN'S ORDERS

1. LABEL BEFORE PLACING IN PATIENT'S CHART ▶
2. INITIAL AND DETACH COPY EACH TIME PHYSICIAN WRITES ORDERS
3. TRANSMIT COPY TO PHARMACY
4. ORDERS MUST BE DATED AND TIMED

Jason Todd

☐ Inpatient ☐ Outpatient

DATE	TIME	ORDERS	TRANS BY
10/13/19	0800	Diagnosis: Acute Lymphocytic Leukemia Weight: 12.73 kg Height: 3'0"	
		Sensitivities/Drug Allergies: Codeine	
		STATUS: ASSIGN TO OBSERVATION [ ]; ADMIT AS INPATIENT [ ]	
		1. Diet: Regular	
		2. Activity: ↑chair three times a day, Ø rigorous play activity	
		3. O_2–Biox to keep sats >93%	
		4. Vital signs: q.4 h.	
		5. I+O q. 8 hours	
		6. Daily WT.	
		7. IVF: $D_5\frac{1}{2}$ NS 25 mL/h	
		8. Allopurinol 50 mg. p.o. three times a day	
		9. Theophylline 100 mg p.o. q.8 h.	
		10. Prednisone 2 mg/kg/day p.o.	
		11. Vincristine 5 mg/m² in 50 mL of NaCl × 1 IV now	
		12. MVI 1 tablet q.day p.o.	
		13. Compazine 0.07 mg/kg I.M. q.day p.r.n. nausea	
		14. Tylenol 120 mg p.o. three times a day p.r.n. pain	
		15. Call physician SBP >140<90, DBP >90<40, Temp. >38.5 °C, SOB, urinary output <200 mL/shift, any problems	
		16. Labs: CBC c̄ diff., A_7, plts., CXR q.day	
		M. Doctor, M.D.	

Do Not Write Orders If No Copies Remain; Begin New Form   Copies Remaining

MEDICAL RECORDS COPY		PHYSICIAN'S ORDERS							T-5
B-CLIN. NOTES	E-LAB	G-X-RAY	K-DIAGNOSTIC	M-SURGERY	Q-THERAPY	T-ORDERS	W-NURSING	Y-MISC.	

1. Transcribe all regularly scheduled medications. Include date, medication, dose, route, interval, and time schedule. *(4 pts)*

	dose	route	interval								
	dose	route	interval								
	dose	route	interval								
	dose	route	interval								
	dose	route	interval								

2. Transcribe all prn medications. Include date, medication, dose, route, interval, and time schedule. *(2 pts)*

	dose	route	interval								
	dose	route	interval								

3. Your patient requires theophylline 16 mg po q 6 h. You have theophylline elixir 11.25 mg/mL available. Give _____ mL. *(1 pt)*

4. Your patient requires the allopurinol dose now. You have allopurinol elixir 100 mg/mL available. Give _____ mL. *(1 pt)*

tient receives prednisone 2 mg/kg/day. You have 10 mg/mL available. Calculate the
se for the patient's weight. Give _____ mL. *(2 pts)*

6. Your patient requires a vincristine dose now. The vincristine is supplied in 50 mL of NaCl to be infused over 60 minutes. Drop factor is 60 gtt/mL. Administer _____ gtt/min. *(1 pt)*

7. Your patient complains of nausea. You have Compazine 1 mg/mL available. How many milliliters will you administer? _____ Mark the syringe at the appropriate amount. *(2 pts)*

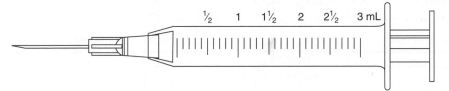

8. Your patient receives D_5 ½ NS at 25 mL/h. How much fluid will your patient receive during each 8-hour shift? _____ mL *(1 pt)*

9. Your patient complains of pain. You have Tylenol elixir 360 mg/2 mL available. How many milliliters will you administer? _____ *(1 pt)*

CASE 5
(18 pts)

Mr. Miller is received on your floor from the recovery room. Refer to the physician's order sheet for the following questions. Show your work where applicable.

	PHYSICIAN'S ORDERS	Mr. Miller
	1. LABEL BEFORE PLACING IN PATIENT'S CHART ▶	
	2. INITIAL AND DETACH COPY EACH TIME PHYSICIAN WRITES ORDERS	
	3. TRANSMIT COPY TO PHARMACY	
	4. ORDERS MUST BE DATED AND TIMED	☐ Inpatient ☐ Outpatient

DATE	TIME	ORDERS	TRANS BY
6/15/19	1600	Diagnosis: S/P ® total hip replacement Weight: 197 lb Height: 6'2"	
		Sensitivities/Drug Allergies: NKDA	
		STATUS: ASSIGN TO OBSERVATION [ ]; ADMIT AS INPATIENT [ ]	
		1. Diet: NPO til fully awake, then clear liquids	
		2. Activity: Bed rest, log roll side-back-side q.2 h.	
		3. Vital signs: q.4 h.	
		4. Overhead frame trapeze	
		5. Abductor pillow while in bed.	
		6. Incentive spirometer q.1 h. while awake.	
		7. Intake and output q.8 h.	
		8. Hemovacs to own reservoirs, record output q.1 h. × 6 h., then q.6 h.	
		9. I+O catheterization q.shift p.r.n. inability to void	
		10. Heparin 5000 units subcutaneous twice a day	
		11. Torecan 10 mg I.M. q.4 h. p.r.n. nausea	
		12. Mylanta 30 mL p.o. p.r.n. indigestion	
		13. Ambien 10 mg. p.o. at bedtime p.r.n. insomnia	
		14. Tylenol c̄ codeine p.o. 2 tabs q.4 h. p.r.n. pain	
		15. Morphine PCA 1 mg I.V. q.10 min to maximum 25 mg/q.5 h. prn for pain	
		16. Dulcolax supp. 1 per rectum every shift prn constipation	
		17. Labs: CBC q.day × 3	
		18. Call orders: Hemovac output >500^{mL}/shift,	
		urinary output<250^{mL}/shift, Temp. >38.5° C, Hgb <10.0,	
		SBP >160<80, DBP >90<50	
		19. IVF: D_5 NS 50^{mL}/h	
		20. Cefuroxime 1g IVPB q.8 h.	
		M. Doctor, M.D.	

Do Not Write Orders If No Copies Remain; Begin New Form   Copies Remaining

PHYSICIAN'S ORDERS					T-5
AGNOSTIC	M-SURGERY	Q-THERAPY	T-ORDERS	W-NURSING	Y-MISC.

1. Transcribe the regularly scheduled medication below. Include date, medication, dose, route, interval, and time schedule. *(2 pts)*

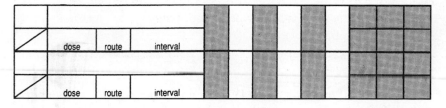

2. Transcribe all prn medications ordered below. Include date, medication, dose, route, interval, and time schedule. *(8 pts)*

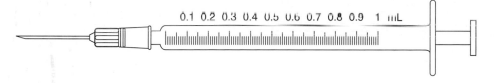

3. Your patient requires 5000 units heparin subcutaneous. You have a vial containing 5000 units/mL. Give _____ mL. Mark the syringe at the appropriate amount. *(2 pts)*

0.1 0.2 0.3 0.4 0.5 0.6 0.7 0.8 0.9 1 mL

4. Your patient requires morphine sulfate via patient-controlled analgesia (PCA) 1 mg every 10 minutes. You have a morphine sulfate syringe with 30 mg/30 mL available. How many milliliters will the patient receive every 10 minutes? _____ mL/10 min *(1 pt)*

5. Your patient complains of nausea and requires Torecan as ordered. You have Torecan 20 mg/2 mL available per vial. Give _____ mL *(1 pt)*

6. Your patient receives D_5 NS at 50 mL/h. How much IV fluid will your patient receive per 8-hour shift? _____ mL/shift Per day? _____ mL/day *(2 pts)*

7. Your patient receives cefuroxime 1 g in 100 mL NS IVPB 30 minutes q 8 h. Drop factor is 60 gtt/mL. _____ mL/h _____ gtt/min *(2 pts)*

CASE 6

(11 pts)

Ms. Keys, admitted with a diagnosis of myocardial infarction, returns from the cardiac catheterization laboratory for a stent placement. Refer to the physician's order sheet and medication profile sheet for the following questions. Show your work where applicable.

PHYSICIAN'S ORDERS

1. LABEL BEFORE PLACING IN PATIENT'S CHART ▶
2. INITIAL AND DETACH COPY EACH TIME PHYSICIAN WRITES ORDERS
3. TRANSMIT COPY TO PHARMACY
4. ORDERS MUST BE DATED AND TIMED

Ms. Keys

☐ Inpatient   ☐ Outpatient

DATE	TIME	ORDERS	TRANS BY
		Diagnosis: MI, s/p stent Weight: 168 lb Height: 5'5"	
		Sensitivities/Drug Allergies: PCN	
3/4/19	1100	1. Transfer to CCU	
		2. Diet: Healthy Heart	
		3. Activity: BR X 6 h, then dangle. If no bleeding from right groin	
		site, up ad lib	
		4. VS q15 min X 4, q30 min X 4, then every hour	
		5. Telemetry	
		6. EKG every morning X 2	
		7. Cardiac profile q8 h X 2 (1800 and 0200)	
		8. O$_2$ 2 L/min	
		9. Tylenol 650 mg po q4 h p.r.n. headache	
		10. ASA 325 mg po daily, start 3/5/19	
		11. Plavix 75 mg po daily, start 3/5/19	
		12. Nitroglycerin drip at 10 mcg/min	
		13. IV heparin per weight-based protocol	
		14. Metoprolol 12.5 mg p.o. twice a day Hold for SBP <80 mm Hg	
		15. Ambien 5 mg p.o. at bedtime p.r.n. insomnia	
		16. Call for chest pain, any concerns	
		M. Doctor, M.D.	

Do Not Write Orders If No Copies Remain; Begin New Form   Copies Remaining

MEDICAL RECORDS COPY			**PHYSICIAN'S ORDERS**					T-5
B-CLIN. NOTES	E-LAB	G-X RAY	K-DIAGNOSTIC	M-SURGERY	Q-THERAPY	T-ORDERS	W-NURSING	Y-MISC.

1. Transcribe each regularly scheduled medication from the physician's order sheet. Include date, medication, dose, route, interval, and time schedule. *(3 pts)*

	dose	route	interval							
	dose	route	interval							
	dose	route	interval							
	dose	route	interval							
	dose	route	interval							

2. Transcribe each prn medication from the physician's order sheet. Include date, medication, dose, route, interval, and time schedule. *(2 pts)*

	dose	route	interval						
	dose	route	interval						

3. The nitroglycerin drip has a concentration of 50 mg/100 mL of 0.9% NS. How many milliliters per hour should the IV pump be programmed for? _____ mL/h *(1 pt)*

4. Follow the heparin protocol in Chapter 16 for the following questions. The patient weighs 76.4 kg.

   a. How many units of heparin should be administered for the bolus? _____ units *(1 pt)*

b. With the following vial of heparin, how many milliliters should the nurse administer?
_____ mL *(1 pt)*

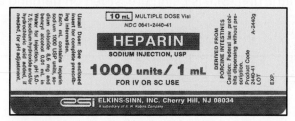

c. For how many milliliters per hour should the IV pump be programmed for the heparin infusion? _____ mL/h *(1 pt)*

5. The metoprolol comes in 25-mg tablets. How many tablets should be administered? _____ *(1 pt)*

6. Ms. Keys complains of a headache after the nitroglycerin is started. The Tylenol comes in 325-mg tablets. How many tablets should the nurse administer? _____ *(1 pt)*

CASE 7 *(5 pts)*

A 5-day-old neonate is admitted to the pediatric unit. She is being breast-fed on demand and supplemented with Enfamil with iron Lipil.

		PHYSICIAN'S ORDERS	

1. LABEL BEFORE PLACING IN PATIENT'S CHART
2. INITIAL AND DETACH COPY EACH TIME PHYSICIAN WRITES ORDERS
3. TRANSMIT COPY TO PHARMACY
4. ORDERS MUST BE DATED AND TIMED

Baby Jackson

☐ Inpatient   ☐ Outpatient

DATE	TIME	ORDERS	TRANS BY
5/1/19	0200	Diagnosis: Fever, poor feeding, jaundice, possible sepsis Weight: 7 lb, 8 oz	
		Sensitivities/Drug Allergies: NKDA	
		STATUS: ASSIGN TO OBSERVATION [ ]; ADMIT AS INPATIENT [ ]	
		1. Admit to pediatric unit	
		2. Cardiac apnea monitor with continuous Biox	
		3. Labs: CBC with diff, Chem 7, Blood cultures ×2, and total bilirubin count @ 0600	
		4. I&O cath for colony count plus micro	
		5. Start IV fluids D_5 45% NS at 12 mL/h continuous until d/c.	
		6. Ampicillin 160 mg IV infuse over 20 minutes per syringe pump q.8 h daily starting today	
		7. Gentamicin 12 mg IV infuse over 30 minutes per syringe pump once daily	
		8. Tylenol elixir 40 mg po q. 6 h. p.r.n. for fever >100.4° F axillary	
		9. Vital signs q.4 h	
		10. Weigh daily	
		11. Strict I&O	
		12. Diet: Breast milk, supplement with Enfamil with iron Lipil po ad lib	
		13. Activity: Up in Mom's arms ad lib	
		14. Call orders: Notify MD for: temp >100.6° or <95° F axillary, pulse >180<100, resp >60<20, any problems or concerns	
		15. Notify MD for sats <92%	
		16. Humidity via isolette	
		M. Doctor, M.D.	

Do Not Write Orders If No Copies Remain; Begin New Form   Copies Remaining

MEDICAL RECORDS COPY	PHYSICIAN'S ORDERS							T-5
B-CLIN. NOTES	E-LAB	G-X-RAY	K-DIAGNOSTIC	M-SURGERY	Q-THERAPY	T-ORDERS	W-NURSING	Y-MISC.

1. Ampicillin is available as 500-mg powder to be reconstituted with 4.8 mL of sterile water for a final dilution of 250 mg/mL. Recommended dosage is 100 to 200 mg/kg/24 h q 6–8 h.

    a. How many milligrams per kilogram per 24 hours of ampicillin is the neonate receiving? _____ mg/kg/24 h b. Is the order safe? _____ c. If yes, how many milliliters are needed to deliver the ordered dose? _____ mL *(3 pts)*

2. The neonate has a body temperature of 100.4° F axillary. Tylenol infant drops come as 80 mg/0.8 mL. How many milliliters are needed to deliver the ordered dose? _____ mL *(1 pt)*

3. This neonate is receiving IV fluids at 12 mL/h. How many milliliters are needed to deliver 6 hours of the ordered fluids? _____ mL *(1 pt)*

CASE 8
(5 pts)

Jeff, a 9-year-old boy, was seen in the local emergency department with fever, vomiting, and severe abdominal pain. After a thorough evaluation Jeff was taken to the operating room for an emergency laparoscopic appendectomy. Jeff's postoperative recovery was uneventful, and he was discharged to home. Refer to the physician's medication discharge orders for the following questions. Jeff weighs 55 pounds.

Physician's discharge medication orders:

1. Acetaminophen 300 mg po elixir q 4–6 h prn for pain or fever.
   (Recommended dosing for acetaminophen is 10 to 15 mg/kg/dose q 4–6 h; maximum 5 doses/24 h)

2. Amoxicillin 600 mg po suspension bid
   (Recommended dosage range of 20 to 50 mg/kg/24 h)

1. Prove mathematically that the ordered dose of acetaminophen is safe to administer. _____
(1 pt)

2. The acetaminophen suspension is available as 160 mg/5 mL. How many milliliters should Jeff receive for the ordered dose? _____ *(1 pt)*

3. What is the best method to deliver the medication to Jeff at home? _____ *(1 pt)*

4. Prove mathematically that the ordered dose of amoxicillin is both safe and therapeutic to administer. _____ *(1 pt)*

5. How many milliliters are needed to deliver the ordered dose of amoxicillin? Amoxicillin is available as 400 mg/5 mL. _____ *(1 pt)*

CASE 9
(5 pts)

Mrs. Taylor, 76, presents to the emergency department with dyspnea and fatigue. The family states that she has a history of heart failure and renal insufficiency and that she is prescribed Lasix 40 mg daily, digoxin 0.25 mg daily, and lisinopril 10 mg daily. Please answer the following questions pertaining to Mrs. Taylor. Show your work where applicable.

1. When assessing Mrs. Taylor's compliance with her prescribed medications, the nurse is aware that the most common medication error for older adults at home is _____. *(1 pt)*

2. Explain how a decrease in cardiac output can affect Mrs. Taylor. _____ *(1 pt)*

3. Mrs. Taylor admits she has been trying to "stretch" her medications, so she has been taking them only every other day. The nurse is aware that the most common reason for patients trying to "stretch" their medications is _____. *(1 pt)*

4. Mrs. Taylor also states that sometimes she can't remember if she has taken her medications. An inexpensive solution to this problem is a _____. *(1 pt)*

5. With discharge teaching, how should the nurse evaluate the effectiveness of the medication teaching? _____. *(1 pt)*

ANSWERS ON PP. 592–595.

evolve   To further test your knowledge base for calculating various dosage problems, refer to the Comprehensive Posttest Section of *Drug Calculations Companion,* Version 5, on Evolve.

ANSWERS

COMPREHENSIVE POSTTEST, pp. 571–591

Case 1, *pp. 571–574*

1. 2 tablets
2. a. Digoxin 0.25 mg
   b. EC ASA 325 mg
   c. Cimetidine 300 mg
   d. Slow-K 10 mEq
3. 400 mL of $D_5\frac{1}{2}$ NS per shift
4.

2/3/19	Percocet 5/500								
	2 dose	p.o. route	q.4 h. interval	prn pain					
2/3/19	Tylenol 650 mg								
	650 mg dose	p.o. route	q.4 h. interval	prn pain or Temp >38° C					
2/3/19	MOM								
	30 mL dose	p.o. route	daily interval	prn constipation					
2/3/19	Mylanta								
	30 mL dose	p.o. route	q.4 h. interval	prn indigestion					
2/3/19	Ambien								
	10 mg dose	p.o. route	at bedtime interval	prn insomnia					

5.

2/3/19	Digoxin							
	0.25 mg dose	p.o. route	daily interval	09				
2/3/19	E.C. ASA 325 mg							
	325 mg dose	p.o. route	daily interval	09				
2/3/19	Cimetidine							
	300 mg dose	p.o. route	Three times daily interval	09	13	17		
2/3/19	Lasix							
	20 mg dose	I.V. route	q.8 h. interval	08		16	24	
2/3/19	Slow-K							
	10 mEq dose	p.o. route	twice daily interval	09		17		

6. Ambien 10 mg po
7. 100 gtt/min
8. Milk of magnesia 30 mL
9. Lasix 20 mg

Case 2, *pp. 575–576*

1. a. Synthroid 0.15 mg
   b. Tagamet 300 mg
2. 1 mL
3. 600 mL/shift
   1800 mL/day if three shifts per day
4. ½ tablet
5. a. Dilaudid
   b. Tylenol
6. 2 mL
7. 2 tablets

8.

2/3/19	Synthroid						09							
	0.15 mg dose	p.o. route	daily interval										
2/3/19	Tagamet						09							
	300 mg dose	p.o. route	daily interval										

Case 3, *pp. 577–578*

1. $FeSO_4$ 0.3 g
2. 325 mL
3. 2 tablets
4.

4/27/19	Perocet 7.5/500											
	7.5/500 dose	p.o. route	q.6 h. interval	prn pain								
4/27/19	Tucks											
	one dose	Peri route	interval	prn @ bedside								
4/27/19	Senokot											
	one tab dose	p.o. route	daily interval	09								
4/27/19	Ibuprofen											
	400 mg dose	p.o. route	q.6 h. interval	prn pain								

Case 4, *pp. 579–581*

1.

10/13/19	Allopurinol					07	1200	1700				
	50 mg dose	p.o. route	3 times daily interval									
10/13/19	Theophylline					06	1400	2200				
	100 mg dose	p.o. route	q.8 h. interval									
10/13/19	Prednisone					09						
	2 mg/kg dose	p.o. route	daily interval									
10/13/19	MVI					09						
	1 tablet dose	p.o. route	daily interval									

2.

10/13/19	Compazine								
	0.07 mg/kg dose	IM route	daily interval	prn nausea					
10/13/19	Tylenol								
	120 mg dose	p.o. route	3 times daily interval	prn pain					

3. 1.42 mL
4. 0.5 mL
5. 25.46, or 25.5 mL rounded
6. 50 gtt/min
7. 0.9 mL

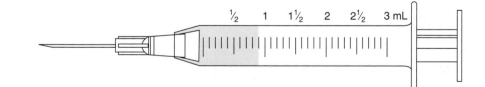

8. 200 mL
9. 0.66 mL, or 0.67 rounded

ANSWERS

Case 5, *pp. 582–584*

1.

6/15/19	Heparin											
⬦	5000 U dose	subcutaneous route	twice daily interval	09		21						
6/15/19	Cefuroxime											
⬦	1 g dose	IVPB route	q.8 h. interval	08	16	24						

2.

6/15/19	Torecan									
⬦	10 mg dose	IM route	q.4 h. interval	prn nausea					
6/15/19	Mylanta									
⬦	30 mL dose	p.o. route	interval	prn indigestion					
6/15/19	Dulcolax Supp.									
⬦	1 dose	pr route	q.shift interval	prn constipation					
6/15/19	Ambien									
⬦	10 mg dose	p.o. route	at bedtime interval	prn insomnia					
6/15/19	Tylenol with codeine									
⬦	2 tabs	p.o. route	q.4 h. interval	prn pain					
6/15/19	Morphine									
⬦	10 mg dose	IV route	q.10 min interval	250 mg/4 h. lockout					

3. 1 mL

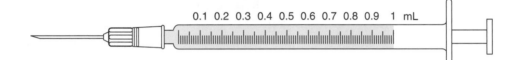

4. 1 mL/10 min
5. 1.0 mL
6. 400 mL/shift
   1200 mL/day
7. 200 mL/h
   200 gtt/min

Case 6, *pp. 585–587*

1.

3/4/19	ASA										
⬦	325 mg dose	p.o. route	daily interval	09							
3/4/19	Plavix										
⬦	75 mg dose	p.o. route	daily interval	09							
3/4/19	Metoprolol										
⬦	12.5 mg dose	p.o. route	2 times daily interval	09		21					

2.

3/4/19	Tylenol									
⬦	650 mg dose	p.o. route	q.4 h. interval	prn headache					
3/4/19	Ambien									
⬦	5 mg dose	p.o. route	at bedtime interval						

3. 3 mL/h
4. a. 5300 units
   b. 5.3 mL
   c. 13 mL/h
5. ½ tablet
6. 2 tablets

Case 7, *pp. 588–589*

1. 2.2 lb:1 kg::7.5 lb:x kg
   2.2x = 7.5
   $$x = \frac{7.5}{2.2}$$
   $x = 3.4$ kg
   a. $\dfrac{160 \text{ mg} \times 3 \text{ doses/24 h}}{3.4 \text{ kg}} = 141.2$ mg/kg/24 h
   b. Yes, the neonate is receiving a dose that is within the recommended dosage range of 100 to 200 mg/kg/24 h.
   c. 250 mg:1 mL::160 mg:x mL
   250x = 160
   $$x = \frac{160}{250}$$
   $x = 0.6$ mL
2. 80 mg:0.8 mL::40 mg:x mL
   80x = 32
   $$x = \frac{32}{80}$$
   $x = 0.4$ mL
3. 12 mL/h × 6 h = 72 mL

Case 8, *p. 590*

1. Jeff is receiving 12 mg/kg/dose of acetaminophen, which is both safe and therapeutic. Recommended dosing for acetaminophen is 10 to 15 mg/kg/dose q 4 h PRN for pain or fever (*Harriet Lane Handbook*).
2. Administer 3.5 mL acetaminophen to deliver the 300-mg ordered dose.
3. Give the parents an oral syringe (5 mL), and mark the syringe at 3.5 mL. Have the parents draw up 3.5 mL in the syringe before discharge.
4. Jeff is receiving 48 mg/kg/24 h, which is within the recommended dosage range of 25 to 50 mg/kg/24 h. It is both safe and therapeutic to administer.
5. Administer 7.5 mL using an oral 10-mL syringe. Teach parents before discharge and have them demonstrate before leaving the children's unit.

Case 9, *p. 591*

1. Omission
2. Decrease the blood flow to the liver and kidneys
3. Inadequate income
4. (2 possible answers) Medication container or a book to record medication administration
5. Have the patient verbally repeat the instructions.

Addends the numbers to be added

Ampule a sealed glass container; usually contains one dose of a drug

Buccal between teeth and cheek

Canceling dividing numerator and denominator by a common number

Capsule a small soluble container for enclosing a single dose of medicine

Complex fraction a fraction whose numerator, denominator, or both contain fractions

Decimal fraction a fraction consisting of a numerator that is expressed in numerals, a decimal point that designates the value of the denominator, and the denominator, which is understood to be 10 or some power of 10

Decimal numbers include an integer, a decimal point, and a decimal fraction

Denominator the number of parts into which a whole has been divided

Difference the result of subtracting

Dividend the number being divided

Divisor the number by which another number is divided

Dosage the determination and regulation of the size, frequency, and number of doses

Dose the exact amount of medicine to be administered at one time

Drug a chemical substance used in therapy, diagnosis, and prevention of a disease or condition

Elixir a clear, sweet, hydroalcoholic liquid in which a drug is suspended

Equivalent equal

Extremes the first and fourth terms of a proportion

Fraction indicates the number of equal parts of a whole

Improper fraction a fraction whose numerator is larger than or equal to the denominator

Infusion the therapeutic introduction of a fluid into a vein by the flow of gravity

Injection the therapeutic introduction of a fluid into a part of the body by force

Integer a whole number

Intramuscular within the muscle

Intravenous within the vein

Invert turn upside down

Lowest common denominator the smallest whole number that can be divided evenly by all denominators within the problem

Means the second and third terms of a proportion

Medicine any drug

Milliequivalent the number of grams of a solute contained in 1 mL of a normal solution

Minuend the number from which another number is subtracted

Mixed number a combination of a whole number and a proper fraction

Multiplicand the number that is to be multiplied

Multiplier the number that another number is to be multiplied by

Numerator the number of parts of a divided whole

Oral dosage a medication taken by mouth

Parenteral dosage a dosage administered by routes that bypass the gastrointestinal tract; generally given by injection

Percent indicates the number of hundredths

Product the result of multiplying

Proper fraction a fraction whose numerator is smaller than the denominator

Proportion two ratios that are of equal value and are connected by a double colon, which symbolizes the word *as*

Quotient the answer to a division problem

Ratio the relationship between two numbers that are connected by a colon, which symbolizes the words *is to*

Reconstitution the return of a medication to its previous state by the addition of water or other designated liquid

Subcutaneous beneath the skin

Sublingual under the tongue

Subtrahend the number being subtracted

Sum the result of adding

Suspension a liquid in which a drug is distributed, must be shaken prior to use

Syrup a sweet, thick, aqueous liquid in which a drug is suspended

Tablet a drug compressed into a small disk

Topical on top of the skin or mucous membrane

Unit the amount of a drug needed to produce a given result

Vial a glass container with a rubber stopper; usually contains a number of doses of a drug

Apothecary System of Measure

The apothecary system of measure is a very old English system and is no longer used for medication ordering and administration. It has been replaced by the metric system.

Physicians occasionally used Roman numerals when writing orders in the apothecary system:

Roman Numeral	Arabic Numeral
i	1
v	5
x	10
l	50
c	100

Addition of Roman numerals is performed when a smaller numeral follows a larger numeral:

$$xi = 11$$
$$xv = 15$$
$$li = 51$$

Addition is performed when a numeral is repeated. However, a numeral is never repeated more than three times:

$$viii = 8$$
$$xii = 12$$
$$ccxi = 211$$

Subtraction is performed when a smaller numeral is placed before a larger numeral:

$$ix = 9$$
$$iv = 4$$
$$ic = 99$$

Subtraction is also performed when a smaller numeral is placed between two larger numerals. The smaller numeral is subtracted from the larger numeral that follows it:

$$xiv = 14$$
$$xxiv = 24$$
$$cxc = 190$$

COMMON APOTHECARY SYSTEM UNITS OF MEASURE

Apothecary Measure of Liquid
16 fluid ounces (fl oz) = 1 pint (pt)
32 fluid ounces (fl oz) = 2 pints (pt) or 1 quart (qt)
4 quarts (qt) = 1 gallon (gal)

APOTHECARY/HOUSEHOLD EQUIVALENTS

Apothecary Measure = Household Measure
8 fluid ounces (fl oz) = 1 standard measuring cup

b indicates boxes, f indicates figures,
and t indicates tables.